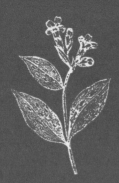

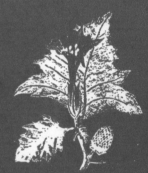

COMMON LUNGWORT.
PULMONARIA OFFICINALIS.

OFFICINAL GUAIACUM.
GUAIACUM OFFICINALE.

COMMON PERUVIAN BARK TREE.
CINCHONA OFFICINALIS.

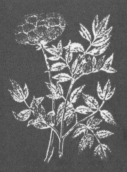

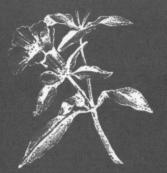

WILD ANGELICA.
ANGELICA SYLVESTRIS.

POMEGRANATE TREE.
PUNICA GRANATUM.

THORN-APPLE.
DATURA STRAMONIUM.

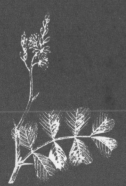

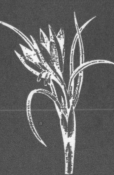

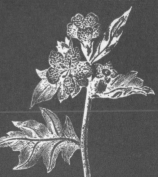

LOGWOOD.
HÆMATOXYLUM CAMPECHIANUM.

SAFFRON.
CROCUS SATIVUS.

HENBANE.
HYOSCYAMUS NIGER.

THE HERBALIST

Medicinal Plants

Plant Vitamins and Minerals

Beverage Teas

Spices and Flavoring Herbs

Plant Colors for Food and Cosmetics

Plant Dyes for Fabrics

Botanicals for Potpourri and Sachets

Dentifrices, Gargles, Cosmetics

Botanical Curios

Smoke Flavoring Botanicals

Assorted other Information

PRINTED AND BOUND BY

RAND MCNALLY & COMPANY, CONKEY DIVISION

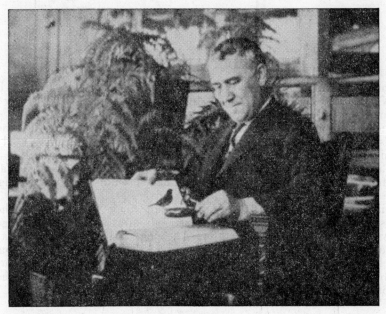

JOSEPH E. MEYER, Author
1878 – 1950

First edition   1918
Second edition 1932
Third edition   1934
Revised and enlarged edition 1960

SPECIAL ATTENTION

The botanical materia medica and recipes of this book are NOT IN-TENDED TO REPLACE THE SERVICES OF PHYSICIANS. By all means see a physician when a condition requires his services.

There is ample proof that botanical medicines have been used for thousands of years, and it is reasonable to believe that they also were used by primitive man to survive diseases, and the rigors of remote ages.

Many botanicals listed in this book are still recognized in United States and foreign pharmacopias. Many of them have been discarded for stronger, more certain, synthetic drugs, or other reasons.

Millspaugh wrote in 1887, regarding Dandelion: "It is one of those drugs, over-rated, derogated, extirpated, and re-instated, time and again by writers upon pharmacology, from Theophrastus, to the present day."

Modern science is now revaluating many of the old-time botanicals, and searching jungles and distant places to seek remedies of aboriginal races. Improved technical methods and equipment is reviving a vast new interest in botanical materia medica.

ANATOMY OF A PLANT
(The Root)

The root of a plant is that portion which is usually found in the earth, the stem and leaves being in the air. The point of union is called the collar or neck of the plant.

The fibrous root is one composed of many spreading branches, as that of barley.

A conical root is one where it tapers regularly from the crown to the apex, as that of the carrot.

A fusiform root is one when it tapers up as well as down, as that of the radish.

A napiform root is one when much swollen at the base, so as to become broader than long, as that of the turnip.

A fasciculated root is one when some of the fibres or branches are thickened.

A tuberiferous root is one when some of the branches assume the form of rounded knobs, as that of the potato.

A palmate root is one when these knobs are branched.

Aerial roots are those emitted from the stem into the open air, as that of Indian corn.

A rhizome, or root stock, is a prostrate stem either subterranean or resting on the surface, as that of calamus, or blood-root.

A tuber is an enlargement of the apex of a subterranean branch of the root, as that of the common potato or artichoke.

A cormus is a fleshy subterranean stem of a round or oval figure, as in the Indian turnip.

A bulb is an extremely abbreviated stem clothed with scales, as that of the lily.

The Stem

The stem is that portion of the plant which grows in an opposite direction from the root, seeking the light, and exposing itself to the air. All flowering plants possess stems. In those which are said to be stemless, it is either very short, or concealed beneath the ground.

An herb is one in which the stem does not become woody, but dies down to the ground at least after flowering.

A shrub is a woody plant, branched near the ground, and 1 to 6 ft. high.

A tree attains a greater height, with a stem unbranched near the ground.

The stem of a tree is usually called the trunk; in grasses it has been termed the culm.

Those stems which are too weak to stand erect are said to be decumbent, procumbent and prostrate.

EPITOME OF BOTANY

That the reader may more intelligently understand the description of the medicinal plants in this book, the author has deemed it prudent to preface the part of this work dedicated to Herbal Materia Medica with a brief analysis of the plant, as made by the botanist. This becomes particularly necessary, inasmuch as a plant cannot be accurately described unless scientific language be employed; but, nevertheless, throughout this whole work it has been the aim of the author to use the plainest language, and not to weary the reader by a pedantic employment of technical terms and scientific language.

Nothing more will be given than the anatomy of the plant, as nothing of systematic botany need be known to the reader to recognize the plant, or to acquaint himself with the medicinal properties thereof. If he has not a common acquaintance with a medicinal plant, but desires it for domestic medication, it is important that he should know that he employs the proper herb, and not use one which simulates it. It has therefore been the aim of the author to give accurate descriptions of the herbs, so that the gatherer may not err in his selection of the plant which his case may need.

Not all parts of the plant are used in medicine—sometimes the seed only; in others the flower, the leaves, root, rhizome; in others two or more of these parts, and, again, in others the whole plant.

Annual plants spring from the seed, make their full growth, and die in one year.

A biennial plant does not flower the first year, but produces leaves only. The second year of its growth it flowers, after which it dies. The carrot and parsnip are examples of biennials.

A perennial plant lives for more than two years. If the plant retains its leaves during the winter, it is known as an evergreen; if the leaves fall upon the approach of cold weather, it is said to be deciduous.

An herb is a plant having a soft stem which dies down to the ground after the plant has reached its full growth.

A shrub is a plant which has a woody stem, grows to a height of twenty-five to thirty feet or less, and branches near the ground.

A tree has a woody stem, is higher than a shrub and does not branch near the ground.

A stolon is a form of a branch which curves or falls down to the ground, where they often strike root.

A sucker is a branch of subterraneous origin, which, after running horizontally and emitting roots in its course, at length rises out of the ground and forms an erect stem, which soon becomes an independent plant, as illustrated by the rose, raspberry, etc.

A runner is a prostrate, slender branch sent off from the base of the parent stem.

An offset is a similar but shorter branch, with a tuft of leaves at the end, as in the houseleek.

A spine is a short and imperfectly developed branch of a woody plant, as exhibited in the honey-locust.

A tendril is commonly a slender leafless branch, capable of coiling spirally, as in the grape vine.

The Leaf

The leaf is commonly raised on an unexpanded part or stalk which is called the petiole, while the expanded portion is termed the lamina, limb or blade. When the vessels or fibres of the leaves expand immediately on leaving the stem, the leaf is said to be sessile. In such cases the petiole is absent. When the blade consists of a single piece the leaf is simple; when composed of two or three more with a branched petiole, the leaf is compound.

The distribution of the veins or framework of the leaf in the blade is termed venation.

A lanceolate leaf has the form of a lance.

An ovate leaf has the shape of ellipsis.

A cuneiform leaf has the shape of a wedge.

A cordate leaf has the shape of a heart.

A reniform leaf has the shape of a kidney.

A sagittate leaf is arrow-shaped.

A hastate leaf has the shape of an ancient halberd.

A peltate leaf is shaped like a shield.

A serrate leaf is one in which the margin is beset with sharp teeth, which point forward towards the apex.

A dentate leaf is one when these teeth are not directed towards the apex.

A crenate leaf has rounded teeth.

A sinuate leaf has alternate concavities and convexities.

A pinnate leaf has the shape of a feather.

A pectinate leaf is one having very close and narrow divisions, like the teeth of a comb.

A lyrate leaf has the shape of a lyre.

A runcinate leaf is a lyrate leaf with sharp lobes pointing towards the base, as in the dandelion.

A palmate leaf is one bearing considerable resemblance to the hand.

A pedate leaf is one bearing resemblance to a bird's foot.

An obovate leaf is one having the veins more developed beyond the middle of the blade.

When a leaf at its outer edge has no dentations it is said to be entire. When the leaf terminates in an acute angle it is acute, when in an obtuse angle it is obtuse. An obtuse leaf with the apex slightly depressed is retuse, or if more strongly notched, emarginate. An obovate leaf with a wider or more conspicuous notch at the apex becomes obcordate, being a cordate leaf inverted. When the apex is cut off by a straight transverse line the leaf is truncate; when abruptly terminated by a small projecting point it is mucronate; and when an acute leaf has a narrowed apex it is acuminate. In ferns the leaves are called fronds.

The Flower

The flower assumes an endless variety of forms, and we shall assume in the dissection merely the typical form of it.

The organs of a flower are of two sorts, viz.: 1st. Its leaves or envelopes; and, 2nd, those peculiar organs having no resemblance to the envelopes. The envelopes are of two kinds, or occupy two rows, one above or within the other. The lower or outer row is termed the Calyx, and commonly exhibits the green color of the leaves. The inner row, which is usually of more delicate texture and forms the most showy part of the flower, is termed the Corolla. The several parts of the leaves of the Corolla are called Petals, and the leaves of the Calyx have received the analogous name of Sepals. The floral envelopes are collectively called the Perianth.

The essential organs enclosed within a floral envelope are also of two kinds and occupy two rows one within the other. The first of these, those next within the petals, are the Stamens. A stamen consists of a stalk called the Filament, which bears on its summit a rounded body termed the Anther, filled with a substance called the Pollen.

The seed-bearing organs occupy the center or summit of a flower, and are called Pistils. A pistil is distinguished into three parts, viz.: 1st, the Ovary, containing the Ovales; 2nd, the Style, or columnar prolongation of the ovary; and 3rd, the Stigma, or termination of the style.

All the organs of the flower are situated on, or grown out of, the apex of the flower-stalk, into which they are inserted, and which is called the Torus or Receptacle.

A plant is said to be monoecious, where the stamens and pistils are in separate flowers on the same individual, dioecious, where they occupy separate flowers on different individuals, and polygamous where the stamens and pistils are separate in some flowers and united in others, either on the same or two or three different plants.

The Fruit

The principal kinds may be briefly stated as follows:

A follicle is the name given to such fruit as borne by the larkspur or milkweed.

A legume or pod is the name extended to such fruit as the pea or bean.

A drupe is a stone fruit, as the plum, apricot, etc.

An achenium is the name of the fruit as borne by the butter-cup, etc.

A cremocarp is the fruit of the Poison Hemlock and similar plants.

A caryopsis is such fruit as borne by the wheat tribe.

A nut is exemplified by the fruit of the oak, chestnut, etc.

A samara is the name applied to the fruit of the maple, birch and elm.

A berry is a fruit fleshy and pulpy throughout, as the grape, gooseberry, etc.

A pome is such as the apple, pear, etc.

A pepo is the name applied to the fruit of the pumpkin, cucumber, etc.

A capsule is a general term for all dry fruits, such as lobelia, etc.

A silique is such fruit as exhibited in Shepherd's purse, etc.

A cone or strobile is a collective fruit of the fir tribe, magnolia, etc.

The Seed

The seed, like the ovule of which it is fertilized and matured state, consists of a nucleus, usually enclosed within two integuments. The outer integument or proper seed coat is variously termed the episperm, spermoderm, or testa.

DEFINITION OF MEDICAL TERMS

Absorbents or Antacids are such medicines that counteract acidity of the stomach and bowels.

Alternatives are medicines which, in certain doses, work a gradual change by promoting the usual functions of different organs.

Anodynes are medicines which relieve pain.

Anthelmintics are medicines which have the power of destroying or expelling worms from the intestinal canal.

Antiscorbutics are medicines which are used in the treatment of scurvy.

Antispasmodics are medicines given to relieve spasm, or irregular and painful action of muscles or muscular fibres.

Aromatics are medicines which have a grateful smell and an agreeable pungent taste.

Astringents are those remedies which, when applied to the body, render the solids dense and firmer.

Carminatives are those medicines which dispel flatulency of the stomach.

Cathartics are medicines which accelerate the action of the bowels, or increase the discharge by stool.

Demulcents are medicines suited to modify the action of acrid and stimulating matters upon the mucous membranes as in the throat, etc.

Diaphoretics are medicines that promote or cause perspirable discharge by the skin.

Diuretics are medicines which increase the flow of urine by their action upon the kidneys.

Emetics are those medicines which produce vomiting.

Emollients are those remedies which, when applied to the solids of the body, render them soft and flexible.

Errhines are substances which, when applied to the lining membrane of the nostrils, occasion a discharge of mucus.

Epispastics are those which cause blisters when applied to the surface of the body, forming sloughs.

Expectorants are medicines capable of facilitating the excretion of mucus.

Narcotics are those substances having the property of diminishing the action of the nervous and vascular systems, and of inducing sleep.

Rubefacients are remedies which excite the vessels of the skin and increase its heat and redness.

Sedatives are medicines which have the power of allaying the action or of lessening the exercise of some particular function.

Sialagogues are medicines which increase the flow of the saliva.

Stimulants are medicines capable of exciting the vital energy, whether as exerted in sensation or motion.

Tonics are those medicines which sharpen the appetite and promote strength and tone.

GATHERING BOTANICAL DRUGS

All roots, barks, herbs, leaves, flowers and bulbs which have a medicinal value are commonly called Botanic Drugs. In the following pages the most important botanical drugs are described, some of the uses for which they have been or may be employed are given, the valuable part of the plant mentioned, the geographical distribution of the plant stated, and directions for gathering, as well as the best time for doing so.

To get the best results from the work of collecting botanical drugs, it is important to handle them properly, as well as to collect at the right time of year. It is also well to see that the articles you collect are not mixed with some of similar appearance. The demand is for pure, clean, properly handled goods, and these only will bring the highest prices.

DIRECTIONS FOR COLLECTING LEAVES

Leaves should always be collected in clear, dry weather, in the morning, after the dew is off. They are at their best when the plant is in bloom and should be collected at this time. Leaves of biennials are most valuable during the second year of their growth. In drying, spread out thinly on a clean floor and stir occasionally until they are thoroughly dry. Remove all stems from leaves and remember that the leaves which are worth most are those which retain their natural green color. Dampness will turn leaves black, so be careful not to let them get damp.

DIRECTIONS FOR COLLECTING HERBS

In collecting herbs, strip off the flowers, smaller leaves, and very small stems and reject the large stem. Dry same as leaves. The large woody stems are of no value.

DIRECTIONS FOR COLLECTING FLOWERS

Flowers are worth the most, from the standpoint of their medical value, immediately upon opening. The directions for collecting leaves also apply to flowers, which sell best when their natural color is preserved in drying.

DIRECTIONS FOR COLLECTING BULBS

Bulbs should be gathered at the time the leaves of the plant die, which is, of course, in the autumn. The outer heavy coat should be removed and the bulb sliced, after which it should be dried by artificial heat, not to exceed 100° F.

DIRECTIONS FOR COLLECTING BARKS

Barks may be gathered either in the fall or spring. Wild Cherry and other rough barks should be rossed before peeling—that is, the rough outer bark must be scraped or shaved off, and the inner bark then peeled. Barks may be dried in sunlight, except green Wild Cherry.

DIRECTIONS FOR COLLECTING SEEDS

Seeds should be gathered as soon as they ripen. Only heavy full developed seeds are of value; others should be removed by winnowing.

VALUE OF BOTANICAL DRUGS

The price of botanical drugs is constantly changing and for this reason it would be useless to mention market values in a book of his kind.

SHIPPING INSTRUCTIONS

Never ship goods to a dealer before getting an order from him.

The more valuable and perishable articles should be shipped in boxes or barrels; other goods may be shipped in bags. See that all goods are dry before shipping; otherwise they will mould while on the road and be worthless when they arrive at their destination. It is always best to correspond with dealers before shipping.

Mark shipments plainly with your name, the name of the consignee and the name of the article or articles contained in the shipment.

Herbal Materia Medica

Every herb employed for a medicinal purpose, whether in its natural state or after having undergone various preparations, belongs to the Herbal Materia Medica, in the extended acceptation of the term. It shall, however, be our purpose here merely to describe each separate herb in its living state, or the medicinal part thereof, and not dwell much upon the forms usually prepared by the apothecary or physician. In this portion of our work we propose to give an account of those herbs which are commonly or popularly known and classified as medicinal in some degree, however slight, or at least have been so regarded at some time or other. But our mention or discussion of a botanical here is not to be understood as a claim or representation that the particular herb actually has the medicinal powers and possibilities with which it has been or still may be credited. Nor is our failure to include some botanical in this book to be taken as an indication of a belief on our part that the botanical is worthless or of little value. To describe all botanicals worthy or capable of classification as medicinal, even in the popular sense, would make this book too voluminous and expensive. Moreover, it is our province or purpose here merely to stimulate interest in the products of field and forest, rather than to pose as an authority or attempt a medical treatise.

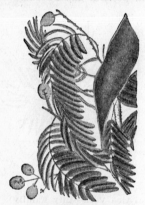

ACACIA VERA
(Pulse Family)

Common Names—Gum Arabic, Egyptian Thorn.

Medicinal Part—The concrete juice or gum.

Description—Acacia Vera is a small tree or shrub, but sometimes attains the height of forty feet. The gum flows naturally from the bark of the trees in the form of a thick and rather frothy liquid and speedily concretes into tears.

Properties and Uses—The gum is nutritive and demulcent and exerts a soothing influence upon irritated mucous surfaces by shielding them from the influence of deleterious agents, atmospheric air, etc.

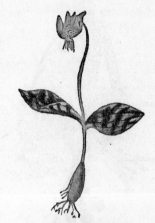

ADDER'S TONGUE
(Erythronium Americanum, Lily Family)

Common Names — Dog-Tooth Violet, Serpent's Tongue, Yellow Snowdrop, Rattlesnake-Violet, Yellow Snakeleaf.

Medicinal Parts—The bulb and leaves.

Description—This is a perennial plant, springing from a bulb at some distance below the surface. The bulb is white internally and fawn-colored externally. The leaves are two, lanceolate, pale green with purplish or brownish spots, and one nearly twice as wide as the other. It bears a single drooping yellow flower, which partially closes at night and on cloudy days. Fruit a capsule.

This beautiful little plant is among the earliest of our spring flowers, and is found in rich open grounds, or in thin woods throughout the United States, flowering in April or May. The leaves are more active than the roots; both impart their virtues to water.

Properties and Uses—It is emetic, emollient, and antiscorbutic when fresh; nutritive when dried. The fresh root simmered in milk, or the fresh leaves bruised and often applied as a poultice, together with a free internal use of an infusion of them, is highly useful in the condition in which such a remedy is indicated. The express juice of the plant, infused in cider, also has been found beneficial.

Dose—One teaspoonful of the dried leaves or two of the root to the cup of boiling water. Drink one cupful a day.

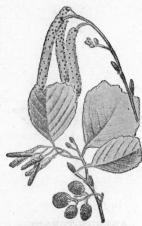

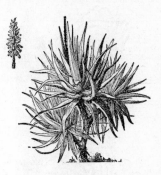

a bland soothing collyrium for bathing the eyes.

Dose—A teaspoonful of the root to a cup of boiling water. Drink cold one or two cupfuls a day, a large mouthful at a time; of the tincture, ½ to 1 fl. dr.

ALMOND
(Amygdalus Dulcis—Rose Family)

Common Names — Jordan Almond, Greek Nuts.

Medicinal Part—Kernels.

Description—The Almond Tree, cultivated from the Orient, is from ten to twenty feet high, with large sessile flowers which appear before the leaves. The leaves are lanceolate, firm, and closely serrate. The fruit with a dry flesh, which finally splits away, freeing the nut, the Almond of commerce.

Properties and Uses—Emollient, demulcent, pectoral and sweet.

ALDER, EUROPEAN
(Alnus Glutinosa—Oak Family)

Common Name—Owler.

Medicinal Part—Bark and leaves.

Description—European Alder is cultivated from Europe. The leaves are round obovate and scalloped and finely sharp-toothed, a tuft of down in the axils of the veins beneath, the young growth and petioles glutinous.

Properties and Uses—Bitters, astringent.

ALTHEA
(Althea Officinalis, Mallow Family)

Common Names — Sweet Weed, Wymote, Marsh Mallow.

Medicinal Part—The root.

Description—Althea is a perennial 2 to 4 feet high, having several wooly stems; leaves 1 to 3 inches long, serrate, both sides pubescent; flowers large, 1 to 2 inches in diameter, purple color.

Properties and Uses — The root is sweet and very mucilaginous when chewed, containing more than half its weight of saccharine viscous mucilage. It is, therefore, emollient, demulcent, pain-soothing and lubricating; serving to subdue heat and irritation, whilst, if applied externally diminishing the irritation. It is for these reasons much employed in domestic poultices, and in decoction as a medicine for coughs due to colds, hoarseness, and as a vaginal douche. Also the decoction acts well as

ALOE
(Aloe Vera—Lily Family)

Common Names—Curacao or Barbadoes Aloes.

Medicinal Part—Fresh and dehydrated juice.

Description—Plant forms a cluster of leaf blades radiating from the base and growing about 18 to 20 inches high. Greenish orange flowers are borne on slender stalks about 30 inches high. The thick blades contain a greenish translucent salve-like juice, much used as a medicinal in the tropics, where the plant is grown. Aloe is easily grown as a house plant.

Properties and Uses—Dehydrated juice used as a purgative. Fresh juice used for minor burns, sunburn, insect bites and other emollient uses.

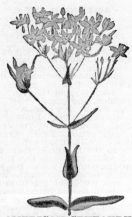

Properties and Uses—It is an excellent tonic. It is also serviceable as a bitter tonic in dyspepsia and convalescence. When administered in warm infusion it has many valuable uses.

Dose—Steep a teaspoonful of the herb, broken into small pieces, into a cup of boiling water, for half an hour. When cold drink 1 or 2 cupfuls a day, a good mouthful at a time. Of the tincture, ½ to 1 fl. dr.

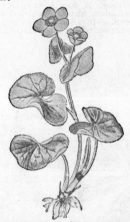

AMERICAN CENTAURY
(Sabbatia Angularis, Gentian Family)
Common Names—Rose Pink, Bitterbloom, Bitter Clover.
Medicinal Part—The herb.
Description—This plant has a yellow fibrous, biennial root, with an erect, smooth, quadrangular stem, with the angles winged, having many opposite branches, and growing from one to two feet in height. The leaves are opposite, fine veined, smooth, entire, from one to five inches in length and from half an inch to one and a half inches wide, clasping the stem. The flowers are numerous, from an inch and a quarter to an inch and a half in diameter, of a rich rose or carnation color, standing, as it were, at the tops of one umbril or tuft, very like those of St. John's Wort, opening themselves in the day time and closing at night, after which come seeds in little short husks, in forms like unto wheat corn. There are three varieties of the Centaury in England, one kind bearing white flowers, another yellow, and another red. All have medicinal properties, although the American variety is considered preferable to the European Centaury.

This plant is common to most parts of the United States, growing in moist meadows, among high grass, on the prairies, and in damp, rich soils, flowering from June to September. The whole herb is used. It has a very bitter taste, and yields its virtues to water or alcohol. The best time for gathering it is during the flowering season.

AMERICAN COWSLIP
(Caltha Palustrus—Crowfoot Family)
Common Names — Marsh Marigold, Meadow Bouts, Water Dragon.
Medicinal Part—Plant.
Description—American Cowslip has a stem one to two feet high, bearing one or more rounded or somewhat kidney-shaped, entire or crenate leaves and a few flowers with showy yellow calyx, followed by a cluster of many-seeded pods. Found in the marshes in the spring.
Properties and Uses—Expectorant and pectoral.

AMERICAN HELLEBORE
(Veratrum Viride, Bunchflower Family)
Common Names—Green Hellebore, Indian Poke, Itch-weed.
Medicinal Part—The rhizoma.
Description—This plant has a perennial, thick and fleshy rhizome, tunicated at the upper part, sending off a multitude of large whitish roots. The stem is from three to five feet high; lower leaves from six inches to a foot long,

7

oval, acuminate; upper leaves gradually narrower, linear, lanceolate, and all alternate. The flowers are numerous and green, part of them barren.

American Hellebore is native to the United States, growing in swamps, low grounds and moist meadows, blossoming in June and July. The roots should be gathered in autumn, and as it rapidly loses its virtues, it should be gathered annually and kept in well-closed vessels. When fresh, it has a very strong, unpleasant odor, but when dried is almost inodorous. It has a sweetish-bitter taste, succeeded by a persistent acridity.

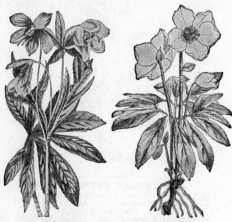

AMERICAN
HELLEBORE

BLACK
HELLEBORE

Properties and Uses—It has many very valuable properties, being preferred to other drugs for various purposes. However, it is too powerful a drug for use without medical supervision.

Dose—Veratrum is usually given in the form of a tincture, the formula being of the dried root, eight ounces to sixteen ounces diluted .835 alcohol, macerating for two weeks, then to be expressed and filtered.

The Helleborus Niger, Black Hellebore, inhabiting the subalpine and southern parts of Europe, was formerly much use, but is now more or less discarded. It has diuretic properties, but as it is very toxic in effects, its use as a home remedy is not advised.

AMERICAN IVY

(Ampelopsis Quinquefolia, GrapeFamily)

Common Names—Woodbine, Virginia Creeper, Five Leaves, False Grape, Wild Wood-vine.

Medicinal Parts—The bark and twigs.

Description—This is a woody vine, with a creeping stem, digitate leaves; leaflets acuminate, petiolate, dentate, and smooth; flowers inconspicuous, greenish, or white; and the fruit a berry acid, dark blue, and small.

The American Ivy is a common, familiar, shrubby vine, climbing extensively, and, by means of its radiating tendrils, supporting itself firmly on trees, stone walls, churches, etc., and ascending to the height of from fifty to a hundred feet. The bark and the twigs are the parts usually used. Its taste is acrid and persistent, though not unpleasant, and its decoction is mucilaginous. The bark should be collected after the berries have ripened. It is like the ivy of England and other countries.

Properties and Uses—Tonic, astringent, and expectorant. It is used principally in form of syrup. An old author affirms that there is a very great antipathy between wine and ivy, and therefore it is a remedy to preserve against **drunkenness,** and to relieve or discourage intoxication by drinking a draught of wine in which a handful of bruised leaves of ivy have been boiled.

Dose—A teaspoonful of the bark or twigs, cut small or granulated to a cup of boiling water. Drink cold during the day, a large mouthful at a time; of the tincture, 5 to 20 min.

AMERICAN SARSAPARILLA

(Aralia Racemosa, Ginseng Family)

Common Names—Spikenard, Spignet.

Medicinal Part—The root.

Description—For a description of American Sarsaparilla, see **Spikenard** on page 240. The foreign Sarsaparilla grows in New Grenada, on the banks of the Magdaline, near Bajorque. Great quantities are sent to Mompox and Carthagena, and from thence to Jamaica and Cadiz.

The Smilax Syphilitca, S. Papyracea, S. Medica, S. China, and S. Sarsaparilla, are all members of the same family of plants, their medicinal qualities are similar, and they form the Sarsaparilla of commerce, with the exception of the S. Sarsaparilla, which is native to the United States, flowering from May to

August. The American plant is the one we Americans should use. The plant extensively known in the South as Bamboo Brier, which is but a species of Sarsaparilla, certainly possesses medicinal qualities equal if not superior to commercial Sarsaparilla.

The Sarsaparilla of commerce consists of very long roots, having a thick bark of grayish or brownish color. They have scarcely any odor, but possess a mucilaginous taste. Those roots that have a deep orange tint are the best, and the stronger the acrid and nauseous qualities, the better are the properties of the root. Water and alcohol extract its medicinal qualities. By chemical analysis it contains salseparin, a coloring matter, starch, chloride of potassium, an essential oil, bassorin, albumen, pectic and acetic acid, and the several salts of lime, potassa, magnesia and oxide of iron.

Properties and Uses—An alterative. When properly prepared it exerts a beneficial influence in some conditions and enjoys repute for particular uses. Its chief use, however, is an adjuvant to other alteratives; its individual properties being too feeble to answer all the conditions required for an alterative.

Dose—A teaspoonful of the root to a cup of boiling water. Drink cold one or two cupfuls a day, a large mouthful at a time; of the tincture, ½ to 1 fl. dr.

AMERICAN SENNA
(Cassia Marilandica, Senna Family)

Common Names—Wild Senna, Locust Plant.

Medicinal Part—The leaves.

Description—This is a perennial herb, growing from four to six feet high, with round, smooth and slightly hairy stems. The leaves have long petioles, ovate at base; each petiole has eight or ten leaflets, which are oblong, smooth, mucronate, an inch or two long and quite narrow. The flowers are bright yellow, and the fruit is a legume from two to four inches long.

The American Senna is to be found from New England to Carolina, growing in rich soils here and there. It flowers from June to September, and the leaves are gathered for their medicinal value while the plant is in bloom. They yield their virtues to alcohol or water.

Properties and Uses—It is one of the most important herbal cathartics furnished by America, and is mentioned here solely on the ground that it appears to be equally valuable as the foreign Senna, or ordinary Senna of the drug-shops, and costs much less.

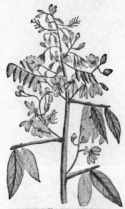

AMERICAN SENNA

Dose — Steep a teaspoonful of the leaves into a cup of boiling water for half an hour. Drink a half cupful upon retiring at night, hot or cold. Or take a mouthful 3 times a day. One or 2 cupfuls may be taken. Of the tincture, ½ to 1 fl. dr.

ANISE
(Pimpinella Anisum, Parsley Family)

Common Name—Anise.

Medicinal Parts—The fruit or seed.

Description—Anise has a perennial, spindle shaped, woody root, and a smooth, erect, branched stem, about ten or twelve inches in height. The leaves are petiolated, roundish, cordate, serrate; flowers small and white, disposed on long stalks. Calyx wanting, or minute. The fruit is ovate, about an eighth of an inch long, dull brown, and slightly downy.

It is a native of Egypt, but now cultivated in many of the warm countries of Europe and America. The Italian Aniseed is commonly used for medicinal purposes. The odor of Anise is penetrating and fragrant, the taste aromatic and sweetish. It imparts its virtues wholly to alcohol, only partially to water.

Properties and Uses—Stimulant and carminative; used in cases of flatulency, colic of infants, and to remove nausea. Some times added to other medicines to improve their flavor or to correct disagreeable effects.

9

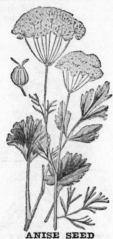

ANISE SEED

Dose—A teaspoonful of this to a cup of boiling water. Drink cold 1 or 2 cupfuls a day. Of the tincture, ¼ to ½ fl. dr.

Medicinal Parts—Root, herb and seed.

Description—This plant is five to six feet high. The root has a purple color; leaves ternate, with large petioles; calyx five-toothed, with equal petals, and the fruit a nut.

The plant is perennial, and grows in fields and damp places, from Labrador to Delaware and west to Minnesota, developing greenish white flowers from May to August. The plant has a powerful, peculiar, but not unpleasant odor, a sweet taste, afterwards pungent; but in drying it loses some of these qualities.

Properties and Uses—It is aromatic, stimulant, carminative, diaphoretic, expectorant and diuretic. It is also used in flatulent colic and heartburn. It is serviceable in promoting elimination through the urine and skin.

Dose—A teaspoonful of seed to a cup of boiling water. Drink cold 1 or 2 cupfuls a day. Of the tincture, ¼ to ½ fl. dr.

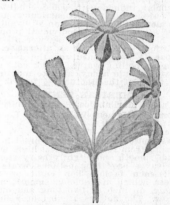

ARNICA
(Arnica Montana)

Common Name—Leopardsbane.

Part Used—Flowers.

Description — Arnica is a northern plant with large, delicate, pure yellow, daisy-like flowers. Its slightly hairy stem grows from 1 to 2 feet tall. The basal leaves are long-petioled, but the stem ones are sessile and opposite, shallow-toothed. At the summit are one to nine flower-heads on slender peduncles. About the central disc are 10 to 14 yellows rays, each with three notches in their ends. Found in Canada and the

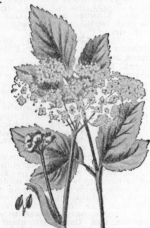

ARCHANGEL
(Angelica Atropurpurea, Parsley Family)

Common Names—Masterwort and Angelica.

mountains of the northern United States.

Properties and Uses — This flower should be used only externally, as it may have serious reaction when taken internally. Arnica tincture is very efficacious in promoting the healing of wounds, bruises, etc. For irritation of the nasal passages and chapped lips there is nothing superior. Arnica may also be used for the above purposes in the form of a salve. The salve is made by heating one ounce of the flowers with one ounce of lard for a few hours.

For external use take two heaping teaspoonfuls of the flowers to a cup of boiling water. Apply cold to the sores or wounds.

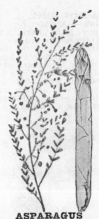

ASPARAGUS
(Asparagus Officinalis—Lily Family)
Common Name—Sparrow Grass.
Medicinal Part—Young shoots.
Description—Cultivated from Europe for its esculent spring shoots, spontaneous about gardens and waste places. Tall, bushy branched, the leaves thread-shaped and the berries red.
Properties and Uses—Edible, diaphoretic, aperient and deobstruent.

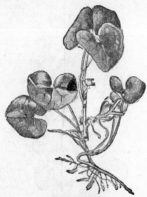

ASARABACCA
(Asarum Europaeum—Birthwort Family
Common Names—European Snakeroot, Public House Plant, Wild Nard.
Medicinal Part—Leaves and root.
Description—An acrid herb found in woods in Europe. Its roots and leaves are aromatic. The leaves are petioled, usually heart-shaped. The flowers are solitary, large and odd.
Properties and Uses—Leaves—errhine, emetic and cathartic. Roots—purgative, emetic and diuretic.

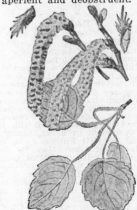

ASPEN, QUAKING
(Populus Tremula—Willow Family)
Common Names—European Poplar.

A related species, Asarum Canadense (Wild Ginger) is found in central parts of the U.S.A., and Canada. Indians used the aromatic roots to flavor mud fish and questionable meats.

Medicinal Part—Bark.

Description—A slender tree with smooth, very light bark. The young foliage is glabrous, petioles very slender, flattened laterally, causing the leaves to quiver in the slightest breeze. The leaves are ovate, short acuminate at the apex, rounded or subcordate at the base.

Properties and Uses—The active principle of the bark is salicin and populin. The bark is used as a febrifuge, antiscorbutic and as a vermifuge by veterinaries.

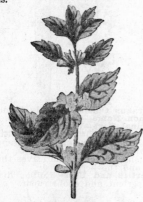

BALM
(Melissa Officinalis, Mint Family)

Common Names—Melissa, Lemon-balm, Garden-balm, Sweet-balm.

Medicinal Part—The herb.

Description—Balm is a perennial herb, with upright, branching, four-sided stems, from ten to twenty inches high. The leaves are broadly ovate, acute, and more or less hairy. The flowers are pale yellow, with ascending stamens. Balm is a native of France, but naturalized in England and the United States. It grows in fields, along roadsides, and is well known as a garden plant, flowering from May to August. The whole plant is officinal or medicinal and should be collected previous to flowering. In a fresh state it has a lemon-like odor, which is nearly lost by drying. Its taste is aromatic, faintly astringent, with a degree of persistent bitterness. Boiling water extracts its virtues. Balm contains a bitter extractive substance, a little tannin, gum and a peculiar volatile oil. A pound of the plant yields about four grains of

the oil, which is of a yellowish or reddish yellow color, very liquid, and possessing the fragrance of the plant in a high degree. The Nepeta Citridora, a powerful emmenagogue, is sometimes cultivated and employed by mistake for Balm. It has the same odor, but may be distinguished by having both surfaces of the leaves hairy.

Properties and Uses—It is moderately diaphoretic. A warm infusion, drank freely, is very serviceable to produce sweating, or as a diaphoretic. When so given it may be rendered more agreeable by the addition of lemon juice. The infusion may be taken at pleasure.

Dose—Two teaspoonfuls to a cup of boiling water. Of the tincture, ½ to 1 fl. dr.

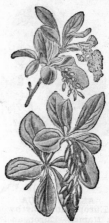

BARBERRY
(Berberis Vulgaris, Barberry Family)

Medicinal Part—Bark and berries.

Description—Barberry is an erect, deciduous shrub, from three to eight feet high, with leaves of an obovate-oval form, terminated by soft bristles, about two inches long, and one-third as wide. The flowers are small and yellow, in clusters, and the fruit bright-red oblong berries, in branches, and very acid.

This shrub is found in the New England states, on the mountains of Pennsylvania and Virginia, among rocks and hard gravelly soil. Occasionally it is found in the West on rich grounds. It flowers in April and May, and ripens its fruit in June. Its active principle is Berberina.

Properties and Uses—It is tonic and laxative. The berries form an agreeable acidulous draught, useful as a refrigerant; the bark of the root is the most active; a teaspoonful of the powder will act as a purgative. A decoction of the bark or berries wil be found of service as a mouth wash or gargle.

Dose—One teaspoonful to a cup of boiling water. Drink 1 or 2 cupfuls a day. Tincture, ½ to 1 fl. dr.

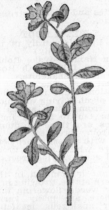

BEARBERRY

(Arctostaphylos Uva-Ursi, Heath Family)

Common Names—Uva-Ursi, Upland Cranberry, Arberry.

Medicinal Part—The leaves.

Description — Bearberry is a small, perennial shrub, having a long fibrous root. The stems are weedy and trailing, bark smooth. The leaves are alternate, evergreen, obovate, acute, and have short petioles. The fruit is a small, scarlet colored drupaceous berry.

This plant is a perennial evergreen, common in the northern part of Europe and America. It grows on dry, sterile, sandy soils, and gravelly ridges. The berries ripen in winter, although the flowers appear from June to September. The green leaves, picked from the stems in the fall and dried in a moderate heat, are the parts used. These leaves are odorless until reduced to powder, when the odor emitted is like that of dried grass. The powder is of a light brown color, tinged with a yellowish green.

The taste is astringent and bitterish. The properties of the leaves are extracted by alcohol or water.

Properties and Uses—Bearberry is especially astringent and tonic, depending upon these qualities for the most of its good effects. It is particularly useful in conditions indicating a diuretic of this particular type, containing tannic acid and arbutin.

Dose—Best results are obtained if the leaves are soaked in sufficient alcohol or brandy to just cover them and taking 1 teaspoonful of the soaked leaves to a cup of boiling water. Drink 2 or 3 cupfuls a day, cold. The tea may be made without the alcohol, of course, if desired. Of the tincture, 10 to 30 min.

BEARSFOOT

(Helleborus Fœtidus)

Common Name—Stinking Hellebore.

Medicinal Part—Root and herb.

Description—This is a European species of Hellebore containing the active principles of Black Hellebore and being the most energetic and active species.

Properties and Uses—Powerful emetic and cathartic and a drastic purgative, vermifuge and anthelmintic.

BEARSWORT

(Meum Athamanticum Jacquin)

Common Names—Baldmoney, Spieknel, Spignel.

Medicinal Part—Root.

Description—A genus of the Umbelliferæ, a native of the mountains of middle and western Europe. The root has an aromatic odor and taste. The fruit or seed is also aromatic.

Properties and Uses — Carminative, aromatic and stomachic.

BELLADONNA

(Atropa Belladonna)

Common Names—Dwale, Black Cherry.

Medicinal Part—The leaves.

Description—This perennial herb has a thick, fleshy, creeping root, and an annual erect leafy stem about three feet high. Leaves ovate, acute, entire, on short petioles, and of a dull green color. The flowers are dark purple, and fruit a many-seeded berry.

This plant is common to Europe, growing among ruins and waste places, blossoming from May to August, and maturing its fruit in September. The leaves should be gathered while the plant is in flower. They yield their virtues to water and alcohol.

Properties and Uses—Belladonna is an energetic narcotic. It is anodyne, antispasmodic, calmative, and relaxant. In the hands of skilled herbal physicians this botanical has great virtues, but it is too powerful and dangerous for general or home use.

Dose — Steep 1 teaspoonful of the leaves into a pint of boiling water. When cold take 1 to 2 teaspoonfuls of the tea 2 or 3 times a day. Of the tincture, ½ to 1 min.

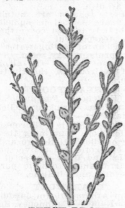

BEECH DROPS
(Orobanche Virginiana, Broomrape Family)

Common Names—Cancer Root.

Medicinal Part—The plant.

Description—This is a parasitic plant, with a smooth, leafless stem from a foot to foot and a half in height, with slender branches given off the whole length of it. The root is scaly and tuberous.

This plant is native of North America, and generally a parasite upon the roots of beech trees, flowering in August and September. The whole plant is of a dull red color, without any verdure. It has a disagreeable astringent taste. It yields its virtues to water and alcohol.

Properties and Uses—An eminent astringent. Locally applied to minor cuts, wounds and bruises.

BENNE
(Sesame Indicum—Pedalium Family)

Common Names—Sesame, Gingili, Teel.

Parts Used—Seeds, leaves, oil. Seeds used in bakery, confections, etc. Oil used in cookery, cosmetics, etc. Leaves—demulcent and emollient.

BENNET
(Geum Urbanum—Rose Family)

Common Names—Yellow Avens, Blessed Herb, Star of the Earth.

Medicinal Part—Root.

Description — Bennett is found in woods, hedges and shady places. It has an erect, hairy stem red at the base with terminal bright yellow drooping flowers. It has a graceful trefoiled leaf and the flower has fine yellow petals which fall off and a small round prickly ball is to be seen.

Properties and Uses—Astringent, tonic and styptic.

BETH ROOT
(Trillium Pendulum, Lily of the Valley Family)

Common Names—Wake Robin, Indian Balm, Ground Lily, Birth Root, Cough Root, Jewsharp, Snakebite.

Medicinal Part—The root.

Description—This is an herbaceous, perennial plant, having an oblong tuberous root, from which arises a slender stem from ten to fifteen inches high. The leaves are three in number, acuminate, from three to five inches in diameter, with a very short petiole. The flowers are white, sepals green, petals ovate and acute, styles erect, and stigmas recurved.

This plant is common in the Middle and Western states, growing in rich soils and shady woods, flowering in May and June. There are many varieties, all possessing analogous medicinal properties. These plants may be generally known by their three net-veined leaves, and their solitary terminal flower, which varies in color in the different species, being whitish-yellow and reddish-white.

Properties and Uses—It is astringent, and when boiled in milk it is of eminent benefit in diarrhoea. The root made into a poultice is very useful in stings of insects. The leaves boiled in lard is a good external application.

Dose—One teaspoonful of the root to a cup of boiling water. Drink hot or cold upon retiring at night. One or two cupfuls may be taken a day. Of the tincture, ¼ to ½ fl. dr.

BILBERRY
(Vaccinium Myrtillus)

Common Names—Whortle Berry, Blue Berry. Burren Myrtle.

Medicinal Parts—Leaves and Berries.

Description—Bilberry is a low shrub growing in sandy regions of the northern parts of the United States. Leaves are obovate, about one inch long, upper surface dark green and shiny. Flowers in May. They are reddish pink or white with red lips; 5 seeds resembling currants in appearance, but of a dark blue or black color, with a purplish bloom.

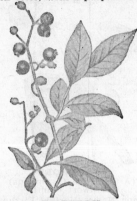

BILBERRY
Properties and Uses—The leaves are strongly astringent and somewhat bitter. They are of great value in diarrhoea. A mixture of equal parts of Bilberry leaves, Thyme and Strawberry leaves make an excellent tea.
Dose—A teaspoonful of the leaves or berries to a cup of boiling water. Drink cold, one or two cupfuls a day, a large mouthful at a time; of the tincture, ½ to 1 fl. dr.

BIRCH
(Betula Lenta)
Common Name—Sweet Birch.
Parts Used—Leaves and bark.
Description—Birch is a medium sized tree, 45 to 50 feet high, ovate in contour, the dark brown trunk fairly straight, often measuring 5 feet in diameter. The upper branches ascending, the lower ones nearly horizontal, slender and often drooping. Bark dark slate gray; brown on younger trees and their slender branches smooth, not peeling, strongly marked with horizontal lines resembling the bark of the cherry tree; on old trees broken into irregular gray brown plates. The leaves grow alternately in pairs; they are pointed-ovate, bright green above, lighter beneath, smooth and more or less heart shaped at the base, finely toothed, sharp pointed. Pistillate catkins about 1 inch long are produced only once in 3 or 4 years; staminate catkins, about 3 inches long; in clusters.

Properties and Uses—The bark is aromatic. Beer is often made from the sap of this tree, and oil wintergreen is distilled from its inner bark and twigs.
The leaves are useful to promote the discharge of the urine and to expel worms.
Dose—One teaspoonful of bark or leaves to a cup of boiling water. Drink 1 or 2 cups a day. Tincture, ¼ to ½ fl. dr.

BIRD CHERRY
(Prunus Padus—Rose Family)
Common Names—Hag Berry, Hoop Ash, Fowl Cherry, Cherry Bay, Cluster Cherry.
Medicinal Part—Bark.
Description—Bird Cherry has long and loose and often drooping racemes. The leaves are oblong. The fruit which ripens in summer has a rough stone.
Properties and Uses—Bark yields oil like Almonds.

BIRD-ON-THE-WING
(Polygala paucifolia—Milkwort Family)
Common Names—Fringed Milkwort, Large flowered Polygala.
Parts Used—Roots.
Description—Small plant, leaf-blades various, lower scale-like; upper elliptic, oval, or ovate; bracts similar to upper leaves. Flowers rose-colored, rose purple, or white. Found in moist woods from Canada to Georgia and Wisconsin, and particularly in the Blue Ridge Mountains of Virginia.
Properties and Uses—Bitter, diaphoretic, expectorant, pectoral.

15

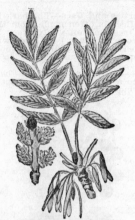

BIRDS TONGUE
(Fraxinus Excelsior)
Common Names—European Ash.
Medicinal Part—Bark.

Description—A tree with opposite and odd-pinnate leaves, and small polygamous flowers appearing before or with the leaves in the spring from the axils of those of the previous season. The fruit is a flat samara, winged at the apex only or all around, usually one seed. The seed is oblong, pendulous.

Properties and Uses—Febrifuge and diuretic.

* * *

"He who lives physically must live miserably. To cut off our days by intemperance, indiscretion, and guilty passions, to live miserably for the sake of gratifying a sweet tooth, or a brutal itch; to die martyrs to our luxury and wantoness, is equally beneath the dignity of human nature, and contrary to the homage we owe to the Author of our being. Without some degree of health, we can neither be agreeable to ourselves, nor useful to our friends; we can neither relish the blessings of divine providence to us in life, nor acquit ourselves of our duties to our Maker, or our neighbor. He that wantonly transgresseth the self-evident rules of health, is guilty of a degree of self-murder; and an habitual perseverance therein is direct suicide, and consequently, the greatest crime he can commit against the Author of his being."—G. Cheyne, M.D. 1725

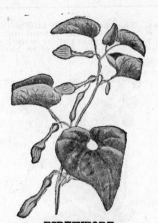

BIRTHWORT
(Aristolochia Clematitus)
Birthwort Family
Common Name—Upright Birthwort.
Medicinal Part—Root.

Description—Birthwort is an herbaceous perennial with an erect stem one or two feet tall. The leaves are dark green, reniform. Petioles shorter than the blades, flowers fascicled in the axels. Tube of the calyx is yellowish green, straight, enlarged around the ovary, the six lobes appendaged.

Properties and Uses — Febrifuge, emetic, stimulant and acrid.

BITTER ROOT
(Apocynum Androsaemifolium, Dogbane Family)
Common Names — Dog's Bane, Milk Weed, Honeybloom.
Medicinal Part—The root.

Description—This is a smooth, elegant plant, five or six feet high, with a large perennial root. The leaves are dark green above, pale beneath, ovate, and about two or three inches long and an inch wide. Corolla pink, calyx five-cleft, and stamens five. Fruit a follicle. Every part of the plant is milky.

This plant is indigenous to the United States, growing in dry, sandy soils, and in the borders of woods, from Maine to Florida, flowering from May to August. When any part of the plant is wounded a milky juice exudes. The large, milky root is the part used for medicinal purposes. It possesses an unpleasant amarous taste. It yields its properties to alcohol, but especially to water. Age impairs its medicinal quality.

Properties and Uses—Emetic, diaphoretic, tonic and laxative. In conjunction with Yellow Parilla it is excellent in dyspepsia. As a laxative it is useful in constipation. As a tonic it stimulates the digestive apparatus, and thus effects a corresponding impression on the general system.

Dose—One teaspoonful of the root to a pint of boiling water. Drink cold two or three tablespoonfuls six times a day. Of the tincture, 5 to 10 min.

the foliage has fallen the twigs should be gathered. Boiling water and diluted alcohol extract their virtues.

Properties and Uses—Formerly this botanical was widely used in a variety of conditions but now is employed chiefly for relief of skin irritation.

Dose—Two teaspoonfuls of the root to a pint of boiling water. Drink cold, 2 or 3 tablespoonfuls six times a day. Of the tincture, 10 to 20 min.

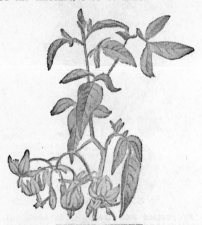

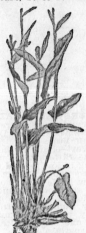

BITTER SWEET
(Amara Dulcis, Solanum Dulcamara, Potato Family)

Common Names — M o r t a l, Woody Nightshade, Felon Wort, Fever Twig, Violet-bloom, Scarletberry.

Medicinal Part—Bark of root and twigs.

Description—Bitter Sweet is a woody vine, with a shrubby stem several feet in length, having an ashy green bark. Leaves acute, and generally smooth, lower one cordate, upper ones hastate. The flowers are purple, and the fruit a scarlet, juicy and bitter berry, which, however, should not be eaten or used.

Bitter Sweet is common to both Europe and America, growing in moist banks, around dwellings and in low damp grounds, about hedges and thickets, and flowering in June and July. The berries ripen in autumn, and hang upon the vines for several months. After

BISTORT
(Polygonum Bistorta)

Common Names—Patience Dock, Snake Weed, Dragonwort.

Medicinal Part—Root.

Description — Bistort has a thick, short-knobbed root, blackish without and of a reddish color within, somewhat crooked with numerous black threads from which leaves spring every year on long foot-stalks. The leaves are somewhat broad and long like a dock leaf, bluish-green, a little purplish underneath. The flowers are pale and borne in a spike. Flowers from May until the first of July.

Properties and Uses—Astringent, diuretic, alterative.

Prince's Pine — Valuable in various conditions. Mixed with Elder Flowers it is said to be very good for skin irritations.

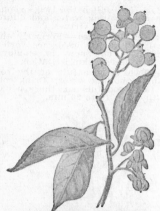

object in the midst of the general nakedness of vegetation. Hence the plant is often called Winterberry.

Black Alder is common throughout the United States and England, growing in moist woods, swamps, etc., flowering from May to July, and maturing its fruit in the latter part of autumn. It yields its virtues to water by decoction or infusion. The bark has a bitterish sub-astringent taste, and the berries have a sweetish taste.

BITTERSWEET—FALSE

(Celastrus Scandens, Stafftree Family)
Common Names—False Bittersweet, Waxwort, Staff Vine.

Medicinal Part—Bark of the root.

Description—Bittersweet is a vine found growing in low ground from Eastern Canada to South Dakota and from North Carolina to New Mexico, with thin ovate-oblong and pointed, finely serrate leaves, racemes of greenish white flowers (in early summer). Often planted for the showy, autumnul fruit.

Properties and Uses—Alterative, diuretic and herpatic.

BLACK ALDER

(Prunos Verticillatus, Holly Family)
Common Names—Winterberry, Feverbush.

Medicinal Parts—The bark and berries.

Description—This is an indigenous shrub of irregular growth, with a stem six or eight feet in height; bark bluish gray and alternate branches. The leaves are ovate, acute at the base, olive green in color, smooth above and downy beneath. Flowers small and white; calyx small and six-cleft; corolla divided into six obtuse segments. The fruit when ripe consists of glossy, scarlet, roundish berries, about the size of a pea, containing six cells and six seeds. Several of these berries are clustered together, so as to form little bunches at irregular intervals on the stem. In the latter part of autumn, after the leaves have fallen, they still remain attached to the stem, and render the shrub a striking

BLACK ALDER

Properties and Uses—It is tonic, alterative and astringent. Two teaspoonfuls of the powdered bark and one teaspoonful of powdered Golden Seal infused in a pint of boiling water, and, when cold, taken in the course of the day, in doses of a wineglassful, and repeated daily, has proved very efficacious in dyspepsia. Externally the decoction forms an excellent local application for irritation of the skin. The berries are cathartic and vermifuge, and form, with cedar apples, a pleasant and effectual worm medicine for children.

Dose—A teaspoonful of the bark or berries to a cup of boiling water. Drink cold 1 or 2 cupfuls a day. Of the tincture, 15 to 30 min.

BLACK COHOSH

(Cimicifuga Racemosa, Crowfoot Family)
Common Names — Rattleroot, Squaw Root, Black Snake Root.

Medicinal Part—The root.

Description—This plant is a tall, leafy perennial herb, with a large knotty root, having long slender fibres. The stem is simple, smooth, and furrowed and from three to nine feet high. The flower is a small and fetid one.

It is a native of the United States, inhabiting upland woods and hillsides, and flowering from May to August. The root is the medicinal part. It contains a resin, to which the names of Cimicifugin or Macrotin have been given; likewise fatty substances, starch, gum, tannic acid, etc. The leaves of Cimicifuga are said to drive away bugs; hence its name from cimex, a bug, and fugo, to drive away.

Boiling water takes up the properties of the root but partially, alcohol wholly.

Properties and Uses—It is a very active and useful remedy in many conditions. It is slightly narcotic, sedative, antispasmodic.

It exerts a tonic influence over mucous and serious tissues, and is a superior remedy in a variety of ailments, according to the Eclectic School of Medicine.

Dose—Two teaspoonfuls of the root to a pint of boiling water. Drink cold, two or three tablespoonfuls six times a day. Of the tincture, 10 to 20 min.

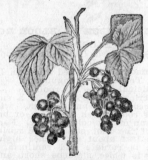

BLACK CURRANT
(Ribes Nigrum, Saxifrage Family)
Common Name—Quinsy Berry.
Medicinal Part—Leaves.
Description—Leaves slightly heart-shaped, sharply 3-5 lobed and doubly serrate; racemes drooping, downy, bearing greenish-white flowers.
Properties and Uses—Diuretic.

Squaw Weed—Diuretic and tonic. Combined with Lily Root it is popular as a tonic for female use particularly.

BLACK INDIAN HEMP
(Apocynum Canabinum)
Common Names—Canadian Hemp, Indian Hemp, Bowman's Root, Rheumatism Weed, Amy Root, Indian Physic.
Part Used—The root.
Description—This plant is a native of America, growing wild in pastures and fields. It stands erect about 3 feet high and exudes a milky juice when broken. The leaves are in pairs exactly opposite each other, attached to the main stem by short stems. They are lanceolate with slightly oval ends, about 4 inches in length; upper surface smooth, lower surface silky hairs. Blooms in July, flowers in clusters, whitish, tinted with green. Seed pods are 6 to 8 inches long and pointed toward the end. The root is from 5 to 6 feet long and about ½ inch thick, dividing near the end into small branches; color yellowish brown, old roots dark brown, wrinkled lengthwise. The fresh root emits a milky juice.

Properties and Uses—Black Indian Hemp contains Apocynin, tannin, resin, starch and bitter extractives. It is diuretic, diaphoretic, expectorant, tonic, and cathartic, but caution should be observed in its use.

Dose—A teaspoonful of the root to a pint of boiling water. Take a teaspoonful of the tea 3 to 8 times a day; of the tincture, 2 to 5 min.

BLACK ROOT
(Leptandra Virginica, Figwort Family)
Common Names—Culver's Physic, Tall Speedwell, Tall Veronica, Leptandra, Culver's Root.
Medicinal Part—The root.
Description—It is perennial, with a simple, straight, smooth, herbaceous stem and grows from three to four or five feet high. The leaves are short, petioled, whorled in fours to sevens, lanceolate, acuminate, and finely serrated. The flowers are white, nearly sessile, and very numerous. Calyx four-parted corolla small and nearly white; stamens, two. The fruit is a many seeded capsule.

This plant is indigenous to the United States, but is to be found in good condition only in limestone countries. It is often discovered in new soil, in moist woods, in swamps, etc., but its medicinal virtues are feeble, excepting when it is found where there is limestone. The root is the part used. It is perennial, irregular, horizontal, woody, and about as thick as the forefinger. It is gathered in the fall of the second year. The fresh root, after having been properly prepared, is what may be relied upon for beneficial effects.

Properties and Uses—The fresh root is too irritant to be used, although a decoction of it may, with care, be employed. The dried root is laxative, cholagogue, and tonic. It is an excellent laxative. As a laxative and tonic it is very useful in conditions associated with torpidity of the liver.

Dose—Steep a heaping teaspoonful of this root cut into small pieces into a cup of boiling water for half hour. When cold drink one cupful a day, a good mouthful at a time. Of the tincture, 10 to 30 min.

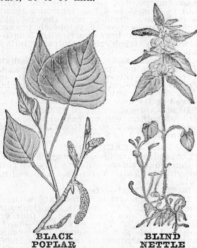

BLACK POPLAR   BLIND NETTLE

BLACK POPLAR
(Populus Nigra, Willow Family)
Common Name—Poplar Buds.
Medicinal Part—The buds.
Description—A medium sized tree, very sparingly planted, with broadly triangular or diamond-ovate, small leaves, which are not deeply toothed and commonly hairy young shoots.
Properties and Uses—Resinous, vulnerary.

BLIND NETTLE
(Laminum Album, Mint Family)
Common Names — Stingless Nettle, White Nettle, White Archangel.

Medicinal Part—The plant.
Description—This plant is found growing in gardens and waste grounds in New England. The plant is hairy, leaves all petioled, ovate and heart-shaped, the flowers are white.
Properties and Uses—Styptic and used as a vaginal douche.

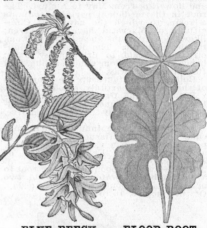

BLUE BEECH   BLOOD ROOT

BLOOD ROOT
(Sanguinaria Canadensis, Poppy Family.)
Common Names—Red Puccoon, Indian Plant, Tetterwort, Sanguinaria.
Medicinal Part—The root.
Description—Blood root is a smooth, herbaceous, perennial plant, with a fibrous root, which when cut or bruised emits an orange-colored juice. For each bud of the root stalk there springs a single leaf about six inches high, and which is cordate and reniform. The flower is white, stamens short, and anthers yellow. The fruit is a two-valved capsule.

Blood Root grows throughout the United States, in shaded woods and thickets, and rich soils generally, and flowers from March to June. Although the whole plant is medicinal, the root is the part chiefly used. The fresh root is fleshy, round and from one to four inches in length, and as thick as the fingers. It presents a beautiful appearance when cut and placed under a microscope, seeming like an aggregation of minute precious stones. The dried root is dark brown outside, bright yellow inside; has a faint virose odor, and a bitter and acrid taste. It may be readily reduced to powder. Its active properties are taken up by boiling water or by alcohol. Age and moisture impair the qualities of the root, and it is of the utmost consequence to get that which has been properly gathered, and not kept too long.

Properties and Uses—The actions of Blood Root vary according to administration. In small doses it stimulates the digestive organs, acting as a stimulant and tonic. It appears to be used chiefly as an expectorant.

Dose—Steep a level teaspoonful of the root into a pint of boiling water for half hour. Strain. When cold take a teaspoonful 3 to 6 times a day. Of the tincture, ½ to 1 min.

BLUE BEECH
(Carpinus Americana, Oak Family)
Common Names—Hornbeam, Water Beech.

Medicinal Part—Leaves.

Description—Low trees or shrubs with furrowed trunks and very hard wood. Found on the banks of streams from New England to Minnesota. Leaves are ovate-oblong pointed doubly serrate leaves, becoming smooth. Flowers with the leaves in spring.

Properties and Uses—Bitter, tonic, anti-periodic and alterative.

BLUE COHOSH
(Caulophyllum Thalictroides, Barberry Family)
Common Names—Papoose Root, Squaw Root.

Medicinal Part—The root.

Description—This is a smooth, glaucous plant, purple when young, with a high, round stem, one to three feet high. Leaves biternate or triternate, leaflets oval, petilate, pale beneath, and from two to three inches long. The flowers appear in May or June.

It is a handsome perennial plant, growing in all parts of the United States, near running streams, and in low, moist, rich grounds; also in swamps and on islands. The seeds, which ripen in August, make a decoction which closely resembles coffee. The berries are dry and rather mawkish. Its active principle is Caulophyllin.

Properties and Uses—It has been employed by eclectic physicians as an emmenagogue. It also possesses diuretic, diaphoretic and anthelmintic properties. It is a valuable remedy, but should be

given in combination with such other remedies as the case requires.

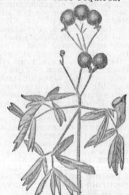

BLUE COHOSH
Dose—A teaspoonful of the root, cut small or granulated, to a cup of boiling water. Drink cold, one cupful during the day, a large mouthful at a time; of the tincture, 5 to 10 min.

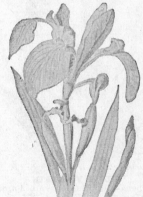

BLUE FLAG
(Iris Versicolor, Iris Family)
Common Names—Iris, Flag Lily, Liver Lily, Water Flag, Snake Lily.

Medicinal Part—The rhizome.

Description — Blue Flag is common throughout the United States, growing in moist places, and bearing blue or purple flowers from May to July. The root has a peculiar odor, augmented by rubbing or pulverizing, and a disagreeable taste. It imparts its virtues to boiling water, alcohol, or ether. The root should be sliced transversely, dried and placed in vessels, well closed and placed in a dark place; it will then preserve its virtues for a long time.

Properties and Uses — This is one among our most valuable medicinal plants, capable of extensive use. It is alterative, cathartic, and has been popular with the Eclectic School of Medicine. Combined with mandrake, poke, black cohosh, etc. It will sometimes salivate, but it need cause no apprehension; and when this effect is established it may be distinguished from mercurial salivation by absence of stench, sponginess of the gums, and loosening of the teeth.

Dose—One teaspoonful of the root to a pint of boiling water. Drink cold, 2 or 3 tablespoonfuls six times a day. Of the tincture, 5 to 10 min.

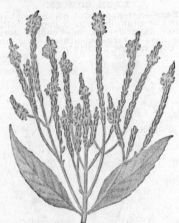

BLUE VERVAIN
(Verbena Hastata, Vervain Family)

Common Names — Wild Hyssop, Simpler's Joy, Indian Hyssop.

Medicinal Part—The root and herb.

Description—Vervain is an erect, tall, elegant and perennial plant, with a four-angled stem tree or four feet high, having opposite branches. The leaves are petiolate, serrate, acuminate and hastate.

The flower is a small purplish blue one, sessile, and arranged in long spikes. Seeds, four.

Vervain is indigenous to the United States, and grows along roadsides and in dry, grassy fields, flowering from June to September. It is also found in England, growing among hedges, by the way-side, and other waste grounds, flowering in July, and the seeds ripening soon after.

Properties and Uses—Vervain is tonic and expectorant. The infusion, taken cold, is said to make a good tonic. Also useful in coughs due to colds.

Dose—Two teaspoonfuls of the herb to a pint of boiling water. Drink cold, two or three teaspoonfuls six times a day. Of the tincture, 10 to 20 min.

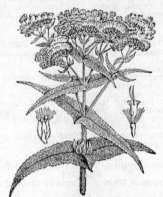

BONESET
(Eupatorium Perfoliatum, Aster Family.)

Common Names—Thoroughwort, Indian Sage, Ague Weed, Crosswort, Eupatorium.

Medicinal Part—The tops and leaves.

Description—Boneset is an indigenous perennial herb, with a horizontal crooked root; the stems being rough and hairy, from one to five feet high, and the leaves veiny, serrate, rough and tapering to a long point. The flowers are white and very numerous.

Boneset grows in low ground, on the borders of swamps and streams, throughout the United States from Canada to Florida, west to Texas and Nebraska, flowering in August and September. Alcohol or boiling water extracts the virtues of the parts used. It

22

has a feeble odor, but a very bitter taste. It contains tannin and the extractive salts of potassa. It is called Boneset on account that it was formerly supposed to cause rapid union of broken bones.

Properties and Uses—It is a very valuable medicinal agent. The cold infusion or extract is tonic and aperient, the warm infusion diaphoretic and emetic. As a tonic it is particularly useful. A strong infusion, as hot as can be comfortably swallowed, is administered for the purpose of vomiting freely. This is also attended sooner or later, by an evacuation of the bowels. During the intermission the cold infusion or extract is given every hour as a tonic The warm infusion is also administered to promote the operation of other emetics.

Dose—Steep a level teaspoonful of the herbs into a cup of boiling water for half hour. Strain. When cold take a teaspoonful three to six times a day. Of the tincture, 10 to 40 min.

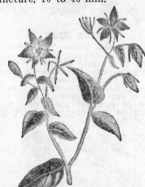

BORAGE

(Borago Officinalis, Borage Family)
Common Names—Burrage, Common Bugloss.

Medicinal Part—Plant.

Description—A spreading, branched plant beset with sharp and whitish spreading bristles. The leaves are oval or oblong-lanceolate and the flowers loosely racemed, handsome, blue or purplish with dark anthers.

Properties and Uses—Borage is a cordial, pectoral and aperient.

The lovely star-like flowers of Borage are used fresh to garnish beverages, green salads, gelatin molds, etc.

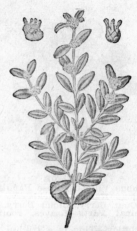

BOX WOOD

(Buxus Sempervirens)
Common Names—Box, Bush Tree.

Medicinal Part—The leaves.

Description—Box Wood is a small, dense-leaved, hard-wood, evergreen tree. The leaves are ovate, deep shining green, becoming red in autumn; flowers pale yellow; and the fruit a six-seeded globular capsule.

The Box Wood tree is a native of the West of Asia, but grows on dry hills and sandy elevations generally in Europe, and but rarely on similar soil in America.

Properties and Uses—It is cathartic, sudorific and alterative, according to some. The preparations of the leaves are excellent for purging the bowels.

* * *

Herbal bath: Add equal amount of borax crystals with fragrant herb or mixture, and place in a silk or nylon bag (or old stocking) and tie with ribbon so that it can be suspended from the hot water tap of the bath. When the water is turned on, the whole atmosphere of the room becomes permeated with the aroma of herbs. The bag can be used repreatedly before becoming exhausted. Any sachet or pot-pourri mixture may be used for fragrant baths. The addition of Khus-Khus roots is desirable, as they help the pot-pourri to retain its perfume for a much longer period.

23

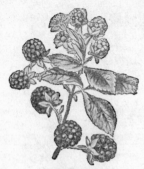

BRAMBLE

(Rubus Villosus, Rose Family)

Common Names—Blackberry, Dewberry, Gout Berry, Cloud Berry.

Medicinal Parts—Leaves, roots and fruit.

Description—This is a trailing plant, with slender branches, growing in sandy or dry soil in the northeastern and middle parts of the United States. The stems are armed with stout recurved prickles. Flowers white, about 1 inch broad. Fruit black, pulpy and delicious to eat, much used for making wine and brandy.

Properties and Uses—This shrub is rich in tannin and is therefore a good astringent and tonic, long a favorite home remedy for diarrhea. Also used by some for offensive saliva.

Dose—A teaspoonful of the root or leaves to a cup of boiling water. Drink cold, one or two cupfuls a day, a large mouthful at a time; of the tincture, ½ to 1 fl. dr.

BRIER HIP

(Rosa Canina.)

Common Names—Sweet Brier, Dog Rose, Witches Brier.

Medicinal Part—The flowers and hips.

Description—Brier is a bushy shrub, 2 to 3 feet high, stems numerous, covered with prickles and a few sharp spines; leaves alternate, imparipinnate, two pairs opposite leaflets, these nearly sessile, ovate, rounded at base, acute at apex, serrate, pale, hairy below, leaf-serratures not edged with glands; flowers large, petals five in the wild state, more when cultivated, rich crimson; fruit (hip) scarlet to orange-red, oblong; containing many 1-seeded achenes, calyx persistent. The petals are usually in small cones, consisting of many imbri-

cated roundish retuse, deep purplish-red, yellow-clawed petals, characteristic, fine rose-like odor; bitterish, slightly acidulous, distinctly stringent taste.

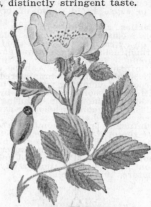

BRIER HIPS

Properties and Uses—The flowers are tonic, mild astringent, and carminative and once were quite commonly used for diuretic purposes. Useful as a flavoring vehicle and for perfumery.

Dose—A teaspoonful of the flowers or hips to a cup of boiling water. Drink cold one or two cupfuls a day, a large mouthful at a time; of the tincture, ½ to 1 fl. dr.

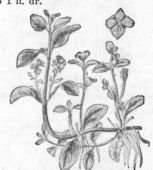

BROOKLIME

(Veronica Beccabunga)

Common Names—Water Pimpernel, Water Purslain, Beccabunga.

Medicinal Part—Herb.

Description—Brooklime grows quite commonly in brooks and ditches as a succulent plant with smooth leaves and small flowers of bright blue, being found in situations favorable to Water Cress. It has a creeping root which sends forth strings at every joint.

Properties and Uses—Anti-scorbutic, diuretic, emmenagogue, and febrifuge.

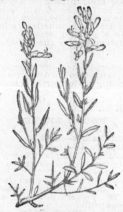

BROOM
(Cytisus Scoparius.)

Common Names—Link, Genista, Banal.

Part Used—Tops.

Description—The Broom is a leguminous shrub, common in our rural districts. It grows 4 to 8 feet high. Leaves are small, alternate, oblong downy, trifoliate. Flowers racemes, brilliant yellow; bloom from May to June. Fruit a pod containing 12 to 18 seeds.

Properties and Uses—The Broom Tops are purgative and act on the kidneys to increase the flow of urine. This tea is of great service. It is often used in equal parts with the root Dandelion for diuretic purpose.

Dose—A teaspoonful of the tops to a cup of boiling water. Drink cold, 1 or 2 cupfuls a day, a large mouthful at a time; of the tincture, ½ to 1 fl. dr.

BRYONIA
(Bryonia Alba)

Common Names—Wild Bryony, White Bryony.

Parts Used—The root.

Description — Bryony is a perennial climber, native of Europe, but culti-

vated here. Leaves heart shaped, 5-lobed; flowers small, greenish white or yellowish; fruit, berries size of a pea, of a black color. Root spindle shaped 1 to 2 feet long, fleshy.

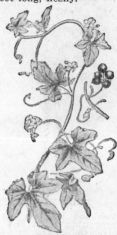

BRYONY

Properties and Uses—The dried root of Bryony is inodorous, bitter and contains bryonin, starch, gum, fat, malates, etc. It yields its properties to alcohol or hot water. Useful in pectoral conditions, as in the spasms of whooping cough. It is very powerful and poisonous in large doses.

Dose—A teaspoonful of the granulated root to a pint of boiling water. Take 1 teaspoonful of this tea at a time as required, every 1 or 2 hours if necessary. Tincture, 5 to 20 min.

BUCK BEAN
(Menyanthes Trifoliata, Buckbean Family)

Common Names—Bogbean, Bog Myrtle, Water Shamrock, Marsh Trefoil.

Medicinal Parts—The root, rhizome and dried leaves.

Description—This is a perennial herb, 8 to 12 feet high. The root is ½ inch thick, long jointed, branching and black. Leaves on petioles 4 to 6 inches long, ternate, leaflets sessile 2 to 3 inches long, obtuse, obovate, entire and sometimes crenate, smooth, pale green. It may be easily recognized growing in water by its large leaves overtopping

25

the surface. The flowers when in bud are of a bright rose color and when fully open have the inner surface of their petals thickly covered with a white fringe often referred to as "white fluff."

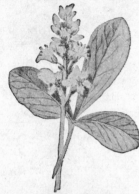

BUCK BEAN

Properties and Uses—A tea of Bog Bean improves digestion and promotes and improves the gastric juices. It is a bitter tonic with cathartic power.

Dose—A teaspoonful of the root, rhizome or dried leaves, cut small or granulated to a cup of boiling water. Drink cold one cupful during the day, a large mouthful at a time; of the tincture, 5 to 20 min.

BUCKHORN BRAKE

(Osmunda Regalis, Royal Fern Family)
Common Names—Male Fern, King's Fern, Royal Flowering Fern.
Medicinal Part—The root.
Description—This Fern has a hard, scaly, tuberous root, quite fibrous and a whitish core in the center. The fronds are three or four feet high, bright green, and doubly pinnate. The numerous leaflets are sessile and oblong, some of the upper ones cut.

This beautiful Fern is found in meadows and low, moist grounds throughout the United States, blossoming in June. The main root or caudex is the official part; it is about two inches long, and has the shape of a buck's horn. It contains an abundance of mucilage, which is extracted by boiling water. The roots should be collected in August, or about the latter part of May, and dried with

great care, as they are apt to become mouldy.

The Osmunda Cinnamonea, or cinnamon-colored Fern, is inferior to the preceding, but is frequently used for the same medical purposes.

Properties and Uses — Mucilaginous, tonic and styptic. Used in coughs resulting from colds, as well as in diarrhea; also used as a tonic during convalescence. One root, infused in a pint of hot water for half an hour, will convert the whole into a thick jelly, very valuable in indicated uses. The mucilage mixed with brandy is a popular remedy as an external application for the muscles of the back.

Dose—Steep a heaping teaspoonful of this root, cut into small pieces, into a cup of boiling water for half hour. When cold drink 1 to 2 cupfuls a day; a good mouthful at a time. Of the tincture, ½ to 1 fl. dr.

BUCHU LEAVES
(Barosma Crenata.)
Common Names—Bookoo.
Medicinal Part—The leaves.
Description—This plant has a slender, smooth, upright, perennial stem, between two and three feet high. The leaves are opposite, flat, about an inch long, ovate or obovate, acute, serrated and dotted. The flowers are pink, and fruit an ovate capsule.

The Buchu Plant is a native of Southern Africa. It does not grow very prolifically. There are two other varieties from which the leaves are taken, and which are of equal value with the Barosma Crenata. The leaves are the parts which are termed officinal. As we get the leaves they are ½ to 1 inch in length, and from a sixth to half an inch in width, elliptical, lanceolate, slightly acute, or shorter and obtuse; their margin is serrated and glandular, upper surface smooth, and of a clear shining green, the under surface paler, with scattered oil points. They have to be kept very carefully, if their odor and virtues are desired to be thoroughly preserved for any reasonable length of time. The leaves of all the varieties are somewhat similar, and possess about the same qualities. They yield their volatile oil and extractive (upon which their virtues are mainly dependent) to alcohol or water.

Properties and Uses—Buchu is aromatic and stimulant, diuretic and diaphoretic. Because of those properties it is a well known remedy in conditions in which it is indicated.

Dose—Steep a teaspoonful of these leaves, broken into small pieces, into a cupful of boiling water for half hour. When cold drink one or two cupfuls a day; a good mouthful at a time. Of the tincture, ½ to 1 fl. dr.

BUFFALO HERB
(Medicago Sativa)
Common Names—Lucerne, Alfalfa.
Medicinal Part—Leaves.
Description—Buffalo Herb is found growing from Maine to Virginia and westward to the Pacific coast. It is from one to one and one-half feet high and flowers from June until August. The leaflets are obovate-oblong, racemes oblong, pod several-seeded, linear, coiled about 2 turns. The flowers are violet purple or bluish.
Properties and Uses—Nutrient and tonic. Contains vitamines and organic minerals.

An infusion of Alfalfa with a bit of mint, makes an excellent tea for daily use. It is one of nature's richest sources of a variety of easily assimilated natural vitamins, minerals and trace elements.

BUGLE WEED
(Lycopus Virginicus)
Common Names—Water Bugle, Gipsy Wort.
Part Used—The herb.
Description—This plant is native to the United States. It has a smooth, obtusely quadrangular stem, ½ to 2 feet high; leaves 2 inches long, illiptic, glanular, flowers purple, 4-lobed, stamens 2, mint odor and bitter taste. The root is perennial, creeping.
Properties and Uses—It is tonic, astringent, sedative and mild narcotic.
Dose—A teaspoonful of the herb, cut small, to a cup of boiling water. Drink cold, one or two cupfuls a day; a large mouthful at a time; of the tincture, ½ to 1 fl. dr.

BUGLOSS
(Anchusa Officinalis, Borage Family)
Common Names—Oxtongue, Garden Alkanet.
Medicinal Part—Herb.
Description — A European biennial plant having narrow, oblong leaves and purple flowers, the latter arranged in racemes.
Properties and Uses—Expectorant, diuretic, diaphoretic and an emollient with a sweetish, mucilaginous taste.

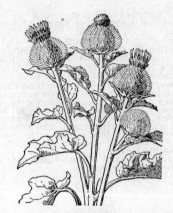

BURDOCK
(Arctium Lappa.)
Common Names—Clotburr, Bardana.
Medicinal Part—Root and seed.
Description—Burdock is a coarse biennial weed growing in the northern parts of the United States, 2 to 6 feet high, branched. Leaves cordate oblong, dentate, rough, petiolate. Flowers purple, from July to September.
Properties and Uses—The root should be dug in the fall or early spring. Only one-year-old roots should be used. It is diaphoretic, diuretic, alterative, aperient and depurative. Of excellent service in a variety of uses. Externally it is valuable in salves or as a wash for burns, wounds and skin irritations.
Dose—A teaspoonful of the root to a cup of boiling water. Drink cold 1 or 2 cupfuls a day. A large mouthful at a time. Of the tincture, ½ to 1 fl. dr.

CARDAMON
(Elettaria Cardamomum)
Part Used—Seeds.
Description — Large perennial plant with long lanceolate blades, smooth and dark green above, pale and finely silky beneath. Small yellowish flowers produced in loose racemes near the ground. Grown mainly in southern india.
Properties and Uses — Carminative, stimulant, aromatic, but rarely used alone. Seeds useful in flatulence because of their warmth.

For other uses see page 180—Spices and Flavoring Herbs; page 197—Botanical Products Used in Potpourri and sachets; page 205—Botanical Breath Sweeteners.

27

for various conditions, such as the spasm of asthma and bronchial irritation.

CARROT
(Daucus Carota, Parsley Family)

Common Names—Bee's Nest Plant, Bird's Nest Root, Queen Anne's Lace.

Medicinal Parts—Root and seed.

Description—The common Wild Carrot is an immigrant from Europe and which makes itself a great nuisance to the farmer. Flowering from June to September, the flowers are lacy and attractive when in their prime. The Umbel is concave like a bird's nest. The leaves are cut into fine divisions; involucre of pinnatifid leaves.

Properties and Uses—Stimulant, diuretic and carminative.

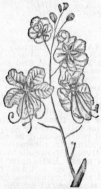

CASSIA FISTULA

Common Names—Purging Cassia, Cassia Stick Tree, Pudding Pipe Tree, Drumstick Tree.

Medicinal Part—Beans.

Description—Small trees or shrubs with evenly pinnate leaves, not sensitive to the touch and mainly yellow flowers. Calyx-teeth nearly equal, mostly obtuse, generally longer than the tube. The pod is flat or terete, often curved, septate or continuous between seeds, the vales elastically dehiscent. Seeds numerous.

Properties and Uses—Mildly cathartic.

Cassia fistula flowers and leaves are also purgative. The bark of the tree is powerfully astringent.

* * * *

"When you are sick of the world of men, turn to the world of plants."—David Fairchild.

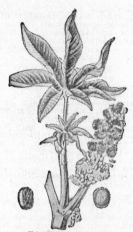

CASTOR BEAN
(Ricinus Communis, Spurge Family)

Common Names—Castor Oil Plant, Palma Christi, Bofareira.

Medicinal Part—Seed yields oil.

Description—A sort of tree but cultivated in temperate climates as a stately annual, for its seeds from which castor oil is expressed and in ornamental grounds for its magnificient foliage. The peltate and palmately cleft leaves are one or two feet broad or even more. Flowers in the late summer.

Properties and Uses—Seeds are cathartic and yield castor oil.

CEDRON SEED
(Cedron Simaba)

Medicinal Part—The seed.

Description—Simaba is a small tree, with an erect stem about half a foot in diameter, branching luxuriantly at the top. Leaves obovate, large and serrated; flowers sessile, pale brown, and the fruit a solitary drupe.

This tree grows in New Granada and Central America. Its value as a medicinal agent has long been known in Costa Rica, Trinidad, etc., and from thence was communicated to scientific gentlemen in France. The seed, which is the part used, is about an inch and a half long, nearly an inch broad, and about half an inch thick. It is hard, but can be easily cut by a common knife. It is inodorous, but tastes like quassia or aloes, and yields its properties to water or alcohol. In South

America the properties of these seeds were known as early as the year 1700. At that time they were applied more especially as an antidote to the bites of poisonous serpents and similar affections.

Properties and Uses—It is an antispasmodic, and one of the most valuable articles of the kind known to educated herbalists. It is very useful in dyspepsia and certain acro-narcotic poisons. Snake bites should at the same time be bathed in the tincture.

Dose—A teaspoonful of the seed to a pint of boiling water. Take a teaspoonful 2 to 6 times a day. Of the tincture, ½ to 2 min.

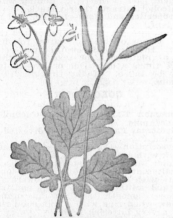

CELANDINE
(Chelidonium Majus, Poppy Family)
Common Names—Tetterwort, Garden Celandine, Great Celandine, Chelidonium.
Medicinal Parts—Herb and root.
Description—This plant is an evergreen perennial, with a stem from one to two feet in height, branched, swelled at the joints, leafy, round and smooth; the leaves are smooth, spreading, very deeply pinnatified; leaflets in from two to four pairs, from one and a half to two and a half inches long, and about two-thirds as broad, the terminal one largest, all ovate, cuneately incised or lobed; the lateral ones sometimes dilated at the lower margin, near the base almost as it auricled; color of all, a deep shining green; the flowers are bright yellow, umbellate, on long, often hairy stocks.

Celandine is a pale green, fleshy herb, indigenous to Europe and naturalized in the United States; it grows along fences, by-roads, in waste places, etc., and flowers from May to October. If the plant be wounded, a bright yellow, offensive juice flows out, which has a persistent, nauseous bitter taste, with a biting sensation in the mouth and fauces. The root is the most intensely bitter part of the plant, and is more commonly preferred. Drying diminishes its activity. It yields its virtues to alcohol and water.

Properties and Uses—It is stimulant, acrid, alterative, diuretic, diaphoretic, purgative and vulnerary. It is used internally in decoction or tincture, and externally in poultice or ointment. As a drastic hydragogue, or purge, it is believed to be fully equal to gamboge. The juice, when applied to the skin, produces inflammations, and even vesications. It has long been known as a caustic for application to warts.

Tetterwort is also used in saltrheum, tetter or ringworm. It has been preferred by some to arnica as a vulnerary; an alcoholic tincture of the root (three ounces to a pint) will be found an unrivalled application.

Dose—Steep one level teaspoonful of the herb broken into small pieces into a cup of boiling water for half hour. When cold drink one cupful a day. Of the tincture, 10 to 15 min.

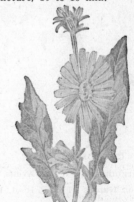

CHICORY
(Chicorium Intybus)
Common Names—Succory, Endive.
Medicinal Part—The root.

Description—Chicory is a perennial herb, native of Europe, but has become thoroughly naturalized in the United States. The stem is stiff, tough, and angular in cross-section; it attains heights of from one to three feet. It is often quite branching, but the branches spring out abruptly so that the effect is not very graceful. The leaves are long-lanceolate. dark gray-green and coarsely toothed The flowers are very beautiful—a violet-blue, approaching a pure blue in color. There are at least two ranks of strap-shaped rays, the inner one much shorter, all toothed at the ends. Succory blooms in dry situations from July until October.

Properties and Uses—A tea made of the dried root is good for sour stomach. It may also be taken whenever the stomach has been upset by any kind of food. The fresh root is bitter and a milky juice flows from the rind, to which is attributed any medicinal virtues it may possess.

Dose—A teaspoonful of the root to a pint of boiling water. Drink cold, a mouthful 2 or 3 times a day.

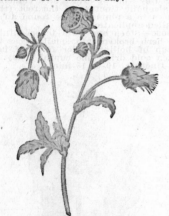

CHOCOLATE ROOT
(Geum Rivale—Water Avens, Geum
Virginianum—White Avens,
Rose Family)

Common Names—Throat Root, Purple Avens, Evans Root.

Medicinal Part—The root.

Description—Geum Rivale, or Purple Avens, is a perennial, deep green herb; woody root; leaves nearly lyrate,

crenate-dentate, and from four to six inches long. The flowers are few and purple in color.

Geum Virginianum, or Throat Root, is also a perennial, with a small crooked root. The stem is two or three feet high. The leaves are pinnate or lyrate; flowers rather small and white; and the fruit an achenium. The former is common to the United States and Europe, flowering in June and July, and the latter only to the United States, flowering from June to August.

These plants, with other varieties, have long been used in domestic practice. The whole herb contains medicinal properties, but the officinal and most efficient part is the root. Boiling water or alcohol extracts their virtues.

Properties and Uses—Is tonic and astringent.

Dose—Steep a teaspoonful of the root into a cup of boiling water, for half hour. Drink a half cupful upon retiring at night cold, or take a mouthful three times a day. One or two cupfuls may be taken. Of the tincture, 10 to 20 min,

COLOCYNTH
(Cucumis Colocynthis)

Common Names — Bitter Cucumber, Bitter Apple.

Medicinal Part—The fruit divested of its rind.

Description—Colocynth is an annual plant, with a whitish root, and prostrate, angular, and hispid stems. The leaves are alternate, cordate, ovate, many-lobed, white with hairs beneath. Flowers yellow and solitary; petals small, and fruit globose, smooth, size of an orange, yellow when ripe with a thin solid rind. and a very bitterish flesh.

This plant is a native of the south of Europe, Africa and Asia. The fruit assumes a yellow or orange color externally during the autumn, at which time it is pulled and dried quickly, either in the stove or sun. That which is deprived of its rind, very white, light, spongy and without seeds, is the best article; all others are more or less inferior in quality.

Properties and Uses—It is a strong hydragogue cathartic, producing copious water evacuations. It should never be used alone, but be combined with other cathartics, as it is too dangerous otherwise. In combination with Black Henbane it loses its irritant properties, and may be so employed whenever its peculiar cathartic effects are desired.

Dose—A teaspoonful of the fruit to a pint of boiling water. A tablespoonful two to four times a day, cold. Of the tincture, 1 to 2 min.

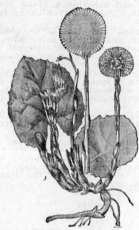

COLTS FOOT
(Tussilago Farfara, Aster Family)

Common Names — Coughwort, Foal's Foot, Horse Hoof, Horse Foot, Bull's Foot, Ginger Root.

Medicinal Part—The leaves.

Description—Colts Foot has a long, perennial, creeping, fibrous rhizome. The leaves are erect, cordate, sharply dentate, smooth green above and pure white and cottony beneath. They do not appear until the flowers are withered, and are from five to eight inches long, and like a colt's foot in shape. The flowers are large and bright yellow.

This plant grows in Europe and the East Indies, from the seashore to elevations of nearly eight thousand feet. It also grows in the United States, in wet places, on the sides of brooks, flowering in March and April. Its presence is a certain indication of a clayey soil. The leaves are rather fragrant, and continue so after having been carefully dried. The leaves are the parts used, though all parts of the plant are active, and should always be employed, especially the leaves, flowers and root. The leaves should be collected at about the period they have nearly reached their full size, the flowers as soon as they commence opening, and the root immediately after the maturity of the leaves. When dried, all parts have a bitter,

mucilaginous taste, and yield their properties to water or diluted alcohol.

Properties and Uses—It is emollient, demulcent and slightly tonic, and is serviceable in coughs associated with colds. It is also used externally in form of poultice.

Dose — Steep a teaspoonful of the leaves into a cup of boiling water for half hour. Drink a half cupful upon retiring at night, hot or cold. Or take a mouthful 3 times a day; one or two cupfuls may be taken. Of the tincture, 1 to 2 fl. dr.

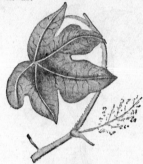

COLUMBO
(Cocculus Palmatus)

Common Name—Kalumb.

Medicinal Part—The root.

Description—Columbo, so important in the present practice of medicine, is a climbing plant, with a perennial root which is quite thick and branching. The root is covered with a thin brown skin, marked with transverse warts. The stems, of which one or two proceed from the same root, are twining, simple in the male plant, branched in the female, round, hairy and about an inch or an inch and half in circumference. The leaves stand on the rounded glandular-hairy footstalks, and are alternate, distant, cordate, and have three, seven or nine lobes and nerves. The flowers are small and inconspicuous.

This plant inhabits the forests near the southeastern coast of Africa, in the neighborhood of Mozambique, where the natives call it Kalumb. The root is dug up in the dry season in the month of March, and is cut in slices, strung on cords, and hung up to dry. The odor of Columbo is slightly aromatic; the taste bitter and also mucilaginous. The root is easily pulverized, put spoils by keeping after having been reduced to a powder. It is best to powder it only as it is required for use.

Properties and Uses—It is a mild, bitter tonic, free from astringency and therefore it can hardly be surpassed as a remedial agent. It is used in many combinations, according to indications.

Dose—Steep a level teaspoonful of the root into a cupful of boiling water for half hour. Strain. When cold take a teaspoonful 3 to 6 times a day. Of the tincture, 5 to 10 min.

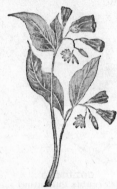

COMFREY
(Symphytum Officinale, Borage Family)
Common Names—Healing Herb, Blackwort, Bruisewort, Wallwort, Gum Plant.
Medicinal Part—The root.
Description—Comfrey has an oblong, fleshy, perennial root, black on the outside and whitish within, containing a glutinous or clammy tasteless juice, with divers very large, hairy, green leaves lying on the ground, so hairy, or so prickly, that if they touch any tender parts of the hands, face or body, it will cause it to itch. The stalks are hollowed and cornered, very hairy, having leaves that grow below, but less and less up to the top; at the joints of the stalk it is divided into many branches, at the ends of which stand many flowers, in order one above another, which are somewhat long and hollow like the finger of a glove, of a pale, whitish color; after them come small black seeds. There is another sort which bears flowers of a pale purple color, having similar medicinal properties.

Comfrey is a native of Europe, but naturalized in the United States, grow·

ing on low grounds and moist places, and flowering all summer. The root is officinal and contains a large amount of mucilage, which is readily extracted by water.

Properties and Uses—The plant is demulcent and slightly astringent. Formerly it was somewhat esteemed as a vulnerary but later used domestically in nasal congestion or catarrh.

It may be boiled in water, wine or made into a syrup, and taken in doses of from a wineglassful to a teacupful of the preparation, two or three times a day.

Externally the fresh root, bruised, forms an excellent application to bruises, fresh wounds, etc.

Dose—Steep a teaspoonful of this root, cut into small pieces, into a cup of boiling water for half hour. When cold drink 1 or 2 cupfuls a day, a good mouthful at a time. Of the tincture, ½ to 1 fl. dr.

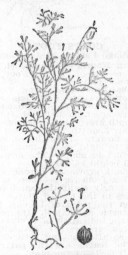

CORIANDER
(Coriander Sativum, Parsley Family)
Common Names—Coriander, Coriander seed herb.
Medicinal Part—Seed.
Description—A low plant with small umbels of few rays flowering in the

summer. Cultivated from the Orient for the aromatic coriander seed.

Properties and Uses—Aromatic, pungent, carminative, cordial, stomachic.

CORSICA MOSS
(Fucus Helminthicorton)

Medicinal Part—The whole plant.

Description—This marine plant has a cartilaginous, tufted, entangled frond, with branches marked indistinctly with transverse streaks. The lower part is dirty yellow, the branches more or less purple.

It is found growing on the Mediterranean coast, and especially on the Island of Corsica. It is cartilaginous in consistence, is of a dull and reddish-brown color, has a bitter, salt and nauseous taste, but its odor is rather pleasant. Water dissolves its active principles.

Properties and Uses—It has been used by some as an anthelmintic for intestinal worms.

Dose—A teaspoonful of the plant, cut small or granulated, to a cup of boiling water. Drink cold one cupful during the day, a large mouthful at a time; of the tincture, 5 to 20 min.

The Fucus Vesiculosis, Sea-Wrack or Bladder Fucus, possesses similar properties.

COTTON ROOT
(Gossypium Herbaceum)

Medicinal Part—The inner bark of the root.

Description—Cotton is a biennial or triennial herb, with a fusiform root, with a round pubescent branching stem about five feet high. The leaves are hoary, palmate, with five sub-lanceolate, rather acute lobes; flowers are yellow, calyx cup-shaped, petals five, deciduous, with a purple spot near the base; stigmas, three or five; and the fruit a three or five-celled capsule, with three or five seeds involved in cotton.

It is a native of Asia, but is cultivated extensively in many parts of the world, and in the southern portions of America more successfully than anywhere else. The inner bark of the recent root is the part chiefly used in medicine. Its active principle, which is that administered by all educated herbal physicians is called Gossypiin.

Properties and Uses—The preparation Gossypiin has been compared by some to ergot but it hardly is worthy of such comparison because of its inferior power. At all events, it should not be employed by the unskilled.

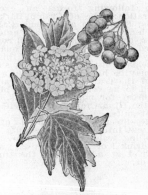

CRAMP BARK
(Viburnum Opulus, Honey Suckle Family)

Common Names—Squaw Bush, High Cranberry, Genuine Cramp Bark.

Medicinal Part—The bark.

Description—It is a nearly smooth and upright shrub, or small tree, usually from five to twelve feet in height, with several stems from the same root branched above; the leaves are three-lobed, three-veined, broadly wedge-shaped, and crenately toothed on the side. The flowers are white, or reddish-white; the fruit ovoid, red, very acid, ripens late, and remains upon the bush after the leaves have fallen. It resembles the common cranberry, and is sometimes substituted for it.

It is indigenous to the northern part of the United States and Canada, being a handsome shrub, growing in low rich lands, woods and borders of fields, flowering in June, and presenting at this time a very showy appearance. The flowers are succeeded by red and very acid berries, resembling low cranberries, and which remain through the winter. The bark is the officinal part, as met with in drug stores. It is frequently put up by shakers, when it is somewhat flattened from pressure. It has no smell, but has a peculiar, not unpleasant, bitterish and astringent taste. It yields its properties to water or diluted alcohol.

Properties and Uses—It has been credited with some virtue as an antispasmodic, and hence commonly known among American practitioners as Cramp Bark.

The following forms an excellent preparation: take of Cramp Bark, two ounces; Scull Cap and Skunk Cabbage, of each one ounce; Cloves, half an ounce; Ginger, two drachms. Have all coarsely bruised, and add to them two quarts of sherry or native wine. Dose of this, half a wineglassful two or three times a day.

It may be here remarked that a poultice of the fruit of the Low Cranberry is said to be very efficacious applied to the throat for minor irritations. Probably the High Cranberry will effect the same results.

Dose—Steep a teaspoonful of this bark, cut into small pieces, into a cup of boiling water for half hour. When cold, drink 1 or 2 cupfuls a day; a good mouthful at a time. Of the tincture, ½ fl. dr.

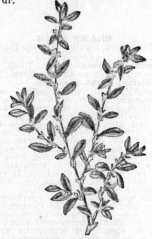

CRAWL GRASS
(Polygonum Aviculare, Buckwheat Family)

Common Names—Common Knotweed, Doorweed, Bird's Knot Grass.

Medicinal Part—Plant.

Description—Crawl Grass is generally prostrate and creeping with bluish-green leaves. It is found growing everywhere in hard soils about yards. The stems and roots are very strong and the leaves are small, oblong or lanceolate, acute or acutish. The sepals are very small, green and pinkish.

Properties and Uses—Astringent and diuretic.

CRAWLEY
(Corallorhiza Odontorhiza, Orchid Family)

Common Names—Dragon's Claw, Coral Root, Chickentoe.

Medicinal Part—The root.

Description—This is a singular, leafless plant, with coral-like root stocks. The root is a collection of small fleshy tubers; the flowers, from ten to twenty in number, are of a brownish-green color, and the fruit a large oblong capsule.

The plant is a native of the United States, growing about the root of trees, in rich woods, from Maine to Florida, flowering from July to October. The entire plant is destitute of verdure. The root only is used for medicinal purposes. It is small, dark brown, resembling cloves, or a hen's claws; has a strong, nitrous smell, and a mucilaginous, slightly bitter astringent taste.

Properties and Uses—It is one of the most prompt and satisfactory diaphoretics in the materia medica; but its scarcity and high price have tended to keep it from coming in general use. It promotes perspiration without producing any excitement in the system. Its chief value is as a diaphoretic.

Combined with Blue Cohosh it forms an excellent agent in indicated conditions.

In fevers Crawley may be advantageously combined with Black Root or May Apple when it is found necessary to act upon the bowels; and mixed with Colic Root is will be found helpful in flatulent and bilious colic.

Dose—Steep a teaspoonful of the root into a cup of boiling water for half hour. When cold drink 1 or 2 cupfuls a day; a good mouthful at a time. Of the tincture, 10 to 20 min. It may be also taken as hot as one can stand it upon retiring at night.

All of the teas in this book should be taken cold, except when otherwise stated.

CROWFOOT
(Ranunculus Bulbosus, Crowfoot Family)

Medicinal Parts—The cormus and herb.

Description—This plant is not to be confounded with the Geranium Maculatum, which is also called Crowfoot. The cormus or root of this herb is a perennial, solid, fleshy, roundish and depressed, sending out radicles from its under sides. The root sends up annually erect hairy stems, six to eighteen inches in height. The leaves are on long petioles, dentate and hairy. Each stem supports several solitary golden-yellow flowers; sepals, oblong and hairy; petals, five; cordate; stamens numerous and hairy.

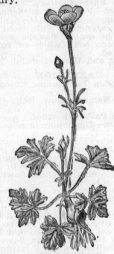

CROWFOOT

This plant is common in Europe and the United States, growing in fields and pastures, and flowering in May, June and July. There are a great many varieties, but all possess similar quali-ties, and designated by the general name of Butter Cup. When any part of these plants is chewed, it occasions much pain, inflammation, excoriation of the mouth, and much heat and pains in the stomach, if it be taken internally.

Properties and Uses—This plant is too acrid to be used internally, especially when fresh. When applied externally it may be employed where conditions of counter-irritation are indicated. Its ac-tion, however, is generally so violent that it is seldom used.

CUBEBS
(Piper Cubeba)
Common Names—Tailed Pepper, Java Pepper.
Medicinal Part—The berries.
Description—This is a perennial plant with a climbing stem, round branches, about as thick as a goose-quill, ash-colored, and rooting at the joints. The leaves are from four to six and a half inches long by one and a half to two inches broad, ovate-oblong, acuminate and very smooth. Flowers arranged in spikes at the end of the branches; fruit, a berry rather longer than that of black pepper.

Cubebs is a native of Java and other islands of the Indian Ocean, growing in the forests without cultivation. The fruit is gathered before fully ripe, and then dried. It affords a volatile oil, which is much used. Cubebs has a pleasant, aromatic odor, and a hot, bit-ter taste.

Properties and Uses — It is mildly stimulant, expectorant, stomachic and carminative. It acts particularly on mucous tissues. It exercises an influence over the urinary apparatus, rendering the urine of deeper color and promoting its flow.

Dose — Steep a teaspoonful of the berries into a cup of boiling water for half hour. Drink a half cupful upon retiring at night, hot or cold. Or take a mouthful three times a day.

CONDURANGO
(Equatoria Garciana)
Common Name—Condor Vine.
Medicinal Part—The bark of the vine.
Description — Condurango, or Condor Vine, a name derived from two words, cundur and angu, whose medicinal pos-sibilities have interested the medical profession, is a climbing vine, resem-bling much in its habits the grape vine of our forests. The vines are from three to five inches in diameter. They are quite flexible when fresh, but when dry very brittle. The bark is externally of a greenish-gray color, and has numerous small warty excrescences. The leaves are large, sometimes reaching six inches in length by five in breadth, opposite, simple, entire dentate, cordate and of a dark green color. The flowers are small, arranged in complete umbels; stamens five; petals five; sepals five, and filaments small. The fruit is a pair of pods and seeds numerous and dark brown. It should be more properly Cun-durangu, as there is no "o" in the lan-guage of the Incas.

This plant is a native of the Andes Mountains in South America, especially in the southern portion of Equador, and found most plentifully in the mountains surrounding the city of Loja. It is gen-erally found on the western exposure of the Andes, at an altitude of 4,000 or 5,000 feet. Its virtues are said to have been known to the Indians of the local-ity for a long time. It is sometimes used in the powdered form combined with sugar and water, so as to form a thick syrup, but the fluid extract (when it can be obtained pure) is a much more convenient form of administering it. A great deal that is spurious is found in the market. It is a singular coincidence that both Quinine and Condurango are found in the same region, and thrive only under the same climatic conditions.

Properties and Uses—While this botanical has been credited with various powers, there is no available evidence that it really has medicinal virtues and each person must rely on his own judgment as to whether Condurango is worthy of a trial for any purpose.

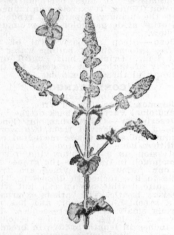

CURLED MINT
(Mentha Crispa, Mint Family)

Common Names—Crisped Leaved or Cross Mint.

Medicinal Part—The herb.

Description—Curled Mint has a rather weak stem usually much branched from 1½ to 3 feet long. Leaves are distinctly petioled, or the uppermost sessile, ovate in outline, mostly acute at the apex, their margins crisped, wavy and incised. Whorls of flowers in dense, thick terminal spikes which become from one to one and one-half inches long in fruit. Found in swamps and roadside ditches.

Properties and Uses—Aromatic, stimulant, stomachic and carminative.

CYANI
(Centaurea Cyanus, Composite Family)

Common Names — Bluebottle, Cornflower, Bachelor's Button.

Medicinal Part—Flowers.

Description—Found in gardens, sparingly running wild. A native plant of Europe but extensively cultivated in this country. The outer flowers are very large and blue with white or rose colored varieties.

Properties and Uses—Cordial, tonic.

DANDELION
(Leontodon Taraxacum, Chicory Family)

Common Names—Blow Ball, Cankerwort.

Medicinal Part—The root.

Description—Dandelion is a perennial top-shaped herb, having a very milky root. The leaves are all radical, shining green in color, sessile and pinnate. The scape or flower stem is longer than the leaves, five to six inches in height, and bearing a single yellow flower. The fruit is an achenium.

This plant is a native of Greece, but is now found growing abundantly in Europe and the United States, in fields, gardens and along roadsides, flowering from April to November. The root only is the officinal part, and should be collected when the plant is in flower. Alcohol or boiling water extracts its properties. The young plant is frequently used as a salad or green, and possesses some slight narcotic properties.

Properties and Uses—The dried root when fresh is a stomachic and tonic, with slightly diuretic and aperient actions. It has long been credited with various beneficial uses as a home remedy.

Dose—Steep a heaping teaspoonful of this root, cut into small pieces, into a cup of boiling water for half hour. When cold drink 1 or 2 cupfuls a day; a good mouthful at a time. Of the tincture, ½ to 1 fl. dr.

DEVILS BIT
(Liatris Squarrosa, Aster Family)

Common Names—Gay Feather, Blazing Star, Rattlesnake Master.

Medicinal Part—The root.

Description—There are three varieties of this plant used in medicine. The above is the most common one. It has a tuberous root and an erect annual stem from two to five feet high, linear leaves and flowers sessile, and of bright purple color.

Liatris Spicata, or Button Snake Root, is very similar to the above.

Liatris Scariosa, or Gay Feather, has a perennial tuberous root, with a stout stem from four to five feet high. The leaves are numerous and lanceolate, lower ones on long petioles.

The two former are natives of the Middle and Southern states, and the latter is found from New England to Wisconsin. These splendid natives flower from August to September. The roots have a hot bitter taste and an agreeable turpentine odor. The virtues are extracted by alcohol.

Properties and Uses—These plants are diuretic, and tonic stimulant. The decoction is very useful for such purposes. As a gargle in throat irritation it is of advantage. These plants have been used for snakebites and other conditions but their virtues are subject to some doubt.

Dose—Steep a heaping teaspoonful of these small pieces into a cup of boiling water for half hour. When cold drink 1 or 2 cupfuls a day, a good mouthful at a time. Of the tincture, ½ to 1 fl. dr.

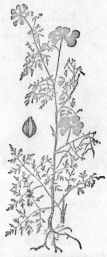

DOG POISON
(Aethusa Cynapium, Carrot Family)

Common Names — Small Hemlock, Fool's Parsley.

Description—An annual herb, erect, leafy, rather slender from one to one and one-half feet high. The leaves are slender-petioled. The flowers are white. Found in waste places.

Properties and Uses—A poison not suitable for domestic use.

DOG WOOD
(Cornus Florida, Dogwood Family)

Common Names—Box Wood, Flowering Cornel, Green Ozier.

Medicinal Part—The bark.

Description—Dogwood is a small indigenous tree from twelve to thirty feet high, with a very hard and compact wood, and covered with a rough and brownish bark. The tree is of slow growth. The leaves are opposite, smooth, ovate, acute, dark green above, paler beneath. The flowers are very small, of a greenish yellow color, and constitute the chief beauty of the tree when in bloom. The fruit is an oval drupe of a glossy scarlet color, containing a nut with two cells and two seeds.

This tree grows in various parts of the United States: it flowers in April and May. The fruit matures in autumn.

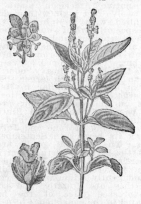

DOG MERCURY
(Mercurialis Perennis)

Common Name—Dog's Cole.

Medicinal Part—Herb.

Description — Dog's Mercury grows commonly in hedges and ditches, occurring in large patches, with egg-shaped, pointed leaves, square stems and light green flowers developed in spikes.

Properties and Uses—Emetic and purgative, but since it is a poison it is unsuited for domestic use.

The wood is used for many purposes. The bark yields its virtues to water and alcohol. The chemical qualities are tannic and gallic acids, resin, gum, oil, wax, lignin, lime, potassa and iron.

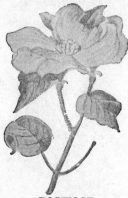

DOGWOOD

Properties and Uses — It is mildly tonic, astringent and slightly stimulant. Sometimes it has been employed as a substitute for Peruvian Bark, when the foreign remedy was not to be obtained. The bark should only be used in its dried state. Cornine, its active principle, seems to have been occasionally used as a substitute for quinine.

Dogwood, or green ozier, exerts its best virtues in the shape of an ointment.

Dose—Steep a teaspoonful of the bark into a cup of boiling water for half hour. Drink a half cupful upon retiring at night, hot or cold. Or take a mouthful three times a day. One or two cupfuls may be taken. Of the tincture, ½ to 1 fl. dr.

DWARF ELDER
(Sambucus Ebulus)

Common Names—Wild Elder, Danewort, Walewort.

Medicinal Parts—Root and bark.

Description—Dwarf Elder is a shrub quite different from the true elder. It grows throughout the eastern and middle states. The fruit is four-seeded, resembling true elderberries, but seldom becomes fully ripe.

Properties and Uses—The properties of the bark and berries are laxative and perhaps diuretic, but the flowers are of doubtful value.

Dose—A teaspoonful of the root and bark to a cup of boiling water. Drink cold 1 or 2 cupfuls a day, a large mouthful at a time; of the tincture, ½ to 1 fl. dr.

DWARF ROSEBAY
(Rhododendron Hirsutum)

Common Name—Alpine Rose.

Medicinal Part—Leaves.

Description—A hairy-leaved species growing in Central Europe. The leaves are oblong and the corolla red or pink red.

Properties and Uses—Stimulant, diaphoretic and diuretic.

ELDER
(Sambucus Canadensis, Honeysuckle Family)

Common Names—Sambucus, American Elder, Sweet Elder.

Medicinal Parts—The flowers, berries and root.

Description—This is a common, well-known native American plant, from five to twelve feet high, with a shrubby stem, filled with a light and porous pitch, especially when young. The bark is rather scabrous and cinerous. The leaves are nearly bipinnate, antiposed. The flowers are numerous, white, in very large level-topped, five-parted cymes, and have a heavy odor. The European Elder, though larger than the American kind, is similar in its general characteristics and properties.

It is an indigenous shrub, growing in all parts of the United States, in low, damp grounds, thickets and waste places, flowering in June and July, and maturing its berries in September and October. The officinal parts are the flowers, the berries and the inner bark.

Properties and Uses—In warm infusion the flowers are said to be diaphoretic and gently stimulant. In cold infusion they are diuretic, and cooling. The expressed juice of the berries, evaporated to the consistence of a syrup, is a valuable aperient and alterative; one ounce of it will purge. An infusion of the young leafbuds is likewise purgative, and sometimes acts with violence. The juice will purge moderately in doses from half a fluid ounce to a fluid ounce. Beaten up with lard or cream, it forms an excelent discutient ointment, of much value in burns and scalds. A tea of the root in half-ounce doses, taken daily, acts as a hydragogue cathartic and stimulating diuretic.

ELECAMPANE
(Inula Helenium, Aster Family)

Common Name—Scabwort.

Medicinal Part—The root.

Description—This plant has a thick top-shaped, aromatic and perennial root, with a thick, leafy, round, solid stem, from four to six feet high. The leaves are large, ovate, dark green above, downy and hoary beneath, with a fleshy mid-rib. The flowers are of a bright yellow color, and the fruit an achenium.

Elecampane is common in Europe and cultivated in the United States. It grows in pastures and alone road-sides, blossoming from July to September. The root is the part used, and should be gathered in the second year of its development and during the fall months. It yields its properties to water and alcohol, more especially to the former.

Properties and Uses—It is tonic and gently stimulant and as such has been widely used by former generations.

Dose—Steep a heaping teaspoonful of this root cut into small pieces into a cup of boiling water for half hour. When cold drink 1 or 2 cupfuls a day; a good mouthful at a time. Of the tincture, ½ to 1 fl. dr.

ERGOT
(Secale Cornatum)

Common Names — Spurred or Smut Rye.

Medicinal Part — The degenerated seeds.

Description—Ergot is the name given to the fungoid, degenerated seeds of the common rye, which is the result of a parasitic plant called Oidium Abortificaciens.

Ergot consists of grains, varying in length, of a violet-black color; odor fishy, peculiar and nauseous. Their taste is not very marked, but is disagreeable and slightly acrid. They should be gathered previous to harvest.

Properties and Uses—Ergot has a remarkable effect upon the human system, and when persisted in for a length of time manifests certain symptoms termed Ergotism. Its chief use as a medicine is to promote uterine contractions.

This is a valuable remedy in the hands of a physician and obstetrician, but is too powerful and dangerous for domestic use or self-medication.

* * * *

"A weed is a plant whose virtues we have not yet discovered."

—Emerson

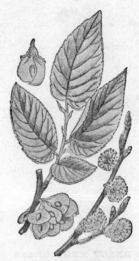

ENGLISH ELM
(Ulmus Campestris, Nettle Family)

Common Names—European Elm.

Medicinal Part—Bark.

Description—A large tree from Europe with rather short horizontal or ascending branches and smooth leaves. Immensely variable under cultivation and known under many names. Flowers early in the early spring and fruit in the early summer.

Properties and Uses—Astringent, demulcent and diuretic.

ENGLISH IVY
(Hedera Helix, Ginseng Family)

Common Names—True or English Ivy.

Medicinal Parts—Leaves and berries.

Description—A woody climber with evergreen, glossy, rounded heart shaped or kidney-shaped and three-lobed or three-angled, often variegated leaves or in some varieties more deeply 3-7 cleft, yellowish green flowers in the summer and blackish berries. Covers shaded walls adhering by its rootlets.

Properties and Uses—Leaves: Stimulant, vulnerary, exanthematous and insecticide. Berries: Emetic and cathartic.

* * * *

"Those who farm and ranch, and live close to the soil, have an outlook on life which is wholesome, and which contributes greatly to our common sense way of life.

—author unknown

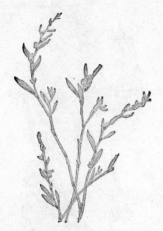

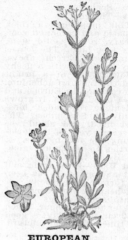

ERECT KNOT GRASS
(Polygonum Erectum, Buckwheat Family)

Common Name—Knotweed.

Medicinal Part—The plant.

Description—Very similar to Crawl Grass but erect instead of prostrate and with flowers on more evident pedicels. Leaves oblong or oval and obtuse. Found growing along roadsides.

Properties and Uses—Mild astringent, vulnerary, styptic, febrifuge.

EUPHORBIA
(Euphorbia maculata—Euphorbia Family)

Common Names—Spreading Spurge, Dysentery-weed, Milk-purslane.

Medicinal part—Herb.

Description—A very common small prostrate weed found along roadsides, cultivated ground, waste places, and along railroads over a large part of the United States and southern Canada. Entire plant generally very red in color. Branches and stem puberulant or pilose. Tiny leaves opposite, elliptic or ovate-elliptic. Tiny flowers inconspicuous. Characteristic 3 seed capsule. Plant has milky juice.

Properties and Uses—Bitter, astringent. This and other species (E. hirta, E. glyptosperma) widely used by Indians, negroes, and West Indians.

EUROPEAN CENTAURY **EUROPEAN SENEKA**

EUROPEAN CENTAURY
(Erythraea Centaurium, Gentian Family)

Common Names — Lesser Centaury, Bitter Herb.

Medicinal Parts—Tops and roots.

Description—An annual plant, erect and branches from six to fifteen inches high. Leaves oblong, apex obtuse, the base narrowed. Stem leaves are smaller distant, rounded at the sessile. The flowers are numerous. Found in waste places from Nova Scotia and Quebec to Massachusetts, Illinois and Michigan.

Properties and Uses—Aromatic, bitter, tonic and febrifuge.

EUROPEAN SENEKA
(Polygala Vulgaris, Milkwort Family)

Common Names—Milkwort, Rogation Flower, Gang Flower.

Medicinal Part—The root.

Description—European Seneka is an herb with opposite leaves. The flowers are rose purple and racemose. Capsule, membranous, compressed, dehiscent along the margin and one seed in each cavity, generally hairy.

Properties and Uses—Stimulant, sialogogue, expectorant, diaphoretic, diuretic and emmenagogue.

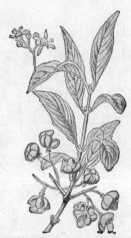

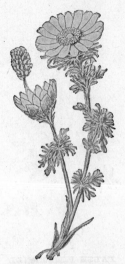

EUROPEAN SPINDLE BUSH
(Euonymus Europeus, Staff Tree Family)

Common Names—Spindle Tree, Louseberry Tree.

Medicinal Part—Bark.

Description—This shrub grows from six to ten feet high, common in parks and gardens, with smaller leaves from one to two inches long, squareish branchlets and green new twigs. The flowers are greenish yellow or creamy white borne at the junction of the leaf with the branch. Fruit a four-lobed, smooth short pod, lusterless crimson red, splitting open and showing the cadmium orange skinned, hard seed within.

Properties and Uses—Tonic, laxative, alterative, diuretic and expectorant.

EUROPEAN WATER HEMLOCK
(Cicuta Virosa, Parsley Family)

Common Names — Cowbane, Water Hemlock.

Description—A perennial marsh herb with simply pinnate stem leaves, the lower and basal ones often pinnatisected and compound large umbels of white flowers. Fruit ovate or oval, somewhat compressed.

Properties and Uses—Too powerful and dangerous for domestic use.

* * * *

"Food must be in the condition in which they are found in nature, or at least in a condition as close as possible to that found in nature."

Hippocrates, 460 B.C.

FALSE HELLEBORE
(Adonis Vernalis, Crowfoot Family)

Common Name—Bird's Eye.

Medicinal Part—Plant.

Description—False Hellebore has a leafy stem about six inches high. Leaves are finely cut into very narrow divisions. The stem bears a large showy flower of 10-20 lanceolate, light yellow petals in the early spring.

Properties and Uses—Narcotic, caustic and vesicant.

EUROPEAN WHITE BEECH
(Fagus Sylvatica, Oak Family)

Common Name—White Beech.

Medicinal Part—Bark.

Description—A tree with fine-grained wood, close and smooth, light gray bark and light horizontal spray. Distinguished from the American Beech by broader and shorter, firmer, more hairy and wavy-toothed leaves, some of the main veins tending to sinuses.

Properties and Uses—Astringent and stimulant.

Cathartic—Steep one teaspoonful Black Butternut Bark, one teaspoonful Ginger, one teaspoonful Senna Leaves, three teaspoonfuls Licorice Root in a cup of boiling water half hour. Dose—one to three teaspoonfuls at bedtime.

41

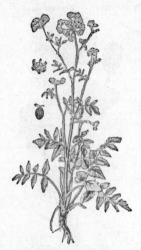

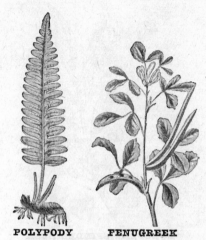

POLYPODY   FENUGREEK

FALSE PIMPERNEL
(Pimpinella Magna)

Common Names—Greater Pimpernel, Pimpinella.

Medicinal Part—Root.

Description—A smooth diffuse little plant four to eight feet high with rounded or oblong leaves found in wet places. Flowers all summer. The flowers are small and purple or bluish.

Properties and Uses—Diuretic, resolvent, astringent, antispasmodic.

FENNEL
(Foeniculum Officinale, Parsley Family)

Common Names—Wild Fennel, Sweet Fennel, Large Fennel.

Medicinal Part—The seed.

Description—Fennel is cultivated from Europe for the sweet, aromatic foliage and fruit. The herb is stout, very smooth and from four to six feet high. The leaves are very numerous and slender with thread-shaped divisions. The umbel is large with no involucre or involucels. The seed is from one-fourth to one-third inch long, ripening in late summer.

Properties and Uses—Aromatic, carminative, pectoral, diuretic and stomachic.

FEMALE FERN
(Polypodium Vulgare, Fern Family)

Common Names—Fern Root, Rock Brake, Rock Polypod, Brake Root, Common Polypody.

Medicinal Parts—The root.

Description—This perennial has a creeping, irregular, brown root. The fronds are from six to twelve inches high, green, smooth and deeply pinnatified. The fruit on the lower surface of the fronds is in large golden dots or capsules.

This fern is common on shady rocks in woods and mountains throughout the United States. The root has a peculiar and rather unpleasant odor, and somewhat sickening taste. Water extracts its properties.

Properties and Uses—This plant is pectoral, demulcent, purgative and anthelmintic. A strong decoction is a good purgative and will expel tenia worms. Dose of the powdered plant, from one to four drachms. Of the decoction of syrup, from one to four fluid ounces, three or four times a day.

FENUGREEK
(Trigonella Foenum Graecum)

Medicinal Part—The seed.

Description—Fenugreek is an annual herb, 1 foot high, cultivated in Europe and the United States; leaves trifoliate, leaflets dentate, flowers yellowish; fruit compressed legume contains 16 seeds.

42

Properties and Uses—A tea of the seed is useful as a gargle for throat irritations. A poultice of the seed is excellent for wounds and minor skin irritations.

Dose—A teaspoonful of the seeds to a cup of boiling water. Drink cold one or two cupfuls a day, a large mouthful at a time; of the tincture, ½ to 1 fl. dr.

FEVERFEW
(Pyrethrum Parthenium, Aster Family)
Common Names — Featherfew, Febrifuge Plant.
Medicinal Part—The herb.
Description—Feverfew is a perennial herbaceous plant, with a tapering root, and an erect, round and leafy stem about two feet high. The leaves are alternate, petiolate, hoary green, with leaflets inclining to ovate and dentate. The flowers are white and compound, and the fruit a wingless, angular and uniform achenium.

The plant is a native of Europe, but common in the United States; found occasionally in a wild state, but generally cultivated in gardens, and blossoms in June and July. It imparts its virtues to water, but much better to alcohol.

Properties and Uses—It is tonic, carminative, emmenagogue, vermifuge and stimulant. The warm infusion is an excellent remedy in ordinary colds and flatulency. The cold infusion or extract makes a valuable tonic. The leaves, in poultice, are an excellent local application. Bees are said to dislike this plant very much, and a handful of the flower-heads carried where they are will cause them to keep at a distance.

Dose—Steep a heaping teaspoonful of this herb into a cup of boiling water for half hour. When cold, drink 1 or 2 cupfuls a day; a good mouthful at a time. Of the tincture, ½ to 1 fl. dr.

FEVER WEED
(Gerardia Pedicularia)
Common Names—Lousewort, Foxglove.
Medicinal Part—The herb.
Description—The stem of this plant is bushy, tall, two or three feet in height. The leaves are numerous, opposite, ovate-lanceolate, flowers large, yellow and trumpet-shaped; calyx five-cleft, corolla yellow, and fruit a two-celled capsule.

This most elegant plant is grown in dry copses, pine ridges and barren woods and mountains, from Canada to Georgia, flowering in August and September. Water or alcohol extracts its virtues.

Properties and Uses—It is diaphoretic and sedative. A warm infusion produces a free and copious perspiration in a short time. Very valuable in ephemeral fever.

Dose—A teaspoonful of the herb, cut small or granulated, to a cup of boiling water. Drink cold, one cupful during the day, a large mouthful at a time; of the tincture, 5 to 20 min.

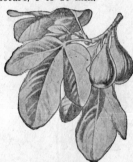

FIG TREE
(Ficus Carica, Nettle Family)
Medicinal Part—The fruit.
Description—The Fig Tree is cultivated from the Levant as a house plant. Figs are single in the axils, pear-shaped and luscious.
Properties and Uses—Laxative, demulcent.

FIGWORT
(Scrophularia Nodosa, Figwort Family)
Common Names—Carpenter's Square, Heal All, Square Stalk.
Medicinal Parts—The leaves and root.
Description—Figwort has a perennial, whitish and fibrous root, with a leafy, erect, smooth stem from two to four feet high. The leaves are opposite, ovate; the upper lanceolate, acute, of deep green color, and from three to seven inches in length. The flowers are small and dark purple in color. The fruit is an ovate-oblong capsule.

This plant is a native of Europe, but it is found growing in the United States from New York to North Carolina and Kansas, in woods, hedges, damp copses, and banks, blossoming from July to October. The plants known by the names of Carpenter's Square, Heal All, Square Stalk, etc. (S. Marilanolica and S. Lanceolatea), and all mere varieties of Figwort, possessing similar medicinal properties. The leaves and root are the officinal parts, and yield their virtues to water or alcohol. The leaves have an offensive odor, and a bitter, unpleasant taste; the root is slightly acrid.

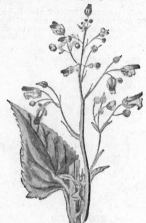

FIGWORT

Properties and Uses—It formerly was employed internally as an alterative and externally as a discutient. Though it has been largely supplanted by laboratory products, this plant possesses many valuable and active medicinal properties. Externally, in the form of fomentation or ointment, it is valuable in bruises, scratches, etc.

Dose—Steep a heaping teaspoonful of the leaves and roots into a cup of boiling water for half hour. When cold drink 1 or 2 cupfuls a day; a good mouthful at a time. Of the tincture, ½ to 1 fl. dr.

FIREWEED
(Erecthites Hieracifolius, Aster Family)

Common Name—Pilewort.

Medicinal Parts—The root and herb.

Description—This plant has an annual, herbaceous, thick, fleshy, branching and roughish stem, from one to five feet high. The leaves are simple, alternative, large lanceolate or oblong (acute, deeply dentate, sessile and light green. The flowers are whitish, and the fruit an achenium, oblong and hairy.

This indigenous rank weed grows in fields throughout the United States, in moist woods, in recent clearings, and is especially abundant in such as have been burned over. It flowers from July to October, and somewhat resembles the Sowthistle. The whole plant yields its virtues to water or alcohol. It has a peculiar, aromatic and somewhat fetid odor, and a slightly pungent, bitter and disagreeable taste.

Properties and Uses—It is emetic and astringent and has been used in diarrhea. It has been employed with some success in the summer complaints of children.

Dose—Steep a heaping teaspoonful of the root and herb into a cup of boiling water for half hour. When cold drink 1 or 2 cupfuls a day; a good mouthful at a time. Of the tincture, ½ to 1 fl. dr.

FIT PLANT
(Monotropa Uniflora, Indian-pipe Family)

Common Names—Ice Plant, Ova-ova, Indian Pipe, Birds Nest, Pipe-plant, Ghostflower.

Medicinal Part—The root.

Description — This plant has dark-colored, fibrous, perennial root, matted in masses like a chestnut vine, from which arise one or more short ivory-white stems, four to eight inches high, adorned with white, sessile, lanceolate leaves.

This singular plant is found from Maine to Carolina, and westward to Missouri, growing in shady, solitary places, in rich moist soil, or soil composed of decayed wood and leaves. The whole plant is ivory-white, resembling frozen jelly, and when handled melts away like ice. It flowers from June to September. It is evidently a parasite of the roots at the base of trees.

Properties and Uses—It is tonic and capable of many beneficial uses. A teaspoonful of this root and one of Fennel Seed to a pint of boiling water makes an excellent eye wash and vaginal douche.

FIT WEED
(Eryngium foetidum—Carrot Family)

Common Names—Shadeau Bennie or Benny.

Medicinal Part—Plant.

Description—Related and similar to water Eryngo, however, much smaller and of prostrate growth. Fit Weed is found in tropical Asia, Africa, South America, West Indies, and has been reported in south-eastern states. The plant has short spiny toothed leaf-blades and small spiny greenish flower heads. The entire plant has a peculiar odor resembling coriander.

Properties and Uses—Reputed to be alterative, febrifuge and sedative.

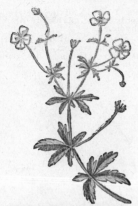

minated with one or two delicate violet blue flowers; these measure about ¾ inches broad; the 5 petals being large, broad and slightly overlapping. The leaves are small, alternate, sharp pointed

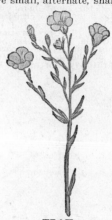

FLAX

FIVE-FINGER GRASS
(Potentilla Canadensis, Rose Family)
Common Name—Cinque-Foil.
Medicinal Parts—The root and leaves.
Description—This perennial plant has a procumbent stem from two to eighteen inches in length. The leaves are palmate, leaflets obovate and flowers yellow on solitary pedicels.

There are two varieties of this plant, the P. Pamilla, which is very small and delicate, flowering in April and May, and growing in dry, sandy soils, and the P. Simplex, a larger plant, growing in richer soils, and flowering from June to August.

Five Finger is common to the United States, growing by roadsides, on meadow banks and waste grounds, and flowering from April to October. The root is the part used. It has a bitterish, styptic taste, and yields its virtues to water.

Properties and Uses—It makes an excellent mouth wash and gargle.

Dose—Steep a teaspoonful of the plant into a cup of boiling water for half hour. Drink a half cupful upon retiring at night hot or cold, or take a mouthful three times a day. One of two cupfuls may be taken. Of the tincture, ½ to 1 fl. dr.

FLAX SEED
(Linum)
Common Names—Linseed, Lint Bells.
Part Used—The ripe seed.
Description—Flax is an annual. The stem is very slender, 1 to 2 feet high and each of its few branches are ter-

and thickly crowded on the stem. They have three longitudinal ribs. This plant is a native of Europe, but may now be found here along roadsides, railroads and waste places.

Properties and Uses—Flax Seed are demulcent and emollient. Useful internally in coughs resulting from colds. Externally the ground seed used in combination with Elm Bark make an excellent poultice for general use in the conditions calling for such a remedy.

Dose—One teaspoonful of the seed to a cup of boiling water. Drink a large mouthful at a time, 3 to 6 times daily.

FOREIGN INDIAN HEMP
(Cannabis Indica)
Common Name—Indian Hemp.
Medicinal Part—The flowering tops.
Description—This is an herbaceous annual, growing about three feet high, with an erect, branched, angular bright green stem. The leaves are alternate, or opposite, on long lax foot-stalks, roughish, with sharply serrated leaflets tapering into a long, smooth entire point. The male flowers are drooping and long, the females simple and erect. The seeds are small, ash-colored and inodorous.

Foreign Indian Hemp, Cannabis Indica, or Cannabis Sativa, is a native of the Caucausus, Persia, but grows in the hilly regions of Northern India. It is cultivated in many parts of Europe and Asia; but medicine of value can only be made from the Indian variety, the active principle of the plant being developed only by the heat of the climate of Hindostan. The dried tops and resin are the parts used. The preparations called Churrus, Gunja, Bhang, Hashish, etc., sold in this country, are mostly feeble imitations of the genuine articles, and are comparatively worthless. Even the

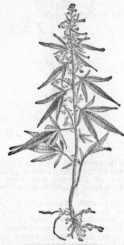

INDIAN HEMP

few specimens of the genuine productions which reach the shops and are sold at high prices are crude and inferior, and a matter of great difficulty to procure the genuine article even direct from dealers in India, unless you have had years of experience as a practicing herbal physician, and have established business connections in various parts of the world as an importer of rare and pure medicinal herbs, barks, roots, resins, etc.

The Cannabis Sativa, or common hemp, possesses similar properties, and can be substituted if the Asiatic hemp is not procurable.

Properties and Uses—It is narcotic, anodyne and antispasmodic. As this is a very powerful drug and poisonous in

overdoses, I would advise all readers to use it only with advice of an experienced physician.

Dose—A teaspoonful of the herb to a pint of boiling water. Take a tablespoonful 2 to 4 times a day, cold. Of the tincture, 2 to 5 min.

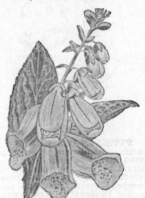

FOX GLOVE
(Digitalis Purpurea)

Common Names—American Fox Glove, Lion's Mouth, Fairy Fingers.

Parts Used—Dried leaves.

Description—Fox Glove is a biennial herb, cultivated for ornament and medicine; stem 2 to 5 feet high, succulent, downy, leafy; flowers July and August; they are tubular, bell shaped, 5 lobed, outside purple; inside sprinkled with black spots upon a white background, mouth hairy; seeds small, numerous, brownish grey inclosed in a 2-celled pyramidal capsule. Leaves 4 to 12 inches long, 2 to 6 inches broad, ovate, dull green, greyish underneath, wrinkled; sparsely hairy above, densely and finely hairy below.

Properties and Uses—The leaves have a slight characteristic odor and a strong, nauseous bitter taste. Only the second year's growth of leaves are used medicinally. They yield the well-known drug, Digitalin.

Fox Glove is very useful in a variety of ailments and conditions. These leaves, however, are very powerful and poisonous and should only be employed by skilled physicians. They are too dangerous for domestic use or self-medication, it acts as a stimulating tonic, antispasmodic and calmative. The infusion and fluid extract contain all the virtues of the plant.

Dose—A teaspoonful of the root, cut small or granulated, to a pint of boiling water. Drink cold, one cupful during the day, a large mouthful at a time.

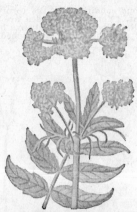

FRAGRANT VALERIAN
(Valeriana Officinalis, Valerian Family)

Common Names—Great Wild Valerian, Vandal Root.

Medicinal Part—The root.

Description—This is a large herb, with a perennial, tuberous, fetid root, most aromatic when growing in dry pastures, and a smooth, hollow, furrowed stem, about four feet in height. The leaves are pinnate, opposite, leaflets, from seven to ten pairs, lanceolate, coarsely serrated and on long footstalks. The flowers are flesh-colored, small and fragrant.

Valerian is a European plant, growing in wet places, or even in dry pastures, flowering in June and July. Several varieties grow in America, and are used, but the English Valerian is by all odds the best. The officinal part is the root. The taste of the root is warm, camphoraceous, slightly bitter, somewhat acrid and nauseous. The odor is not considerable; it is fetid, characteristic and highly attractive to cats and, it is said, to rats also. Besides valerianic acid the root contains starch, albumen, valerianin, yellow extractive matter, balsamic resin, mucilage, valerianate of potassa, malates of potassa and lime, and phosphate of lime and silica.

Properties and Uses—Valerian excites the cerebro-spinal system. In large doses it causes headaches, mental excitement, visual illusions, giddiness, restlessness, agitation and even spasmodic movements. For these reasons it should be used with caution. In medicinal doses

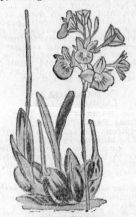

FUMITORY
(Fumaria Officinalis, Poppy Family)

Common Names—H e d g e Fumitory, Earth Smoke.

Medicinal Part—The leaves.

Description—Fumitory is an annual, glaucous plant, with a sub-erect, much-branched, spreading, leafy and angular stem, growing from ten to fifteen inches high. The leaves are mostly alternative. Culpepper, who knew the plant which is now used, better than anybody else, said that "at the top of the branches stand many small flowers, as it were in a long spike one above another, formed like little birds, of a reddish purple color, with whitish bellies, after which come small round husks, containing small black seeds. The root is small, yellow and not very long, and full of juice when it is young." The fruit, or nut, is ovoid or globose, one-seeded or valveless. The seeds are crestless.

Fumitory is found growing in cultivated soils in Europe and America, and flowers in May, June and July. The leaves are the parts used. Culpepper recommended the whole plant, but the modern decision is to use the leaves, gathered at the proper time, alone. They have no odor, but taste bitter under all circumstances. They are to be used when fresh, and possess the same qualities as Culpepper affixes to the fresh root, viz.: malate of lime and bitter extractive principles.

Properties and Uses—Its virtues appear to be those of a gentle tonic and alterative, and in large doses it seems to have laxative and diuretic properties. An infusion of the leaves is usually given in a wineglassful every four hours.

Dose—Steep a heaping teaspoonful of these leaves into a cup of boiling water for half hour. When cold drink 1 or 2 cupfuls a day, a good cupful at a time. Of the tincture, ½ to 1 fl. dr.

GALANGAL
(Alpinia Galangal)

Common Name—Catarrh Root.

Medicinal Part—The root.

Description—Galangal is a native of China. The rhizome cylindrical, branched 2 inches long, about ½ inch thick, annulate from leaf sheaths, rust brown in color, inside yellowish, fibrous, with many resin cells; odor and taste ginger like.

Properties—Galangal is a stimulant and aromatic, somewhat similar to ginger, which will indicate its uses.

Dose—A teaspoonful of the root, cut small or granulated, to a cup of boiling water. Drink cold one cupful during the day, a large mouthful at a time; of the tincture, 5 to 20 min.

GARDEN NIGHT SHADE
(Solanum Nigrum)

Medicinal Part—The leaves.

Description—This is a fetid, narcotic, bushy herb, with a fibrous root, and an erect, branching, thornless stem one or two feet high. Leaves are ovate, dentated, smooth and the margins have the appearance as if gnawed by insects. Flowers white or pale violet; fruit, a berry.

This plant is also called Deadly Nightshade, but is not to be confounded with Belladonna. It is found growing along old walls, fences and in gardens, in various parts of the United States, flowering in July and August. The leaves yield their virtues to water and alcohol.

Properties and Uses—It is somewhat narcotic and sedative, producing, when given in large doses, sickness and vertigo. One to three grains of the leaves, infused in water, should produce a copious perspiration and purge on the day following. They have been freely used

in various conditions in the form of an ointment. Very small doses are taken internally. These should always be prescribed, and their effects watched by a

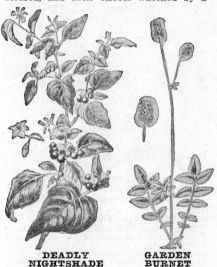

DEADLY NIGHTSHADE **GARDEN BURNET**

physician. It is better to use the plant only in the form of an ointment. The berries are poisonous.

Dose—A teaspoonful of the leaves, cut small, to a quart of boiling water. Take a teaspoonful at a time as required; of the tincture, ½ to 1 min.

GARDEN BURNET
(Sanguisorba Officinalis, Rose Family)

Common Names—Italian Burnet, Italian Pimpernel.

Part Used—Plant.

Description—Garden Burnet is common in old gardens. The plant is nearly smooth, growing in tufts; leaves of many small ovate and deeply toothed leaflets. The stems are about a foot high, bearing a few heads of light green or purplish monoecious flowers in summer, the lower flowers with numerous drooping stems, several of the uppermost with pistil, the style ending in a purple, tufted stigma.

Properties and Uses—Astringent and tonic.

48

sweetish, and then purely intensely and permanently bitter. It imparts its virtues readily to cold or hot water, alcohol, wine, spirits or sulphuric ether.

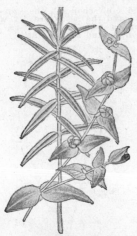

GARDEN SPURGE
(Euphorbia Lathyris, Spurge Family)
Common Names—Mole Plant, Caper Spurge.
Medicinal Parts—Root and seed.
Description—Cultivated from Europe in country gardens; glaucous, erect stem from two to three feet high with thick leaves, those of the stem lance-linear, floral ones oblong-ovate and heart shaped. The umbel is four rayed, then forking; glands short horned.
Properties and Uses—Root: Cathartic. Seed: Cathartic and emmenagogue.

GENTIAN
(Gentiana Lutea, Gentian Family)
Medicinal Part—The root.
Description—This plant has a long, thick cylindrical, wrinkled, r i n g e d, forked, perennial root, brown externally and yellow within, with a stem three or four feet high, hollow and erect; leaves ovate-oblong, five-veined, pale, bright green; the blossoms are large, of a bright yellow, in many flowered whorls, and the fruit is a capsule, stalked, oblong and two-valved.
This plant is common in Central and Southern Europe, especially on the Pyrenees and Alps, being found from 3,000 to 5,000 feet above sea level. The root affords the medicinal portion, and is brought to America chiefly from Havre and Marseilles. It has a feeble aromatic odor, and a taste at first faintly

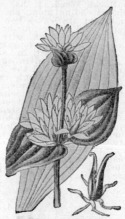

GENTIAN LUTEA

Properties and Uses—It is a time-honored tonic, improves the appetite and promotes digestion.
Dose—Of the powder, ten to thirty grains; of the extract, one to ten grains; of the infusion, a tablespoonful to a wineglassful; of the tincture, one or two teaspoonfuls.
Gentiana Catesbei, or the blue or American Gentian, has a perennial, branching, somewhat fleshy root, with a simple, erect, rough stem, eight or ten inches in height, and bears large blue flowers. It grows in the grassy swamps and meadows of North and South Carolina; blossoming from September to December. The root is in some respects superior to the foreign gentian, and may be used as a substitute for it in the same doses and preparations.
Gentiana Quinqueflora, or Five Flowered Gentian, sometimes called Gall-Weed, on account of its intense bitterness, is very useful. The plant is found from Vermont to Pennsylvania, and a variety of it is common throughout the western states. It grows in woods and pastures, and flowers in September and October. It may be regarded as a valuable tonic, and deserves further investigation of its therapeutic properties.

There is another kind of gentian (Gentiana Ochroleuca), known by the names of Marsh Gentian, Yellowish White Gentian, Straw Colored Gentian and Sampson Snake Weed. It has a stout, smoothish, ascending stem, one or two inches in height, its leaves two to four inches long, and three-fourths to an inch and a half in width, with straw-colored flowers two inches long by three-quarters thick, disposed in a dence, terminal cyme, and often in auxcymes. It is found in Canada and the Southern and Western States, though rarely in the latter, blossoming in September and October; the root is the officinal part, although the tops are often employed. They are bitter, tonic and astringent.

To two ounces of the tops and roots pour a pint and a half of boiling water, and when nearly cold add a half-pint of brandy. Dose, from one to three tablespoonfuls every half hour, gradually increasing as the stomach can bear it, lengthening the intervals between the doses.

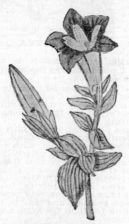

GENTIAN, BLUE
(Gentiana Catesbaei)

Common Names—Blue Bells, Southern Gentian, Rough Gentian.

Medicinal Part—Root.

Description—A perennial plant with an erect stem with short, erect axillary branches from one to two and one-half feet high. Leaves are lanceolate, ovate lanceolate or oblong. The corolla is blue and club shaped. The capsule is stiputate and the seeds broadly winged.

Properties and Uses—Bitters, stomachic, emetic and anthelmintic.

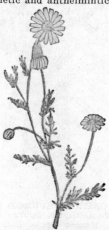

GERMAN CHAMOMILE
(Matricaria Chamomilla, Aster Family.)
Medicinal Part—The flowers.

Description—This is a perennial herb with a strong fibrous root. The stems in a wild state are prostrate, but in gardens more upright, about a span long, round, hollow, furrowed, and downy; the leaves pale green, pinnate, sessile, with thread shaped leaflets. The flower-heads terminal, rather smaller than the daisy, and of yellow color, or whitish.

Chamomile is indigenous to Southern Europe; we have also a common or wild Chamomile (Anthemis Cotula) growing in the United States, but it is not considered as good as the German Chamomile for medicinal purposes, which is the kind I use. The white flowers are the best; they have an aromatic, agreeably bitter taste, and peculiar odor. They yield their properties to alcohol and water.

Properties and Uses—Chamomile is a tonic; one or two teacupfuls of the warm infusion will usually vomit. The cold infusion is highly useful. The oil is carminative and antispasmodic, and is used in flatulency, colic, cramp in the stomach.

A poultice of Chamomile may be applied to external uses.

Dose—Steep a teaspoonful of the flowers into a cup of boiling water for half hour. Drink a half cupful upon retiring at night, hot or cold. Or take a mouthful 3 times a day, 1 or 2 cupfuls may be taken. Of the tincture ½ to 1 fl. dr.

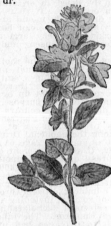

GERMANDER
(Teucrium Canadensis, Mint Family)
Common Names—Wood Sage, Wood Sage Germander.
Medicinal Part—The plant.
Description — Germander is found growing in low grounds. The plant is from one to three feet high, downy with ovate-lanceolate leaves, serrate, downy beneath. The flowers are pale purple or rarely white collected on a spike and blooming in late summer.
Properties and Uses—Stimulant, aromatic and bitter.

GILLENIA
(Gillenia Trifoliata—Rose Family.)
Common Names—Indian Physic, American Ipecac, Western Dropwort.
Medicinal Part—The bark of the root.
Description—Gillenia is an indigenous, perennial herb, with an irregular, brownish, somewhat tuberous root, having many long knotted, stringy fibres. The several stems are from the same root, about two or three feet high, erect, slender, smooth, and of a reddish or brownish color. The leaves are alternate, subsessile; leaflets lanceolate, acuminate, sharply dentated flowers are white with a reddish tinge; and the fruit a two-valved, one-celled capsule, seeds are oblong, brown and bitter.

This species is found scattered over the United States from Canada to Florida, on the eastern side of the Alleghanies, occurring in open hilly woods, in light gravelly soil. The period of flowering is in May, and the fruit is matured in August. The root yields its virtues to boiling water and alcohol.

Properties and Uses—It is emetic cathartic, diaphoretic, expectorant and tonic. It resembles ipecac in action. It is useful in costiveness. May be used where emetics are required.

Dose—A heaping teaspoonful of the bark of the root to a pint of boiling water. Take a tablespoonful 2 to 4 times a day, cold. Of the tincture 2 to 5 min.

GINSENG
(Panax Quinquefolium.)
Common Names—Chinese Seng, Ninsin, Five Fingers, Seng.
Part Used—The dried root.
Description—Ginseng is a perennial herb propagated by seed only. Seedlings appear about the last of April or first of May. At first they somewhat resemble newly sprouted beans. They send up the two cotyledons with a stem bearing three green leaves, seldom rising more than two or three inches above the ground. The work of the plant during the first year is to develop the bud at the crown of the root, which is to produce the next season's stem and leaves. In the autumn the stem dies and breaks off, leaving a scar at the side, which is the bud for next season. In the spring of the second year this bud produces a straight erect stem, at the top of which from two to three leaf stems appear and from five to eleven leaflets. Occasionally a stem root will send up more than one stem, each developing a top. The flower stem does not appear the first year, and with but few exceptions does it appear until the third year. The seed stem which puts forth from the middle of the stem, the first year about an inch in length, increasing until it reaches the extreme height of from four to eight inches.

The stem bears an umbel of small greenish-yellow flowers on little stalks, from one-half to an inch long, the whole forming a compact cluster or umbel. The number of flowers on each umbel varies from three to more than one hundred. Like everything else, with this plant, there is a great variation in the number of flowers with the individuals, with age and environment. The flower stem appears soon after the plant unfolds, but it matures the bloom from the first of June to July. Berries form on each stem of the umbel, and ripen sometimes as early as the latter part of July, continuing on up to frost. The berries are a bright crimson with a shiny surface, and each berry is from one to four-seeded. The fruit is edible and has a taste similar to the root.

Ginseng is a very shy plant and possesses many peculiar traits. It loves seclusion, and hence is found mostly in unfrequented localities. It is found growing almost entirely in the shade, the sunshine being nearly always fatal. The seed germinate in eighteen months instead of six, as is the case with ordinary plants. The berries, on the same umbel, vary greatly in time of ripening, number of seed and shape of berries.

The root when deprived of top or bud will lay in the ground all summer, forming a new bud for the next spring's growth. The roots may be divided at the neck and treated the same as budless plant, and in the following spring each will send up a new top. The plant is very hardy and may be cultivated with profit, but must be grown in the shade.

The best location is a northern slope, though most any may be used. Soil should be thoroughly enriched by stirring in leaf mould, stable manure, etc. As the amount of ground occupied by a nursery would be very small. You can take almost any soil and give it the proper qualities, but the deeper the soil, the better, as it will hold the moisture longer and drain itself better. Moisture is necessary to the plants, but a heavy, clammy, water soaked soil will not do, and a hard sub-soil of clay is likely to be too wet in the spring and too dry in the summer.

After you have your beds once prepared and planted, you have but little cultivation to do, except keeping the weeds pulled out and see that no enemies bother, such as man, beast or insects, and notice that your plants are kept in healthful condition.

Roots for market should be dug in the fall, as they are not so full of sap, and will lose less in weight. After plants get seven or eight years old, other roots start from near the top that take the strength from the old roots, which soon become soft and spongy and of little value for drying. The small top roots can be cut off and used and will grow good plants.

In digging be careful not to break or bruise the roots. Use a spading fork or some similar tool. After they are dug wash immediately before the dirt becomes dry and hard.

They can be dried in or around the stove or in open air. If roots are not thoroughly dried, they mould and spoil.

After drying put in clean boxes and ship to market. In every large city you will find dealers in Ginseng and Golden Seal.

Properties and Uses—The root of ginseng is used for medicinal purposes, to some extent in this country, but chiefly in China. It is therefore an article of export, brought up by dealers in this country for that purpose. While an official drug in this country according to the United States Pharmacopoeia, from 1840 to 1880, it is at present classed among the unofficial Drug-plants and quoted as such on Page 51 of Bulletin No. 89, U. S. Department of Agriculture, Bureau of Plant Industry.

There are more than 400,000,000 Chinese and Koreans who place a high value on it as a remedy for many ills from the humblest citizen through all the grades of society, including the most profound esteemed scholarship, high officials and Emperor. The inhabitants of China have for ages had unlimited faith in the medicinal power of ginseng.

It was formerly thought that they used it in their religious rites in a superstitious manner, but this has been investigated and found to be erroneous, as they use it altogether as a medicine. Besides using it in many ailments a few of the wealthy use it as preventative, while in Southern China, owing to the heat and moisture of their climate, ginseng is taken infused with most of their drinks and taken even with some of their solid foods as a precautionary measure.

GLOBE FLOWER
(Cephalanthus Occidentallis, Madder Family.)

Common Names—Button Bush, Pond Dogwood, Button Wood Shrub.

Medicinal Part—The bark.

Description—This is a handsome shrub, growing from six to twelve or more feet high, with a rough bark on the stem, but smooth on the branches. The leaves are opposite, oval, acuminate, in whorls of three, from three to five inches long by two to three wide. The flowers are white, and resemble those of the sycamore, and the fruit a hard and dry capsule.

This plant is indigenous, and found in damp places, along the margins of rivers, ponds, etc., in Canada to Florida and California, flowering from June to September. The bark is very bitter, and yields its virtues to water and alcohol.

Properties and Uses—The bark is tonic and the root said to be diaphoretic. The inner bark of the root forms an agreeable bitters and is employed as such. It deserves more notice than it receives.

Dose—Steep a teaspoonful of the granulated bark into a cup of boiling water for half hour. Strain. Take a tablespoonful 3 to 6 times a day. Of the tincture 5 to 10 min.

GOATS RUE
(Galega Officinalis.)
Medicinal Part—The herb.

Description—This is a perennial herb growing in the south of Europe and cultivated here. When bruised it emits a disagreeable odor. Its taste is unpleasantly bitter and rough and when chewed it stains the saliva yelowish brown.

Properties—It is supposed to have cathartic properties, either in the leaves or roots.

Dose—A teaspoonful of the herb, cut small or granulated, to a cup of boiling water. Drink cold, one cupful during the day, a large mouthful at a time; of the tincture 5 to 20 min.

GOLDEN ROD
(Solidago Odora.)
Common Name—Sweet Scented Golden Rod. Blue Mountain Tea.
Part Used—The leaves.

Description—This species of Golden Rod has a perennial creeping root and slender erect stem, 2 to 3 feet high, leaves sessile, linear-lanceolate, rough at the margin, elsewhere smooth and covered with pellucid dots. Flowers of a deep golden yellow color, arranged in terminal, panicled racemes. Grows in woods and fields throughout the U. S. Flowers from August to October. The leaves have a fragrant odor and a warm aromatic agreeable taste.

Uses—Golden Rod is aromatic, moderately stimulant and carminative when cold. Diaphoretic when taken in warm infusion. Excellent to disguise the taste of medicinal herbs.

Dose—A teaspoonful of the leaves to a cupful of boiling water. Drink cold one or two cupfuls a day, a large mouthful at a time.

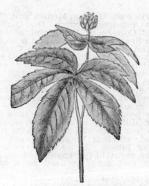

GOLDEN SEAL
(Hydrastis Canadensis, Crowfoot Family.)
Common Names—Yellow Puccoon, Ground Raspberry, Tumeric Root, Hydrastis, Yellow Root, Orangeroot.
Medicinal Part—The root.

Description—This indigenous plant has a perennial root or rhizome, which is tortuous, knotty, creeping, internally of a bright yellow color, with long fibers. The stem is erect, simple, herbaceous, rounded, from six to twelve inches high, bearing two unequal terminal leaves. The two leaves are alternate, palmate, having from three to five lobes, hairy, dark-green, cordate at base, from four to nine inches wide when full grown. The flower is a solitary one, small, white or rose-colored, and the fruit resembles a raspberry, is red, and consists of many two-seeded drupes. It is found growing in shady woods, in rich soils, and damp meadows from Southern New York to Minnesota, south to Georgia and Missouri, but principally in Ohio, Indiana, Kentucky and West Virginia. It flowers in May and June. The root is the officinal part. Its virtues are imparted to water or alcohol. The root is of a beautiful yellow color, and when fresh is juicy, and used by the Indians to color their clothing, etc.

Properties and Uses—The root is a powerful tonic, at the same time exerting an especial influence upon the mucous surfaces and tissues, with which it comes in contact. Internally, it may be used wherever tonics are required. In some instances it proves laxative, but without any astringency, and seems to rank in therapeutical action between rhubarb and blood-root.

A writer on Materia Medica and Therapeutics connected with the Jefferson Medical College of Philadelphia says of Golden Seal: "Very useful as a stomach tonic and in atonic dyspepsia. Constipation, dependent upon different deficient secretions, with hard and dry stools, may be overcome by the remedy."

From the foregoing it must be readily seen how strongly indicated is its use and applicability in catarrhal conditions, of the nasal passages.

This powder may be used in a number of different ways. A teaspoonful placed in a pint of boiling water makes a most efficient vaginal douche and soothing lotion. It may be snuffed up into the nostrils for nasal congestion or catarrh and may be used as a mouth wash.

As a dye, Golden Seal imparts to linen, a rich durable light yellow of great brilliancy, which might probably by proper mordants give all the shades of that color, from pale yellow to orange. With Indigo, it is said to impart a fine green to wool, silk and cotton.

Dose—Place one teaspoonful of the powdered root into a pint of boiling water. Let stand until cold. Drink 1 or 2 teaspoonfuls 3 to 6 times a day.

GOLD THREAD

(Coptis Trifolia, Crowfoot Family.)

Common Names—Mouth Root, Canker Root, Yellow Root.

Medicinal Part—The root and plant.

Description—This plant has a small, creeping, perennial root, of a bright yellow color; the stems are round, slender, and at the base are invested with ovate, acuminate, yellowish scales. The leaves are evergreen on long, slender petioles; leaflets roundish, acute at base, small and smooth and veiny and sessile. The flower is a small starry white one, and the fruit an oblong capsule, containing many small black seeds.

Gold Thread is found growing in dark swamps and sphagnous woods in the northern parts of the United States, and in Canada, Greenland, Iceland, and Siberia. It flowers early in the spring to July. The root is the medicinal part, and autumn is the season for collecting it.

Properties and Uses—It is a pure and bitter tonic, somewhat like quassia, gentain and columbo, without any astringency. It may be beneficially used in all cases where a bitter tonic is required, and is decidedly efficacious as a wash or gargle, when a decoction. In

irritation of the mouth, equal parts of Gold Thread and Golden Seal, made into a decoction, in many instances will destroy the appetite for alcoholic beverages.

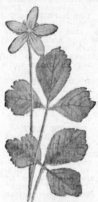

GOLD THREAD

Dose—Steep a teaspoonful of the granulated root into a cup of boiling water, for half hour. Strain. Take a tablespoonful 3 to 6 times a day. Of the tincture 5 to 10 min.

GOOSE GRASS

(Galium Aparine, Madder Family.)

Common Names—Cleavers, Cleaverwort, Bed Straw, Catchweed.

Medicinal Part—The herb.

Description—It is an annual succulent plant, with a weak, procumbent, quadrangular, retrosely-prickled stem, which grows from two to six feet high, and is hairy at the joints. The leaves are one or two inches in length, rough on the margin and tapering to the base. The flowers are white, small and scattered.

This plant is common to Europe and the United States, growing in cultivated grounds, moist thickets, and along banks of rivers, and flowering from June to September. In the green state the plant has an unpleasant odor; but it is inodorous when dried, with an acidulous, astringent, and bitter taste. Cold or warm water extracts the virtues of the plant, boiling water destroys them. The roots dye a permanent red.

Properties and Uses—It is somewhat refrigerant and diuretic, and will be found beneficial in conditions calling for such a combination of qualities.

The plant called Galium Tinctorium, or Small Cleaver, is said to be nervine, anti-spasmodic, expectorant, and diaphoretic. The plant has a pungent, aromatic, pleasant, persistent taste.

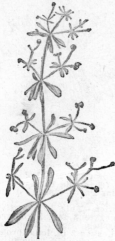

CLEAVERS

Dose—An infusion may be made by steeping an ounce of the herb in a pint of warm water for two hours, of which from two to four fluid ounces may be given three or four times a day when cold. It may be sweetened with sugar or honey. Of the tincture ½ to 1 fl. dr.

GOUANIA
(Gouania luploides—Rhamnaceae Family)

Common Names—Tooth Brush Tree, Chaw stick.

Part Used—Woody stems.

Description—A shrubby vine, found in the tropics. Leaves alternate, petiolate, entire or dentate. Small flowers in clusters.

Uses—Frayed stems used by natives as tooth brushes. The pulverized stems make an excellent natural dentrifice, having a bitterish-sweet flavor, and produces a smooth soap-like froth. An old record states that pieces of Gouania stem put into liquor, causes fermentation, and also imparts a pleasant bitter flavor to cooling drinks.

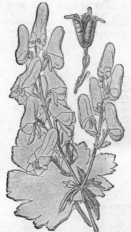

GREAT YELLOW WOLFSBANE
(Aconitum Lycoctonum, Crowfoot Family)

Medicinal Part—The plant.

Description—Great Yellow Wolfsbane has a knobby root and showy yellow flowers. The large upper sepal from its shape is called the hood or helmet. The leaves are palmately divided.

Properties and Uses—A narcotic and a poison.

GROUND IVY
(Nepeta Glechoma, Mint Family.)

Common Names — Gill-go-by-the-ground, Ale Hoof, Cats' Foot, Turnhoof, Field-balm.

Medicinal Part—The leaves.

Description—This plant is a perennial gray, hairy herb, with a procumbent creeping stem, varying in length from a few inches to one or two feet. The leaves have petioles, cordate, and hairy on both sides. The flowers are bluish purple. The corolla is about three times as long as the calyx. This plant is common in the United States and Europe, where it is found in shady places, waste grounds, dry ditches, etc. It flowers in May or August. The leaves impart their virtues to boiling water by infusion. They have an unpleasant odor, and a harsh, bitterish, slightly aromatic taste.

Properties and Uses—It is stimulant, tonic and pectoral, and is useful in many conditions. An infusion of the leaves is very beneficial in lead-colic, and painters sometimes make use of it. The fresh juice snuffed up the nose often relieve nasal congestion and headache.

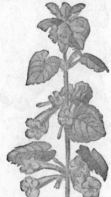

GROUND IVY

Dose—A teaspoonful of the leaves to a cup of boiling water. Drink cold 1 or 2 cupfuls a day. Of the tincture ¼ to ½ fl. dr.

GUAIAC
(Guaiacum Officinale.)

Common Name—Lignum Vitae.
Medicinal Part—The wood and resin.
Description—This is a tree of slow growth, attaining a height of from thirty to forty feet; stem commonly crooked; bark furrowed; wood very hard, heavy, the fibres crossing each other diagonally. Leaves light blue, and the fruit an obcordate capsule.

This tree is an inhabitant of the West Indian Islands, and on the neighboring part of the continent. The wood is used by turners for making block-sheaves, pestles, etc., and is very hard and durable. Both the wood and resin are used in medicine. Alcohol is the best solvent.

Properties and Uses—The wood or resin, taken internally, commonly excites a warmth in the stomach, a dryness of mouth, or thirst. It is an acrid stimulant. If the body be kept warm while using the decoction, it is diaphoretic; if cool, it is diuretic.

Dose—Steep a teaspoonful of the wood, granulated, into a cup of boiling water for half hour. Strain. Take a tablespoonful 3 to 6 times a day. Of the resin 2 to 5 grains.

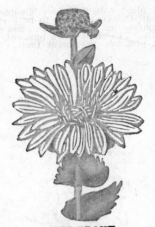

GUM PLANT
(Grindelia Robusta.)

Medicinal Part—The dried leaves and flowering tops.
Description—This is a native perennial herb, 1 to 3 feet high, growing in salt marshes and along mountain ranges. Leaves 2 in. long, broadly spatulate, oblong, sessile, sharply serrate, pale green smooth, finely dotted; heads many-flowered, resinous-viscid; flowers yellow, odor balsamic. Should be collected as soon as in full bloom.

Uses—Grindelia has been used for the spasm of asthma and whooping cough, for bronchial irritation and nasal congestion. It seems to be a stimulating expectorant. Should however, only be used in small doses or it will irritate the kidneys. Externally in solution it is useful in burns, blisters, etc.

Dose—A teaspoonful of the leaves and flowering tops, cut small or granulated to a cup of boiling water. Drink cold one cupful during the day, a large mouthful at a time; of the tincture 5 to 20 min.

HAIRCAP MOSS
(Polytrichium Juniperum, Haircap Moss Family.)

Common Names—Bears Bed, Robin's Eye, Ground Moss.
Medicinal Part—The whole plant.
Description—This is an indigenous plant, having a perennial stem, slender, of a reddish color, and from four to seven inches high; leaves lanceolate.

and somewhat spreading. The fruit a four-sided oblong capsule.

This evergreen plant is found in high, dry places, along the margins of dry woods, mostly on poor sandy soil. It is of darker green color than the mosses in general. It yields its virtues to boiling water.

Properties and Uses—This plant is not much known as a remedial agent, but has been credited with some diuretic power. It causes no nausea or disagreeable sensations in the stomach, and may be used with the hydrogogue cathartics with advantage.

Dose—1 teaspoonful to a cup of boiling water. Drink one or two cupfuls a day a few swallows at a time. Tincture ½ to 1 fl. dr.

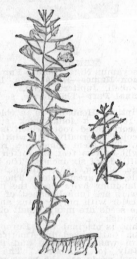

HEDGE HYSSOP
(Gratiola Officinalis, Figwort Family)
Medicinal Part—Plant.

Description — A rather insignificant plant found in low wet places, flowering all summer. Stems generally diffusely branched sometimes creeping at the base. Sterile filaments minute or hardly any. The corolla is whitish with yellowish tube.

Properties and Uses—Acrid, drastic, vermifuge, diuretic and narcotic.

HELONIAS
(Helonias Dioica, Aster Family)
Common Names—False Unicorn Root, Drooping Star Wort.
Medicinal Part—The root.
Description—This is an herbaceous perennial plant, with a large bulbous root, from which arises a very smooth angular stem one or two feet in height. The cauline leaves are lanceolate, acute and small; the radical leaves (or those springing from the root) are broader and from four to eight inches in length. The flowers are small, very numerous, greenish-white, disposed in long, terminal, nodding racemes, resembling plumes. The fruit is a capsule.

This plant is indigenous to the United States, and is abundant in some of the Western states, growing in woodlands, meadows and moist situations, and flowering in June and July.

Properties and Uses—In large doses it is emetic, and when fresh, sialagogue. In doses of ten or fifteen grains of the powdered root, repeated three or four times a day, it has been found beneficial in loss of appetite and for the removal of worms. The plant will kill cattle feeding on it and the decoction, insects, bugs and lice.

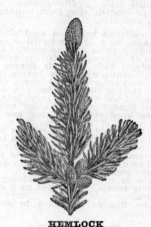

HEMLOCK
(Tsuga Canadensis.)
Common Name—Tanners Bark.
Description—Hemlock grows 50 to 100 feet high, trunk 3 to 6 feet diameter,

bark dull gray brown, perpendicularly seamed, coarse, with large plate-like scales, very red beneath. Twigs extremely soft, and slender, downy, light brown; needles often less than ½ inch long; cones small ½ to ¾ inch long, broad ovoid, stalked and pendent; grows in swamps, mountain slopes, ravines, rocky woods.

Properties and Uses—Hemlock bark is a powerful astringent. Hemlock Pitch, also known as Canada Pitch, is a gentle rubefacient, similar to Burgundy Pitch. Oil from this tree, or Hemlock Oil, is used in liniment.

HENNA

(Lawsonia alba—Lythraceae or Loostrife)

Common Names—Mignonette Tree, Reseda.

Part Used—Leaves.

Description—A rather common shrub, in the tropics where it is grown as a hedge, because of its dense growth. Leaves are elliptical, greyish-green, glabrous and from 1½ to 2 inches long. The highly scented flowers, cinnabar red, are less than a half inch in width, and in many-flowered panicles from 8 to 12 inches long. Fruits globular, shiny green or reddish. The bush is native of Africa and Asia.

Uses—Henna has been used since remote ages as a dye, and still is one of the most popular dyes in modern times. People of ancient civilizations dyed the manes and tails of their horses with Henna. Arabs dye their beards, nails, palms, and soles with the leaves of this bush. Henna alone produces a bright orange-red on white or gray hair, and various shades of red on other hair, depending upon the hair color, and upon the amount of dye used. As a weak rinse, it is used only to enliven brown type hair. It may be mixed with Indigo and other dyeing botanicals for special colors and effects. Henna is used in the Orient to dye wool and silk, as well as a skin dye and hair dye.

Henna is astringent—containing considerable tannin. It is used as a gargle in India.

Henna flowers are used in making perfume.

Self love, my liege, is not so vile a sin as self neglecting.—King Henry V, Act 2, Scene 4—Shakespeare.

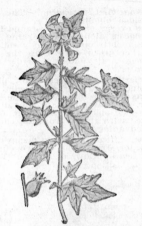

HENBANE

(Hyoscyamus Niger, Potato Family)
Common Names—Hogs Bean, Devil's Eye, Henbell, Jupiter's Bean.
Medicinal Part—The leaves, seed and root.

Description—Henbane is a biennial plant. It has a long thick spindle-shaped corrugated root, which is of a brown color externally, but whitish internally. The stem sometimes reaches the height of two feet, but often stops at an altitude of six inches. The leaves are large, oblong, acute, alternate, and of a pale, dull green color. They have long, glandular hairs upon the midrib. The flowers are funnel-shaped, of a dull yellow color with purple veins and orifice. The seeds are many, small obovate and brownish.

Henbane is original with Europe, but has been naturalized in America. It grows in waste grounds, and flowers from July to September. The root, leaves and seeds are the parts medicinally used. The leaves are collected in the second year, when the plant is in flower; the seeds are gathered when perfectly ripe. It grows more plentifully than elsewhere in America, in the waste grounds of old settlements, in graveyards and around the foundations of ruined houses. Bruise the recent leaves, and they emit a strong narcotic odor, like tobacco. Dry them and they have little smell or taste. Their virtues are **completely extracted by diluted alcohol.** The active principle of Henbane is called

Hyosciamia, but all the recognized preparations are now known by the general name of Hyoscyamus.

Properties and Uses—Henbane is a narcotic, and if improperly and injudiciously used, is "dangerously" poisonous. All narcotics are "dangerously" poisonous if dangerously administered. Nature grows wild some of her most potent medicinal herbs, and those which, if used by persons who understand them, may be very useful and beneficial but which also may be destructive if applied and administered by parties who have not thoroughly studied their properties. Medicinally used, Henbane is calmative, anodyne, and antispasmodic and the leaves make fine external preparations for various purposes. Henbane, however, is solely for the physician or skilled herbalist and should be avoided by all other persons.

Dose—A teaspoonful of the leaves cut small to a pint of boiling water. Take one teaspoonful at a time as required of the tincture 2 to 5 min.

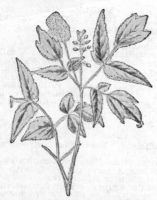

HERB CHRISTOPHER
(Actaea Spicata, Crowfoot Family)

Common Names—Baneberry, Rattlesnake Herb.

Medicinal Part—The root.

Description — Herb Christopher is found growing in rich woods. The leaflets are of the thrice ternate leaves ovate, sharply cleft, and cut-toothed. The flowers are borne on a very short, ovate raceme or cluster on slender pedicels. The red berries ripen in late summer.

Properties and Uses—Vulnerary and astringent.

HIGH MALLOW
(Malva Sylvestris, Mallow Family.)

Common Names—Cheese Flower.

Medicinal Part—The herb.

Description—This plant is a perennial and has a round stem two or three feet high, and a tapering, branching, whitish root. The leaves are alternate, deep green, soft, and downy. The flowers are large, numerous and of purple color; calyx five-cleft; petals five; stamens,, indefinite; pollen large, whitish.

The mallow is a native of Europe, but is naturalized in this country. It grows abundantly in fields, waysides, and waste places, and flowers from May to October. The whole plant, especially the root, abounds in mucilage.

Properties and Uses—It apparently possesses properties common to mucilaginous herbs, and an infusion thereof forms an excellent demulcent in coughs, due to colds, irritations of the air-passages, etc. In conditions of external irritation, the bruised herb forms an excellent application, making, as it does, a natural emollient.

Dose—A teaspoonful of the herb to a cup of boiling water. Drink cold 1 or 2 cupfuls a day; a large mouthful at a time; of the tincture ½ to 1 fl. dr.

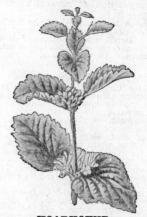

HOARHOUND
(Marrubium Vulgare, Mint Family.)

Common Name—Marrubium.

Medicinal Part—The herb.

Description—This well known herb has a fibrous perennial root, and numerous annual, bushy stem, leafy, and branching from the bottom to one or two feet in height. The leaves are roundish-ovate, rough and veiny above, wooly on the under surface, one or two inches in diameter; the flowers small and white.

Hoarhound is a native of Europe, but has been naturalized in the United States, where it is very common, especially from Maine southward to Texas and westward to California and Oregon. It grows on dry, sandy fields, waste grounds and road sides, flowering from June to September. The entire plant has a white or hoary appearance; the whole herb is medicinal, and should be gathered before its efflorescence. It has a peculiar, rather agreeable, vinous balsamic odor, and a very bitter, aromatic, somewhat acrid and persistent taste. Its virtues are imparted to alcohol or water.

Properties and Uses—A stimulant, tonic, expectorant, and diuretic. It is used in the form of syrup, in ordinary colds and coughs, as well as hoarseness. The warm infusion will promote perspiration and flow of urine, and is used with great benefit. The cold infusion is an excellent tonic and will act as a purgative in large doses. It enters into the composition of several syrups and candies.

Dose—A teaspoonful of the herbs, cut small or granulated to a cup of boiling water. Drink cold, one cupful during the day, a large mouthful at a time; of the tincture 10 to 60 min.

HOG PHYSIC
(Lobelia Cardinalis—Lobelia Family)

Common Names—Cardinal Lobelia, Cardinal Flower, Red Cardinal.

Medicinal Parts—Herb.

Description—A beautiful herb, quite common in moist places from Canada to Florida, and west to the Mississippi River. The plant forms a single stalk generally from 16 to 24 inches high. Lower leaves are elliptic to elliptic-spatulate, serrate or dentate. The intense red flowers were used by rustics as a dye.

Medicinal Uses—Said to have virtues similar to Lobelia inflata. A beautiful blue flowering variety (Lobelia siphilitica) is reputed as an emetic, cathartic and diuretic.

NOTE: The name "Hog Physic" is used only by rustics. I made use of the name merely to have this lovely plant fit in with Joseph E. Meyer's original common name arrangement of plants.

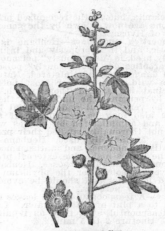

HOLLYHOCK
(Althea Rosea, Mallow Family)

Common Names—Althea Rose, Malva Flowers.

Medicinal Part—Flowers.

Description—Hollyhock has a tall and simple stem, hairy. The flowers are large on very short peduncles forming a long spike. The corolla is of all shades of rose, purple, white or yellow, single or double, three to four inches broad.

Properties and Uses—Emollient, demulcent and diuretic.

HOPS
(Humulus Lupulus.)

Medicinal Part—The strobiles or cones.

Description—This well-known twining plant has a perennial root, with many annual angular stems. The leaves are opposite, deep green, serrated, venated, and very rough. The flowers are numerous and of a greenish color. Fruit a strobile. This plant is found in China, the Canary Islands, all parts of Europe, and in many places in the United States. It is largely cultivated in England and the United States for its cones or strobiles, which are used medicinally, and in the manufacture of beer, ale and porter. The odor of hops is peculiar and somewhat agreeable, their taste slightly astringent and exceedingly bitter. They yield their virtues to boiling water, but a better solvent than water is diluted alcohol. Lupulin is the yellow powder procured by beating or rubbing the strobiles, and then sifting out the grains which form about one-seventh part of the hops. Lupulin is in globose kidney shaped grains, golden yellow and somewhat transparent, and preferable to the hops itself. Lupulite is the bitter principle of hops, and is obtained by making an aqueous solution of Lupulin.

Properties and Uses—Hops are tonic, hypnotic, febrifuge, antilithic, and anthelmintic. They are principally used

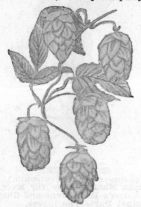

HOPS

for their sedative or hypnotic action—producing sleep, removing restlessness, and abating pain, but sometimes failing to do so. A pillow stuffed with hops is a favorite way for inducing sleep. The tea or tincture is used and does not disorder the stomach nor cause constipation, as with some preparations. Externally, in the form of a fomentation alone, or combined with Boneset or other bitter herbs, it has proved beneficial as an application for bruises, etc. An ointment made by boiling two parts of Stramonium leaves and one of Hops in lard, is an excellent application in skin irritation and itching.

Dose—A teaspoonful of the flowers cut small or granulated to a cup of boiling water. Drink cold one cupful during the day, a large mouthful at a time; of the tincture 5 to 20 min.

Hop Pillow: Fill a small pillowcase with Hops, which have been sprinkled with alcohol, to bring out the active principle.

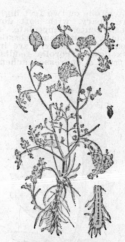

HORSEBANE
(Oenanthe Phellandrium)
Common Names—Water Fennel, Water Dropwort.
Medicinal Part—The plant.
Description—Horsebane is to be found growing wild in swamps. The root is fibrous and the flowers are white.
Properties and Uses—Narcotic, alterative. Supposed to be poisonous.

HORSEMINT
(Monarda Punctata.)
Part Used—The leaves and tops.
Description—This is a perennial plant of the mint family, growing 2 to 3 feet high; stems branched, downy leaves 2 to 3 inches long, lanceolate, serrate, punctate, flowers yellowish, spotted red with pinkish bracts, downy calyx 5 toothed.
Properties and Uses—Horsemint is aromatic, pungent and bitter and contains volatile oil. It is useful as a carminative, and diuretic in flatulent colic, nausea, etc.
Dose—One teaspoonful of the granulated leaves or tops to a cupful of boiling water. Drink one or two cupfuls a day as required. Tincture 10 to 40 min.

HOUND'S TONGUE
(Cynoglossum Officinale, Borage Family.)
Common Name—Gypsy-flower.
Medicinal Parts—The leaves and root.
Description—This biennial plant has

61

an erect stem one or two feet high. The leaves are hoary, with soft down on both sides, acute, lanceolate, radical ones petiolate, cauline ones sessile, with cordate bases. The flowers are in clusters, calyx downy, corolla reddish purple, and fruit a depressed achenium.

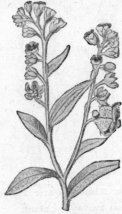

HOUND'S TONGUE

Hound's Tongue grows on the roadsides and waste places of both Europe and America. The leaves and the root are the parts used in medicine. The root upon being gathered, emits an unpleasant heavy odor, which vanishes when it is dried. Its taste is bitter and mawkish. The fresh root is spoken of by several herbalists as being better than the desiccated or dried, but this probably arises from the fact that the roots they used had not been gathered at the proper time, dried in the correct way, or kept in a skilful manner. The dried root is quite as active as the fresh, if prepared by a person who knows its qualities.

Properties and Uses—Hound's Tongue has been used as a demulcent and sedative in coughs resulting from colds, as well as in diarrhea, and it has been employed as a poultice for burns and bruises, but there is some evidence that it is a rather dangerous herb internally and should be avoided, especially by the unskilled.

Cynoglossum Morrisoni, or Virginia Mouse-Ear, Beggars' Lice, Dysentery Weed, etc., is an annual weed with an erect hairy, leafy stem, two to four feet high. Leaves three to four inches long, oblong, lanceolate; flowers very small, white, or pale blue. It grows in rocky grounds and among rubbish. It is efficacious in diarrhea. The root may be chewed or given in powder or infusion.

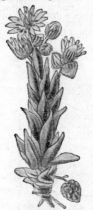

HOUSE LEEK
(Sempervivum Tectorum.)

Common Names—Live for Ever, Sengreen, Aaron's Rod. Hens-and-Chickens.

Medicinal Part—The leaves.

Description—House-Leek has a fibrous root, with several tufts of oblong, acute, extremely succulent leaves. The stem from the center of these tufts is about a foot high, erect, round and downy; flowers large, pale rose-colored, and scentless. Offsets spreading.

This perennial plant is a native of Europe, and is so succulent that it will grow on dry walls, roofs of houses, etc. It flowers in August. It is much cultivated in some places. The leaves contain super-malate of lime.

Properties and Uses—The fresh leaves are useful as a refrigerant when bruised, and applied as a poultice in burns, stings of insects and other irritated conditions of the skin. The leaves have been sliced in two, and the inner surface applied to warts. The leaves also possess an astringent property, serviceable in many cases.

Dose—A teaspoonful of the leaves cut small or granulated to a cup of boiling water. Drink cold, one cupful during the day, a large mouthful at a time; of the tincture 5 to 20 min.

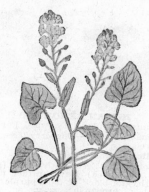

the leaves is hot, spicy, and somewhat bitter, and yield their virtues to water and alcohol. They contain yellow oil and sulphur.

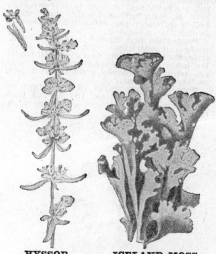

HORSE RADISH
(Cochlearia Armoracia.)
Medicinal Part—The root.

Description—The root of this plant is perennial, sending up numerous very large leaves from the midst of which a round, smooth, erect, branchy stem rises 2 or 3 ft. high. The radical leaves are lanceolate, waved, scalloped on the edges and stand up on strong foot stalks. Those of the stem are much smaller, without foot stalks; flowers numerous, white. The pod is small divided into 2 cells each containing from 4 to 6 seeds. The root is long and tapering; conical at top, fleshy, whitish externally and whitish within of a strong pungent odor when scraped or bruised and of a hot biting taste.

Properties—The fresh root is far more powerful than the dried. It is useful in stimulating the stomach and promoting secretion, as of the urine. Externally it is rubefacient.

Dose—A teaspoonful of the root to a cup of boiling water. Drink cold 1 or 2 cupfuls a day, a large mouthful at a time; of the tincture, ½ to 1 fl. dr.

HYSSOP
(Hyssopus Officinalis, Mint Family.)
Medicinal Parts—The tops and leaves.

Description—Hyssop is a perennial herb, with square stems, woody at the base and a foot or two in height, with rod-like branches. The leaves are opposite, sessile, linear, and lanceolate, green on each side; flowers, bluish-purple, seldom white; stamens four.

It is an inhabitant of Europe and this country, being raised principally in gardens, and flowers in July. The taste of

HYSSOP   ICELAND MOSS

Properties and Uses—Stimulant, aromatic, carminative, and tonic. It has been used in throat irritation, as a gargle with sage. As an expectorant it is beneficial in coughs, due to colds. The leaves have been applied to bruises.

Dose—A teaspoonful of the leaves to a cup of boiling water. Drink cold one or two cupfuls a day, a large mouthful at a time; of the tincture ½ to 1 fl. dr.

ICELAND MOSS
(Cetraria Islandica.)
Common Name—Eryngo-Leaved Liverwort.

Medicinal Part—The plant.

Description—Iceland Moss is a perennial, foliaceous plant from two to four inches high; a native of Britain and the northern countries of Europe, particularly Iceland. It is diversified in its color, being brownish or grayish-white in some parts, and of a reddish hue in others. It is without odor, with a mucilaginous, bitter, somewhat astringent taste, and when dry the lichen is crisp, cartilaginous and coriaceous, and is convertible into a grayish-white powder. It swells up in water, absorbing more than its own weight of that fluid, and communicating a portion of its bitterness to it, as well as a little mucilage; when long chewed it is converted into a mucilaginous pulp, and when boiled in water the decoction becomes a firm jelly on cooling.

Properties and Uses—It is demulcent, tonic and nutritious. Boiled with milk, it forms an excellent nutritive and tonic. Its tonic virtues depend upon its cetrarin, which, if removed, renders the lichen merely nutritious.

Dose—A teaspoonful of the plant to a cup of boiling water. Drink cold 1 or 2 cupfuls a day, a large mouthful at a time.

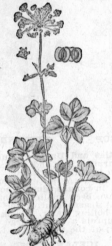

IMPERIAL MASTERWORT
(Imperatoria Ostruthium)

Common Names—Masterwort, Pellitory of Spain.

Medicinal Parts—Root and seed.

Description—Imperial Masterwort has a stout stem, hollow and erect from two to five feet tall. Leaves ternately divided into very broad stalked ovate to obovate segments which are often three parted nearly or quite to the base, sharply and unequally serrate, and often incised. Compound umbels of white flowers. The seed is broad and flat.

Properties and Uses—Aromatic, stimulant, cordial, diaphoretic, emmenagogue.

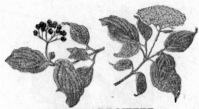

INDIAN ARROWEED
(Cornus Sanguinea, Dogwood Family)

Common Names—Dogberry Tree, Gutter Tree.

Medicinal Part—Bark.

Description—Erect with ovate (sometimes variegated) leaves rather downy beneath, and black or dark purple fruit. Branches brownish, gray or green streaked. Leaves loosely pubescent below. The flowers in the late spring are greenish in a head or close cluster surrounded by a showy corolla-like, four-leaved involucre.

Properties and Uses—Wash for mangy dogs.

INDIAN BLACK DRINK
(Ilex Vomitoria—Holly Family)

Common Names—Yaupon Holly, Emetic Holly.

Parts Used—Smoked Leaves.

Description—Rarely small trees—more often shrubs, found in the southeastern part of the U.S., mainly in lowlands and woods. Leaves evergreen and leathery. Small white flowers followed by red globose fruits. Branches often used for Christmas decorations.

Excerpt from an old record: "When the time of year drew near, Indians of the South East assembled, according to a custom of long standing, from parts far and wide, at some chosen place where the plant grew in abundance. Here they built a great fire, and hung over it a kettle. Into this, with water they then threw quantities of the Yaupon's leaves. As soon as they had sufficiently brewed, they began drinking the beverage, and were soon in consequence violently sick. But still they were undeterred. Again they drank with the same result, and so for two or three days they continued drinking and being sick, or until they deemed their systems to be sufficiently cleansed. After this they returned to their several habitations each carrying on the way, a branch of the holly."

Use—Emetic as a strong black brew. Used as a beverage when brewed like tea.

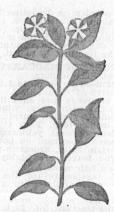

INDIAN CHICKWEED
(Stellaria Media, Pink Family)

Common Names—Chickweed, Starwort.

Description—This plant is an annual or biennial weed, from six to fifteen inches in length, with a prostrate, brittle and leafy stem. The leaves are ovate-cordate; the lower ones on hairy petioles. The flowers are small and white, petals two-parted, stamens three, five or ten. It is a common plant in Europe and America, growing in fields and around dwellings, in moist, shady places. It flowers from the beginning of spring 'til the last of autumn. The seeds are eaten by poultry and birds. The whole herb is used when recent.

Properties and Uses—It is a cooling demulcent. The fresh leaves bruised and applied as a poultice to external conditions will produce decided beneficial results, to be changed two or three times a day. An ointment made by bruising the recent leaves in fresh lard may be used as a cooling application to skin irritations.

INDIAN TURNIP
(Arum Triphyllum, Arum Family)

Common Names—Wake Robin, Jack in the Pulpit, Dragon Root.

Medicinal Parts—The cormus or root.

Description—This plant has a round, flattened, perennial rhizome; the upper part is tunicated like an onion. The leaves are generally one or two, standing on long, sheathing footstalks; leaflets oval, mostly entire, acuminate, smooth and paler on the under side.

It inhabits North and South America, is found in wet locations, and flowers from May to June. The whole plant is acrid, but the root is the only part employed. It is of various sizes, turnip shaped, dark and corrugated externally and milk-white within, seldom exceeding two and a half inches in diameter. When first dug it is too fiercely acrid for internal employment, as it will leave an impression upon the tongue, lips and fauces, like that of a severe scald, followed by inflammation and tenderness,

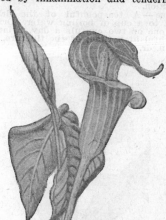

INDIAN TURNIP

which, however, may be somewhat mollified by milk. It exerts no such influence upon the external skin, except upon long and continued application. The root loses its acrimony by age, and should always be used when partially dried. In addition to its acrid principle, it contains a large proportion of starch, with a portion of gum, albumen and saccharine matter. When the acrid matter is driven off by heat, the root yields a pure, delicate, amylaceous matter, resembling arrow root, very white and nutritive.

Properties and Uses—It is acrid, expectorant and diaphoretic, but never should be employed in a fresh or unprepared state or by one unfamiliar with its peculiarities, as it is violently irritating to mucous membrane if improperly used.

IRISH MOSS
(Chondrus Crispus)
Common Name—Pearl Moss.
Part Used—The dried plant.
Description—Irish Moss grows on submerged rocks, to which it is attached by a small disk; when fresh the cartilaginous frond measures 6 to 12 inches long, more or less greenish but turning purple upon drying unless bleached; taste mucilaginous, saline.
Properties—Irish Moss is demulcent, nutrient, dietetic, useful in diarrhea, etc. It may be employed in the form of a decoction.
Dose—A teaspoonful of the dried plant to a cup of boiling water. Drink cold one or two cupfuls a day, a large mouthful at a time; of the tincture, ½ to 1 fl. dr.

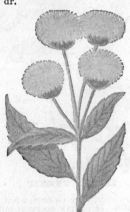

IRON WEED
(Veronia Fasciculata, Composite Family)
Medicinal Part—The root.
Description—This is an indigenous, perennial, coarse, purplish-green weed, with a stem from three to ten feet high. The leaves are from four to eight inches long, one or two broad, lanceolate, tapering to each end. Corolla showy, and dark purple.

This is a very common plant to the Western States, growing in woods and prairies, and along rivers and streams, flowering from July to September. The root is bitter, and imparts its virtues to water and alcohol.
Properties and Uses—It is a bitter

tonic. In powder or decoction the root is beneficial in indicated uses.
Dose—A teaspoonful of the root to a cup of boiling water. Drink cold 1 or 2 cupfuls a day, a large mouthful at a time; of the tincture, ½ to 1 fl. dr.

JABORANDI-PILOCARPUS
Part Used—The leaflets.
Description—This shrub is 4 to 5 feet high, a native of Brazil, S. A., growing in forest clearings and on hill slopes; bark smooth with grey white dots. Flowers small, pinkish purple, leaflets 2½ to 5 inches long, 1 to 1½ inches broad, oblong or oval, yellowish green; shining, veins prominent on both sides, taste bitterish, salty, aromatic pungent.
Uses—The leaves are highly recommended as a hair wash.
Dose—A teaspoonful of the leaflets, cut small or granulated to a cup of boiling water. Drink cold, one cupful during the day, a large mouthful at a time; of the tincture, 5 to 20 min.

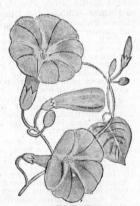

JALAP
(Ipomoea Jalapa)
Medicinal Part—The root.
Description—Jalap has a fleecy, tuberous root, with numerous roundish tubercles. It has several stems, which are smooth, brownish, slightly rough, with a tendency to twine. The leaves are on long petioles, the first hastate, succeeding ones cordate, acuminate, and mucronate. The calyx has no bracts, corolla funnel-shaped, purple and long. Fruit a capsule.

66

This plant grows in Mexico, at an elevation of nearly six thousand feet above the level of the sea, near Chicanquiaco and Xalapa, from which it is exported, and from which last named place it also receives its name. It is generally imported in bags, containing one or two hundred pounds. It is soluble in water and alcohol.

Properties and Uses—Jalap is irritant and cathartic, operating energetically, and produces liquid stools. It is chiefly employed when it is desired to produce an energetic influence on the bowels, or to obtain large evacuations. In intestinal irritations it should not be used.

Dose—A teaspoonful of the root, cut small or granulated, to a cup of boiling water. Drink cold, one cupful during the day, a large mouthful at a time; of the tincture, 1 to 5 min.

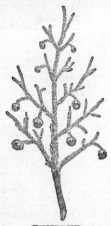

JUNIPER
(Juniperus Communis, Pine Family)

Medicinal Part—The berries.

Description—This is a small, evergreen shrub, never attaining the height of a tree, with many very close branches. The leaves are attached to the stem in threes. The fruit is fleshy, of dark-purplish color, ripening the second year from the flower. This shrub is common on dry, sterile hills from Canada south to New Jersey, west to Nebraska, and in the Rocky Mountains to New Mexico.

The peasantry in the south of France prepare a sort of tar, which they call "huile de cade," from the interior reddish wood of the trunk and branches, by a distillation per descensum. This is our popular Juniper Tar.

Properties and Uses—Juniper Berries are gently stimulant and diuretic, imparting to the urine the smell of violets and producing occasionally, when largely taken, disagreeable irritation in urinary passages. They are chiefly used as an adjuvant to more powerful diuretics. They may be given in substance, triturated with sugar, in the dose of one or two drachms three or four times a day. But the infusion is more convenient. It is prepared by macerating an ounce of the bruised berries in a pint of boiling water, the whole of which may be taken in the course of twenty-four hours. Extracts are prepared from the berries, bruised, and given in the dose of one or two drachms; but, in consequence of the evaporation of the essential oil, they are probably not stronger than the berries in substance.

Dose—A teaspoonful of the berries to a cup of boiling water. Drink cold 1 or 2 cupfuls a day, a large mouthful at a time; of the tincture ½ to 1 fl. dr.

JAMAICA GINGER
(Zingiber Officinale)

Medicinal Part—The root.

Description—This is perennial herb, stem barren, leafy 3 to 4 ft. high, entirely covered with leaf sheaths, solid, round; leaves 6 to 12 inches long, 1 to 1½ inches wide; flowering stalk 6 to 12 inches long, terminating in a spike of 2 or 3 dingy yellow flowers. Rhizomes 2 to 4 inches long, ½ inch broad and 1-6 to 1-3 inch thick, fibrous, whitish or pale buff; agreeable aromatic pungent taste.

Properties—Ginger is useful in flatulent, colic and in conditions calling for a warming and carminative effect.

Dose—A teaspoonful of the root, cut small or granulated to a cup of boiling water. Drink cold, one cupful during the day, a large mouthful at a time; of the tincture 5 to 20 min.

KAVA KAVA
(Piper Methysticum)

Common Name—Ava Root.

Medicinal Part—The root.

Description—Kava-Kava is a species of Piper and is native of the Sandwich Islands. The root is used for making a beverage by the natives called Kava.

Properties—The root has a lilac odor and bitter taste; it is tonic, stimulant, diuretic and diaphoretic.

Dose—A teaspoonful of the root, cut small or granulated, to a cup of boiling water. Drink cold one cupful during the day, a large mouthful at a time; of the tincture, 5 to 20 min.

KIDNEY LIVER-LEAF
(Hepatica Americana, Crowfoot Family)

Common Names — Noble Liverwort, Liver Leaf.

Medicinal Part—The plant.

Description—This is a perennial plant, the root of which consists of numerous strong fibres. The leaves are all radical, on long, hairy petioles, smooth, evergreen, cordate at base, the new ones appearing later than the flowers. The flowers appear almost as soon as the snow leaves the ground in the spring. Fruit an ovate achenium.

Hepatica Acutaloba, or Heart Liver-Leaf, which possesses the same medicinal qualities, differs from the above in having the leaves with three ovate pointed lobes, or sometimes five-lobed. They both bear white, blue or purplish flowers, which appear late in March or early in April.

These plants are common to the United stated, growing in woods and upon elevated situations—the former, which is the most common, being found on sides of hills, exposed to the north, and the latter on the southern aspect. The plants yield their virtues to water.

Properties and Uses—It is a mild, mucilaginous astringent, and is freely used in infusion, in such conditions as coughs due to colds.

Dose—A teaspoonful of the leaves to a cup of boiling water. Drink cold one or two cupfuls a day, large mouthful at a time; of the tincture, ½ to 1 fl. dr.

KNOT WEED
(Polygonum Persicaria, Buckwheat Family)

Common Names—Ladies Thumb, Spotted Knot Weed, Heartease.

Medicinal Part—The whole herb.

Description—The Knotweed is almost identical with Water Pepper, except that its leaves and the entire plant are often larger and the flowers are a pale pink, or purple, while those of Water Pepper are greenish white.

Properties and Uses—Knot Grass is said to be very efficacious as a diuretic; the juice is used for wounds, cuts, bruises, etc.

Dose—A teaspoonful of the herb to a cup of boiling water. Drink cold one or two cupfuls a day, a large mouthful at a time; of the tincture, ½ to 1 fl. dr.

KOLA NUTS
(Cola Acuminata)

Medicinal Part—The seed or nuts.

Description—Kola is a tree native of West Africa, 50 to 60 feet high, smooth stem; leaves 6 to 8 inches long, lance-olate-ovate, acuminate; flowers yellowish, fruit yellowish brown, 5 segments, rough woody, follicle 4 to 5 inches long, segment one to three seeded. Seed 1½ inches long and 1 inch thick, flattened.

Properties—The seed contains caffeine, theobromine, tannin and starch. They are stimulant, tonic, nervine, diuretic, astringent, resembling cocoa in aiding endurance of fatigue without food; useful in neuralgia and headache.

Dose—A teaspoonful of the seed or nuts cut small or granulated, to a cup of boiling water. Drink cold one cupful during the day, a large mouthful at a time; of the tincture, 5 to 20 min.

KOUSSO
(Brayera Anthelmintica)

Medicinal Part—The flowers.

Description—This is a tree, growing about 20 feet high, with round rusty branches. The leaves are crowded, alternate; leaflets oblong, acute and serrate; flowers small, greenish, and becoming purple.

This tree grows upon the table-lands of Northeastern Abyssinia, at an elevation of several thousand feet. The flowers are the parts used. They are gathered when in full bloom, and are used in their fresh state, but are equally valuable when properly dried. After drying they are powdered, and in this form they the mixed with warm water and administered. The value of this medicine has been known for a long time, having been introduced in the French practice over 60 years ago. It is quite difficult to procure even the adulterated or spurious article in America or England; the genuine is not to be obtained at any price in the drug stores.

Practices and Uses—In large doses it will produce heat of the stomach, nausea, and sometimes vomiting, and occasionally will act powerfully on the bowels, but this is only when injudiciously taken. Its chief property has been reported to be the destruction and expulsion of worms, especially the tapeworm. Taken in the proper dose, it seems to have no general effect, but operates wholly and solely upon the worms. The dose of the powdered flowers in infusion is half an ounce to half a pint of warm water. It must be reduced for children. If the medicine does not operate in four hours, drink a tablespoonful of castor-oil. Of the tincture, 1 to 4 drachms may be taken.

KUEMMEL
(Carum)

Common Name—Caraway.

Medicinal Part—The seed.

Description—This is a biennial herb, with a hollow stem, growing 1 to 3 feet high. Leaves bi- or tripinnate, deeply incised. Flowers, small white, May to June. Fruit two-seeded cremocarp, oblong, flattened about 1/6 inch long.

Properties—The seeds are carminative, and stomachic. They are useful in flatulent colic, especially in infants, and as a corrective to nauseous purgatives, and as a spice in cakes, etc.

Dose—A teaspoonful of the seed, cut small or granulated, to a cup of boiling water. Drink cold, one cupful during the day, a large mouthful at a time; of the tincture, 5 to 20 min.

KHUS-KHUS
(Andropogon zizanioides—Grass Family)

Common Names—Cus-Cus, Vetiver, Vetivert.

Part Used—Roots.

Description — Tall upright, narrow blade grass, forming large clumps. Fibrous roots acquire a sandalwood-like fragrance upon drying. Khus-Khus is grown throughout the tropics, as a terracing plant to prevent washouts. Grass is also used to make thatch roofs for native huts. In India the roots are much used for "tats" for shading verandas, these being kept moist during hot weather by sprinkling with water, after which they emit a fragrant odor.

Dried roots are used in the manufacture of a fine perfume, and in the crude state, kept with clothes, to keep insects away.

Small bundles of Khus-Khus are sold in most tropical native markets. Like Ginger and other botanicals, the finest quality roots are only grown on certain soils.

Khus-Khus is a valuable fixative for dry types of perfumes, such as Potpourri and Sachets. See pages 198 and 229.

* * * *

"Calamus would be a useful addition to many of the compound infusions of vegetable stomachics. It is so favourite a remedy with the native practitioners of India, in the bowel complaints of children, that there is a penalty incurred by any druggist who will not, in the middle of the night, open his door and sell it, if demanded."
—Pharmacologia by J. A. Paris, M.D., 1833.

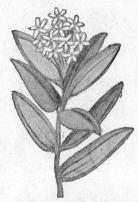

LABRADOR TEA
(Ledum Latifolium, Heath Family)

Common Name—Continental Tea.

Part Used—The leaves.

Description—Labrador Tea is an erect shrub from one to three feet high. Its habitat is in bogs or damp thickets. The narrowly oblong leaves are green above, have the edges rolled back and are covered beneath with a rusty wool.

Properties and Uses—Pectoral and stimulant and sometimes used as a table tea.

LAD'S LOVE
(Artemisia Abrotanum—Compositae Family)

Common Names — Southernwood, Old Man, Old Woman.

Part Used—The Herb.

Description—Related to Wormwood. A favorite plant in old European monasteries and Castle gardens. Used as a border plant because of its upright and dense growth. The soft finely divided leaves are silvery grey, and have a refreshing lemony scent that is disagreeable to bees and other insects. The French call this plant Garderole, and use it to protect their woolens from insects.

Properties and Uses—Used in Italy as a culinary herb, the young shoots being used for flavoring cakes, and other foods. The herb is aromatic, astringent, bitter and tonic. _____

To be happy, we must be true to nature, and carry our age along with us.—Hazlit.

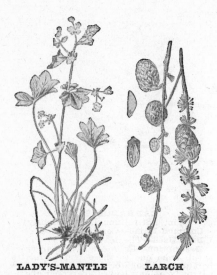

LADY'S-MANTLE   LARCH

LADY'S-MANTLE
(Alchemilla Vulgaris, Rose Family)
Medicinal Part—Plant.
Description—Lady's-Mantle is a low herb, not showy, with somewhat downy, rounded, slightly 7-9 lobed leaves, chiefly from the root, on long stalks, and loose corymbs or panicles of small light green flowers through the summer.
Properties and Uses—Astringent.

LARCH
(Larix Europaea, Pine Family)
Common Names—European Larch.
Medicinal Part—The bark.
Description—A fine fast growing tree with leaves about 1 inch long and cones an inch long, of numerous scales. The flowers are borne in the spring before the leaves appear. The catkins are borne from lateral spurs or broad buds.
Properties and Uses—Laxative, diuretic and alterative.

LARKSPUR
(Delphinum Condolida, Crowfoot Family)
Common Names—Lark Heel, Knight's Spur.
Medicinal Parts—The root and seeds.
Description—Larkspur is an annual herb, with a simple slender root, a leafy stem, from a foot and a half to two feet high, with alternating spreading branches. The leaves are sessile; flowers bright blue and purple.

Delphinum Staphisagria, or Stavesacre, which possesses the same properties as Larkspur, but to a greater degree, is an elegant upright herb, about the same height as Larkspur. Leaves broad, palmate, and petioled. Flowers bluish gray. Fruit a capsule.

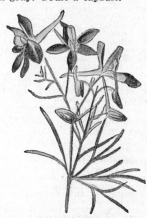

LARKSPUR

Larkspur is a native of Europe, but has become naturalized in the United States, growing in woods and fields. Stavesacre is native to Europe, growing in waste places.
Properties and Uses—Has been credited with some medicinal powers and apparently used to kill domestic vermin. As it is a powerful herb it should not be employed as a medicine unless ordered by a physician.

LARGE-FLOWERED EVERLASTING
(Gnaphalium Margaritacea—Aster Family)
Common Names—Pearly Everlasting, Cotton Weed, Ladies Tobacco.
Parts Used—Leaves and flowers.
Description—Plant resembles Life Everlasting, Gnaphalium polycephalum—flowers are more showy.
Medicinal Uses—Astringent, expectorant, diaphoretic, aromatic, vulnerary. Pioneers used both varieties as aromatic stuffing for pillows.

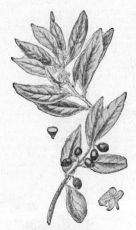

LAUREL BAY
(Laurus Nobilis)

Common Names — Bay Tree, Bay Laurel, Indian Bay.

Medicinal Part—The leaves.

Description—Laurel Bay is a native of Asia Minor. It often grows as a bush about fifteen feet high, but sometimes becomes a tree 30 to 50 feet high.

Properties and Uses—Aromatic, stomachic, astringent, carminative.

LAVENDER
(Lavandula Vera and Lavandula Spica)

Medicinal Parts—The flowers.

Description — Lavandula Vera is a small shrub from 1 to 2 feet high, but sometimes attaining 6 feet. The leaves are oblong-linear or lanceolate, entire, opposite, and sessile. The flowers are of lilac color, small and in whorls.

Lavandula Spica is more dwarfish and more hoary than the first. Leaves oblong-lanceolate. This plant is not used in medicine, but furnishes the oil of Spike, much used in the preparation of artistical varnishes and by porcelain painters.

Lavandula Vera grows in the dry soils of Southern Europe, and flowers in July and August. It is largely cultivated in this country. The whole plant is aromatic, but the flowers are the parts used, and should be gathered shortly after their appearance, and carefully dried. The disease to which this plant is subject can only be prevented by not allowing them to grow too closely together.

Lavender flowers have a strong fragrant odor, and an aromatic, warm bitterish taste. They retain their fragrance after drying. Alcohol extracts their virtues, and a volatile oil upon which their odor depends rises with that liquid in distillation. The oil may be procured separately by distilling the flowers with water. Hagan obtained from a pound of the fresh flowers from half a drachm to two drachms of the oil.

LAVENDER

Properties and Uses — The products obtained by its distillation are much used in perfumery, and as adjuvants to other medicines, which they render at the same time more acceptable to the palate, and cordial to the stomach. Lavender is an aromatic stimulant and tonic, extremely useful in certain conditions, but seldom given in its crude state.

Dose—A teaspoonful of the flowers, cut small or granulated to a cup of boiling water. Drink cold, one cupful during the day, a large mouthful at a time.

LAVENDER COTTON
(Santolina chamaecyparissus— Composite Family)

Common Names — French Lavender, Santolina.

Part Used—Herb.

Description—Not related to true Lavender. A small silvery greyish plant much used in old-fashioned gardens as an edging or bordering plant. Leaves are finely cut, and have an odor somewhat like Chamomile. The plant bears small yellow flowers, that resemble clusters of buttons.

Uses—Once used as a vermifuge for children. Oil used in perfumery.

In Colonial times, bouquets were made up with branches tied up with ribbons, and placed amongst linens, etc., to keep away moths.

A green species of Santolina (S. viride) is used only as a border plant for the ornamental garden.

* * *

GRASS is the forgiveness of Nature—her constant benediction. Fields trampled with battle, saturated with blood, torn with the ruts of cannon, grown green again with grass, and carnate is forgotten. Streets abandoned by traffic become grass grown, like rural lanes, and are obliterated. Forests decay, harvests perish, flowers vanish, but grass is immortal.—Anon.

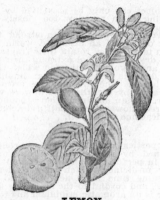

LEMON

(Citrus Limonum, Rue Family)
Medicinal Part—The fruit.

Description—The Lemon is a small tree, native to Eastern Asia, but grown extensively in Florida and California for fruit. Fruit is too common to need any description.

Properties and Uses—Acidulous, refrigerant and anti-scorbutic.

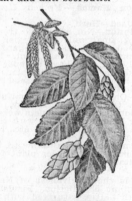

LEVER WOOD

(Astrya Virginica, Birth Family)
Common Names— Iron Wood, Hop Hornbeam, Deerwood.
Medicinal Part—The inner wood.
Description—This small tree of from 25 to 30 feet in height is remarkable for its fine, narrow, brownish bark. The wood is white, hard and strong; leaves oblong-ovate, acuminate, serrate, and somewhat downy. Flowers, fertile and sterile, green and appear with the leaves.

The inner wood and bark are the parts in which reside the curative virtues, and the latter, which are immense, readily yield to water. The tree flowers in April and May, and is common to the United States. The bark and wood should be gathered in August and September.

Properties and Uses—Lever Wood is said to have tonic properties and to be somewhat alterative.

Dose— A teaspoonful of the inner wood cut small or granulated to a cup of boiling water. Drink cold one cupful during the day, a large mouthful at a time; of the tincture, 5 to 20 min.

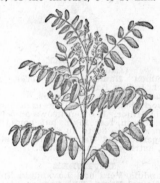

LICORICE ROOT

(Glycyrrhiza Glabra)
Common Name—Sweet Wood.

Part Used—The dried root.

Description—Licorice is a perennial herb, 2 to 5 feet high. Leaflets in pairs of 4 to 7, ovate, smooth, glutinous, beneath, dark green; flowers yellowish white or purplish, pulse shaped racemes, fruit legume 1 inch long, brown ovate, flat, 1 to 6 seeded; root grayish brown or dark brown, wrinkled lengthwise, internally yellow, taste sweetish.

Properties—Licorice is demulcent, expectorant and laxative.

Dose—A teaspoonful of the dried root to a cup of boiling water. Drink cold one or two cupfuls a day, a large mouthful at a time; of the tincture, ½ to 1 fl. dr.

72

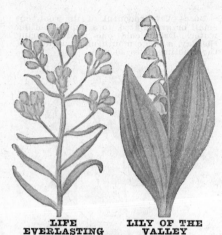

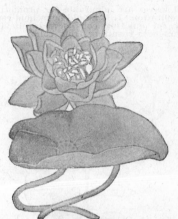

LIFE EVERLASTING

LILY OF THE VALLEY

LIFE EVERLASTING
(Gnaphalium Polycephalum, Aster Family)

Common Names — Old Field Balsam, Indian Posy, Sweet Scented Life Everlasting, White Balsam.

Medicinal Part—The herb.

Description—This indigenous herbaceous annual has an erect, whitish, woolly, and much branched stem, 1 to 2 feet high. The leaves are alternate, sessile, lanceolate, acute, and entire; flowers tubular and yellow.

Properties and Uses—It is an astringent. Irritations of the mouth and throat are said to be relieved by chewing the leaves and blossoms; and the leaves applied to bruises and other local irritations, are very efficacious.

LILY OF THE VALLEY
(Convallaria Majalis, Lily Family)

Common Name—May Lily.

Medicinal Part—Root.

Description—As a garden flower, this species is familiar to nearly everyone. It is a delicately beautiful plant, very rich in fragrance and very hardy. The bell-shaped flowers are white and grow in a one-sided raceme at the top of the scape, the base of which is sheathed by the two large, broad, oblong-pointed, parallel-veined leaves. It flowers in May and June.

Properties and Uses — Mucilaginous and sweet.

LILY ROOT
(White Pond Lily, Castalia Odorata, Water Lily Family)

Common Names—Sweet-scented Water Lily.

Medicinal Part—The root.

Description — This plant grows in ponds and bears a white flower. It is common in ponds, marshes and sluggish streams from Canada to Florida and Louisiana.

Properties and Uses—Astringent and demulcent. Good as a gargle for mouth and throat irritations and as a vaginal douche.

LINDEN
(Tilia)

Common Name—Lime Tree.

Parts Used—Flowers and leaves.

Description—The American and European Linden are of the same species and differ only slightly in their appearance. The European is smaller and its leaves are smaller. The flowers possess no petal-like scales attached to the stamens as in the American.

The American Linden Basswood, as it is commonly known, is 50 to 70 feet high. Bark deep brownish gray, scored perpendicularly with elongated fissures. The leaves perfectly heart-shaped, 4 to 7 inches long, coarsely double toothed; flowers sweet-scented, 5 white petals and sepals, a scale alternating with each petal. Fruit shape and size of a pea, commonly called Monkeys Nuts.

Properties — The flowers and leaves are stomachic. A tea of Linden flowers

73

and leaves are admirable for promoting perspiration. It is an old household remedy for quieting coughs and relieving hoarseness resulting from colds.

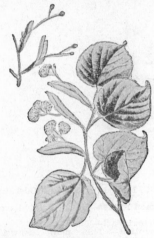

LINDEN

Dose — A teaspoonful of the flowers and leaves to a cup of boiling water. Drink cold one or two cupfuls a day, a large mouthful at a time; of the tincture, ½ to 1 fl. dr.

LION'S ROOT
(Nabulus Albus, Chicory Family)
Common Names—White Lettuce, Rattle Snake Root, White Canker Weed.
Medicinal Part—The plant.
Description—This indigenous perennial herb has a smooth stem, stout and purplish, from 2 to 4 feet high. Radical leaves angular-hastate, cauline ones lanceolate, and all irregularly dentate.
This plant grows plentifully in moist woods and in rich soils, from New England to Iowa, and from Canada to Carolina. The root, leaves and juice of the plant are employed.
Properties and Uses—A decoction of the root taken internally will operate most favorably in cases of dysentery. The milky juice of the plant is taken internally, while the leaves, steeped in water, are applied as a poultice (and frequently changed) for the bite of a serpent.

Dose—A teaspoonful of the root, cut small or granulated, to a cup of boiling water. Drink cold one cupful during the day, a large mouthful at a time; of the tincture, 5 to 20 min.

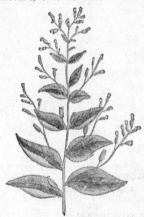

LOBELIA
(Lobelia Inflata, Bell Flower Family)
Common Names—Indian Tobacco, Wild Tobacco, Gagroot, Vomitroot, Bladderpod.
Medicinal Parts—The leaves and seeds.
Description—Lobelia is an annual or biennial indigenous plant, with a fibrous root, and an erect, angular, very hairy stem, from 6 inches to 3 feet in height. The leaves are alternate, ovate-lanceolate, serrate, veiny, and hairy; flowers small, numerous, pale blue; fruit a two-celled ovoid capsule, containing numerous small brown seeds.
Lobelia flowers from July to November, and grows in nearly all parts of the United States, in fields, woods and meadows. The whole plant is active, and the stalks are used indiscriminately with the leaves by those who are best acquainted with its properties. The root is supposed to be more energetic, medicinally, than any other part of the plant. The proper time for gathering is from the last of July to the middle of October. The plant should be dried in the shade, and then be preserved in packages or covered vessels, more especially if it be reduced to powder. It was used in domestic practice by the people of New England long before the time of Samuel Thompson, its assumed discoverer.

Properties and Uses—Lobelia is too dangerous for internal use by the unskilled. But it may be employed externally in the form of an ointment when combined with soothing barks, and roots. In that form it has value in indicated conditions.

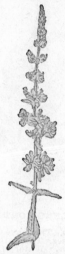

LOOSESTRIFE
(Lythrum Salicaria, Loosestrife Family)

Common Names—Sage Willow, Rainbow Weed, Purple Willow Herb.

Medicinal Part—Herb.

Description—Loosestrife grows from two to four feet high and branches toward the top. The many purple flowers, making up the spike, each have six long petals and are trimorphous. The leaves are broad-lanceolate and often with a heart-shaped base. Found locally in swamps and on marshy borders.

Properties and Uses — Mucilaginous, astringent, demulcent.

Indian Sagwa—Take 1 tablespoonful Gentian Root, 1 of Mayapple, 1 of Rhubarb, 1 of Yellow Dock, 4 of Dandelion, 1 of Sacred Bark and 4 of Swamp Sassafras. Place this mixture in 2 quarts of water. Boil down to 1 quart. Dose, 1 or 2 tablespoonfuls 3 times a day.

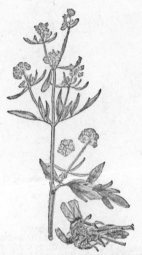

LOVAGE
(Ligusticum Levisticum, Parsley Family)

Common Names—Lavose, Sea Parsley.

Medicinal Part—The root.

Description—Lovage is a tall, very smooth, sweet aromatic herb with large ternately or pinnately decompound leaves, coarse wedge-oblong and cut or lobed leaflets, a thick root and small, many-flowered umbels.

Properties and Uses—Stimulant, carminative, emmenagogue, stomachic, aromatic.

LOVE VINE
(Cuscuta Americana—Dodder Family)

Common Name—Dodder.

Medicinal Part—Entire Plant.

Description—A parasitic plant that resembles a mass of tangled golden threads growing over plants, bushes, and small trees. Plant has no leaves—flowers are small, globular and in clusters. The plant tastes saline and slightly acrid, without odor. It dyes red.

Properties and Uses—Antiscrofulous, laxative, hydragogue.

Another species—Cuscuta Gronovii is found in North Carolina. It appears to thrive particularly on wheat and clover. Properties similar to Cuscuta Americana.

A European species (Cuscuta epithymum) is reputed also to have similar properties.

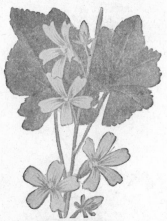

LOW MALLOW
(Malva Rotundifolia, Mallow Family)
Common Names—Maller, Cheese Plant.
Medicinal Part—The whole herb.

Description—The family name Mallow is derived from the Greek malassein "to soften," as alluding to the demulcent qualities of these mucilaginous plants. The common Low Mallow is a well-known roadside plant, with large downy leaves, and streaked trumpet-shaped purple flowers, which later on furnish round button-like seeds, known to the rustics as "pick-cheeses," whilst beloved by schoolboys, because of their nutty flavor, and called by them "Bread and Cheese."

Properties and Uses—Demulcent and emollient in conditions indicating those properties.

Dose—A teaspoonful of the herb to a cup of boiling water. Drink cold one or two cupfuls a day, a large mouthful at a time; of the tincture, ½ to 1 fl. dr.

LUNGWORT
(Pulmonaria Officinalis)
Common Name—Maple Lungwort.
Medicinal Part—The leaves.

Description—This rough plant has a stem about one foot high. The radical leaves ovate, cordate; cauline one, ovate and sessile. Flowers blue; calyx, five-angled, corolla, funnel-shaped; stigma, emarginate; and the fruit a roundish obtuse achenium.

Lungwort is a herbaceous perennial, growing in Europe and this country in

northern latitudes. In Europe it is a rough-leaved plant, but in this country the entire plant is smooth, which exhibits the peculiar climatic influences. It is showy, and freely cultivated. It

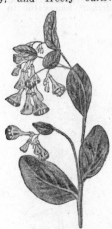

LUNGWORT

flowers in May. The leaves are used for medical purposes. They are without any particular odor. Water extracts their properties.

Properties and Uses—It is demulcent and mucilaginous, and in decoction used in indicated ailments, but its virtues are not clear.

Dose—A teaspoonful of the leaves to a cup of boiling water. Drink cold 1 or 2 cupfuls a day, a large mouthful at a time; of the tincture, ½ to 1 fl. dr.

LYCOPODIUM
(L. Clavatum)
Common Names—Club Moss, Vegetable Sulphur.
Medicinal Parts—Spores and the moss.

Description—This is a low creeping perennial, stem 2 to 10 feet long, slender, tough, flexible, woody; branches ascending; leafy peduncle 4 to 6 inches long, with 1 to 2 linear cylindrical spikes 1 to 2 inches long; leaves linear and awl-shaped, ¼ inch long, dense, light green, tipped with a fine bristle, as are also the numerous bracts on the flowering spikes. The spores are obtained by cutting off the tops when the fruit spikes are nearly ripe; afterward the spores are shaken out and sifted.

Properties—The Moss formerly was considered diuretic but has fallen into disuse in this age of laboratory products.

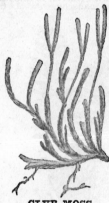

CLUB MOSS

Dose—A teaspoonful of the Moss cut small or granulated to a cup of boiling water. Drink cold one cupful during the day, a large mouthful at a time; of the tincture, 5 to 20 min.

MADDER
(Rubia Tinctorum)
Medicinal Part—The root.

Description—This plant has a perennial, long cylindrical root, about the thickness of a quill, and deep reddish-brown. It has several herbaceous, brittle stems. The leaves are from four to six in a whorl, lanceolate, mucronate, 2 or 3 inches long, and about one-third as wide. Flowers small and yellow.

Madder is a native of the Mediterranean and Southern European countries. The drug is chiefly imported from Holland and France. The root is collected in the third year of the plant, when it is freed from its outer-covering and dried. It is valued as a dye-stuff for its red and purple.

Excerpt from Lee's "Trees, Plants and Flowers" (1854); "The most remarkable circumstances attending Madder root, is that it makes the bones of all animals who feed on it of a fine red. The beaks and claws of birds also become colored." See pages 188 and 218.

MAD DOG WEED
(Alisma Plantago)
Common Name—Marsh Plantain.
Medicinal Part—The leaves.

Description—This perennial herb has all radical, oval, oblong, or lanceolate leaves, from 4 to 6 inches in length, on long radical petioles. The flowers are small and white, and the fruit a three-cornered achenium.

It inhabits the North American continent as well as Europe, grows in watery places and flowers in July.

Properties and Uses—It was once considered a remedy for various ailments, but seems to have lost much if not all of its reputation as a medicinal agent. It may be used in the form of an infusion of the leaves, which must be dried and powdered.

Dose—A teaspoonful of the leaves to a cup of boiling water. Drink cold 1 or 2 cupfuls a day, a large mouthful at a time; of the tincture, ½ to 1 fl. dr.

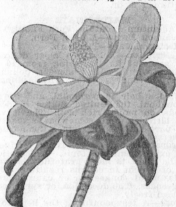

MAGNOLIA
(Magnolia Glauca, Magnolia Family)
Common Names—White Bay, Beaver Tree, Sweet Magnolia.
Medicinal Part—The bark.

Description—This tree varies in height from 6 to 30 feet, being taller in the South than in the North. The leaves are alternate, petioled, entire, and of elliptical shape. The flowers are large and solitary, and of grateful odor. The fruit is a cone.

The therapeutical virtues of these trees are found in the bark and fruit.

The bark of both the trunk and the root is employed. The odor is aromatic, and the taste bitterish, warm and pungent. It is gathered during the spring and summer. It has smooth and ash-colored bark, elegant, odoriferous, cream-colored flowers, and can be found in morasses from Massachusetts to the Gulf of Mexico. It flowers from May to August. There are other varieties which do not require especial mention or description.

Properties and Uses—The bark is an aromatic, bitter tonic with diaphoretic properties. It is used sometimes as a substitute for Peruvian Bark, as it can be continued for a longer time and with more safety. Properly prepared it may be used as a substitute for tobacco, and will help break the habit of tobacco-chewing.

Dose—A teaspoonful of the bark, cut small or granulated, to a cup of boiling water. Drink cold one cupful during day, a large mouthful at a time; of the tincture, 1 fl. dr.

MAIDENHAIR
(Adiantum Pedatum, Fern Family)
Common Name—Maiden Fern.
Medicinal Part—The herb.

Description—This is a most delicate and graceful fern, growing from 12 to 15 inches high, with a slender, polished stalk. Front pedate with pinnate branches.

Maiden hair is perennial, and grows throughout the United States in deep woods, on moist, rich soil. The leaves are bitterish and somewhat aromatic, and part with their virtues upon being immersed in boiling water.

Properties and Uses—It is refrigerant, expectorant and tonic. A decoction of the plant is most gratefully cooling and of benefit in coughs resulting from colds, nasal congestion or catarrh, and hoarseness. The decoction, or syrup, can be used freely.

Dose—A teaspoonful of the herb to a cup of boiling water. Drink cold 1 or 2 cupfuls a day, a large mouthful at a time; of the tincture, ½ to 1 fl. dr.

MALE FERN
(Aspidium Filix Mas, Fern Family)
Common Name—Aspidium.
Medicinal Part—The rhizome.

Description—Male Fern has a large, perennial, tufted, scaly rhizome, sending forth yearly several leaves, three or four feet high, erect, oval, lanceolate, acute, pinnate, bright green, and leafy nearly to the bottom; their stalks and midribs having tough, brown, and transparent scales throughout. Leaflets numerous, crowded, oblong, obtuse and crenate throughout.

Male Fern grows in all parts of the United States and Europe. The root has a dark brown epiderm, is almost inodorous, and a nauseous sweet taste. It

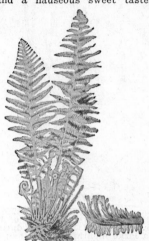

MALE FERN

contains a green fat oil, gum, resin, lignin, tannic acid, pectin albumen, etc. It should be gathered from June to September. After gathering, it should be carefully prepared, as on the preparation its virtues depend. It loses its virtues in two years if not properly preserved.

Properties and Uses—It has been used from time immemorial for the expulsion of worms, especially tapeworms. It was used as such by Pliny, Dioscorides, Theophrastus, and Galen. It is said to have been the celebrated secret remedy of Madame Nouffer, the widow of a Swiss surgeon, who sold her secret to Louis XVI for 18,000 francs. It really seems to be anthelmintic, and worthy of all the high commendation it has received from ages past up to the present time.

However, due to certain allergy reactions, it is not now recommended for self medication, except on prescription of a physician.

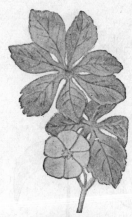

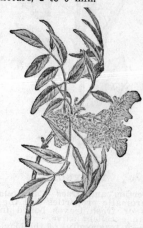

thartic, emetic, alterative, anthelmintic, hydragogue, and sialagogue. It is an active and certain cathartic. It can also be used as an alterative. In constipation it acts upon the bowels without disposing them to subsequent costiveness. It is one of the ingredients of our Calumet Laxative Compound.

Dose—A teaspoonful of the root, cut small to a pint of boiling water. Take one teaspoonful at a time as required; of the tincture, 2 to 5 min.

MANDRAKE
(Podophyllum Peltatum, Barberry Family)

Common Names—May Apple, Wild Lemon, Raccoon Berry.

Medicinal Part—The root.

Description—This plant, which is illustrated by a cut, is an indigenous perennial herb, with a jointed, dark-brown root, about half the size of the finger, very fibrous, and internally yellow. The stem is simple, round, smooth, erect, about a foot high, dividing at the top into two petioles, from 3 to 6 inches long, each supporting a leaf. The leaves are large, palmate, oftener cordate, smooth yellowish-green on top, paler beneath. The flower is solitary in the fork of the stem, large white, and somewhat fragrant. The fruit is fleshy, of a lemon color, and in flavor resembles the strawberry.

The Mayapple is found throughout the United States, in low, shady situations, rich woods, and fields, and flowers in May and June. The fruit matures in September and October. It is scarcer in New England than elsewhere. The Indians were well acquainted with the virtues of this plant. The proper time for collecting the root is in the latter part of October or early part of November, soon after the fruit has ripened. Its active principle is Podophyllin, which acts upon the liver in the same manner but far superior to mercury, and with intelligent physicians it has dethroned that noxious mineral as a cholagogue.

Properties and Uses—Mayapple is ca-

MANNA TREE
(Fraxinus Ornus—Olive Family)

Common Names—Flowering Ash, European Manna Tree.

Medicinal Part—Manna.

Description—Manna tree has light and tough wood, dark-colored buds and small insignificant flowers appearing in spring with or rather before the leaves of the season, from separate buds in the axils of the leaves of the preceding year. Petals four, either distinct or slightly united, or sometimes only two, narrow, greenish; leaflets five-nine, lanceolate or oblong, small. Fruit terete at the base, winged from the other end.

Properties and Uses—Manna is laxative.

MARYGOLD
(Calendula)

Common Names—Calendula, Pot Marigold, Marybud, Holigold.

Parts Used—Leaves and Flowers.

Description—Calendula is an annual

herb, 1 to 2 feet high, stem angular, roughish-hairy, leaves toothed, spatulate, oblanceolate; flower heads terminal two inches broad, yellow or orange yellow color.

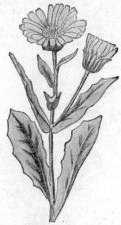

MARYGOLD

Properties and Uses—Calendula has some aromatic properties and the dried flowers or fresh leaves boiled in lard make an excellent salve.

Dose—A teaspoonful of the leaves and flowers, cut small or granulated, to a cup of boiling water. Drink cold, one cupful during the day, a large mouthful at a time; of the tincture, 5 to 20 min.

MARYLAND CUNILA
(Cunila Origanoides—Mint Family)

Common Names—American or Mountain Dittany, Stone Mint, Wild Basil.

Medicinal Parts—Leaves and flowers.

Description—An attractive small bushy plant found growing in woods, thickets, and open hillsides, often in somewhat acid soil, from North Florida to Texas, Missouri, and to New York. The entire plant is aromatic. The purplish pink flowers literally cover the plant and are a favorite of bees.

Properties and Uses—Used both by the American Indians and early settlers from Europe for common colds, and as a beverage. The warm tea is diaphoretic.

Darlington's Flora Cestrica recommends this native American herb as a pleasant tea. The aroma of this herb resembles a mixture of Thyme and Bay.

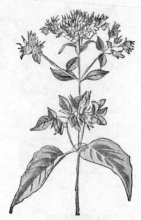

MARJORAM
(Origanum Vulgare)

Parts Used—The herb.

Description—This is a perennial native herb growing 12 to 18 inches high; stem square, purplish, downy; leaves 1 inch long, ovate, entire, pellucid, punctate, hairy beneath; flowers pale purple, calyx 5-toothed, corolla two-lipped, 4 stamens.

Properties and Uses—Wild Marjoram has an aromatic, pungent bitter taste. It is carminative and tonic and as such useful in upset stomach and associated conditions. The oil is used in liniments.

Dose—One teaspoonful to a cup of boiling water. Drink cold, one or two cupfuls a day; tincture, 10 to 30 min.

MATICO
(Piper Angustifolium)

Medicinal Part—The leaves.

Description—This is a tall shrub, presenting a singular appearance from its pointed stem and branches. The leaves are harsh, short-stalked, oblong-lanceolate, and acuminate. Flowers hermaphrodite.

This plant grows at Huanaco and elsewhere in Peru. The dried leaves are the parts used, and have a strong fragrant odor, and a warm, aromatic taste. They contain a dark-green resin, chlorophyll, brown and yellow coloring matter, gum nitrate of potassa, maticine, a volatile oil, salts, and lignin. The plant has long been used by the Indians of Peru for various purposes.

Properties and Uses—Matico is an aromatic stimulant with astringent properties that indicate its internal use in such conditions as diarrhea. Externally it may be used as a local application.

Dose—A teaspoonful of the leaves to a cup of boiling water. Drink cold 1 or 2 cupfuls a day, a large mouthful at a time; of the tincture, ¼ to ½ fl. dr.

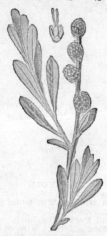

MEADOW FERN
(Myrica Gale—Sweet Gale Family)
Common Names—Sweet Gale, Gale Fern, Bog Myrtle, Sweet Willow.
Medicinal Part—Leaves and buds.
Description—Meadow Fern is found in cold bogs growing from one to four feet high with pale wedge-lanceolate leaves, serrate towards the apex; little nuts, crowded as if winged by a pair of scales. Flowers in the spring with the leaves or earlier.
Properties and Uses—Stimulant, alterative, depurative and vulnerary.

MEADOW LILY
(Lilium Candidum)
Medicinal Part—The root.
Description—The thick stem of this plant is from 3 to 4 feet high and arises from a perennial bulb or root. Leaves scattered, lanceolate, and narrowed at the base. Flowers are large, snow-white and smooth inside.
The Meadow Lily is an exotic. It is a native of Syria and Asia Minor. The flowers are regarded as being very beautiful, but are not used for medicinal purposes. The plant is principally cultivated for the flowers. The bulb is the part used for its curative properties. Water extracts its virtues.

Properties and Uses—It is mucilaginous, demulcent, tonic and astringent. Boiled in milk, it is also useful for external purposes, etc.

Dose—A teaspoonful of the root, cut small or granulated, to a cup of boiling water. Drink cold, one cupful during the day, a large mouthful at a time; of the tincture 5 to 20 min.

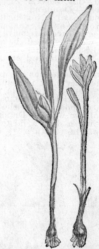

MEADOW SAFFRON
(Colchicum Autumnale)
Common Name—Colchicum.
Medicinal Parts — The cormus and seeds.
Description—The cormus of this plant is large, ovate, and fleshy. The leaves are dark-green, very smooth, obtuse, above a foot long, an inch and a half broad, keeled, produced in the spring along with the capsules. Flowers several, bright-purple, with a white tube appearing in the autumn, without the leaves. Fruit a capsule, seeds whitish and polished.
It grows in meadows and low, rich soils in many part of Europe, and is common in England. The plant is annual or perennial, according to the man-

ner in which it is propagated. The root resembles that of the tulip, and contains a white acrid juice. The bulb should be gathered about the beginning of July, and the seeds early in August. Colchicia is the active principle.

Properties and Uses—It is sedative, cathartic, diuretic, and emetic, but great care should be used in its employment, as serious results may follow an overdose.

MEXICAN DAMIANA
(Turnera Aphrodisiaca—Turneraceae)
Common Name—Damiana.
Part Used—The leaves.

Description — Damiana is a small, shrubby plant of Northern Mexico, Lower California and Texas, growing in dry soil. Leaves are alternate ¾ to one inch long, wedge-shaped base, toothed obovate, light green, with whitish hairs, warm mint-like taste and aroma similar to oranges when dry.

Properties—The leaves are tonic stimulant and laxative. It is reputed to be peculiarly effective as a tonic when used in combination with Palmetto Berries.

Dose—A teaspoonful of the leaves to a cup of boiling water. Drink cold one or two cupfuls a day, a large mouthful at a time; of the tincture, ½ to 1 fl. dr.

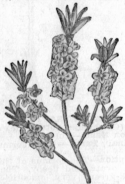

MEZEREON
(Daphne Mezereum—Mezereum Family)
Common Names—Spurge Olive, Spurge Flax, Wild Pepper.
Medicinal Part—Bark.

Description—Mezereon is a low shrub from one to three feet high, with purple-rose-colored (rarely white) flowers in lateral clusters on shoots of the preceding year, in early spring, before the lanceolate very smooth green leaves. The berries are red.

Properties and Uses—Acrid, stimulant, alterative, diuretic and cathartic.

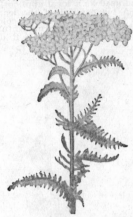

MILFOIL
(Achillea Millefolium, Aster Family)
Common Names—Thousand Seal, Nosebleed, Yarrow.
Medicinal Part—The herb.

Description—Milfoil, also called Thousand Seal, is from 10 to 20 inches high, with a simple stem, branching at the top, and many long, crowded, alternate and dentate leaves spread upon the ground, finely cut, and divided into many parts. The flowers are white or rose-colored, and arrayed in knots from divers green stalks, which arise from among the leaves. Fruit an oblong, flattened achenium.

Milfoil inhabits Europe and North America; it is found in pastures, meadows, and along road sides, flowering from May to October. The plant possesses a faint, pleasant, peculiar fragrance, and a rather sharp, rough, astringent taste, which properties are due to tannic and achilleic acid, essential oil, and bitter extractive, alcohol or water being its proper menstrum.

Properties and Uses—It belongs to the aromatic class of sudorific tonics. Achilles is supposed to be the first that left the virtues of this herb to posterity, hence the active principle of this plant is called Achilleine, which is much used in the South of Europe.

Dose—A teaspoonful of the herb, cut small or granulated, to a cup of boiling water. Drink cold, 1 cupful during the day, a large mouthful at a time; of the tincture 5 to 20 min.

MILK THISTLE

(Carduus Marianus—Compositae Family)

Common Names—St. Mary's Thistle, Holy Thistle.

Part Used—Herb and seeds.

Description — Native of Europe, but now found in parts of the U.S. Plant grows from 2 to 3 feet high. The shiny leaves mottled with white veins give it a striking appearance. Lobes of the lower leaves are broad, and tipped with sharp, prickly spines. Upper leaves clasp the stem by prickly auricles. The large purple flower heads are borne on terminal branches. The fruit is an achenium. Milk Thistle was often mentioned by the prophets in the Bible.

Properties and Uses—Leaves are reputed to be bitter and tonic. Seeds were held in high repute by Dioscorides and other early writers—then more or less neglected throughout the ages until the turn of the century, when Finely Ellingwood, M.D., mentions them in his excellent book—Materia Medica Therapeutics.

MILK WEED

(Euphorbia Corollata, Spurge Family)

Common Names — Large Flowering Spurge, Blooming Spurge, Bowman's Root, Emetic Root, Snakemilk, Milk Ipecac.

Medicinal Part—The bark of the root.

Description—This is a perennial plant with a round, slender, erect stem, one or two feet high, with a yellowish, large, and branching root. The leaves are scattered, sessile, oblong-obovate, smooth in some plants, very hairy in others, and from one to two inches in length. Flowers are white and showy, and fruit a three-celled capsule.

This plant grows plentifully in Canada and the United States, in dry fields and woods, and flowers from June to September. The bark of the root is the part used. The plant is readily detected by a milky fluid which exudes from the stem, when that is broken. This liquid, if applied to warts or wens, is of great benefit, in most cases banishing the offensive excrescences.

Properties and Uses—It is emetic, diaphoretic, expectorant, and perhaps epispastic. As an emetic the powdered bark of the root (say from 15 to 20 grains) is mild, pleasant, and efficacious.

Dose—As an expectorant it is administered three grains at a time, mixed with honey, molasses, or sugar, as a cathartic, from four to ten grains are required.

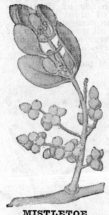 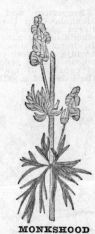

MISTLETOE   MONKSHOOD

MISTLETOE

(Viscum Album, Loranthaceae Family.)

Common Names—Bird Lime, All Heal, Devil's fuge.

Medicinal Parts—Young twigs and leaves.

Description—This is an evergreen parasite growing on the branches of deciduous trees. Its roots penetrating through the bark into the wood.

Properties and Uses—While this herb is credited with beneficial stimulating properties of a high order when properly administered, it might have a contrary effect if improperly used; therefore I recommend only 1 teaspoonful to a pint of boiling water.

MONKSHOOD

(Aconitum Napellus.)

Common Names—Wolf's Bane, Aconite.

Medicinal Parts—The leaves and root.

Description—This plant has a small, napiform root, and simple, straight, erect-stems, about five feet high. The leaves are alternate, petioled, dark-green above, paler beneath. The flowers are large, deep bluish-purple, sometimes white, and hairy; fruit a capsule.

This perennial herb is a native of most parts of Europe, growing in wooded hills, and plains, and is much cultivated in gardens. It flowers in May and June. All parts of the plant contain powerfully poisonous properties; but the root is the part most generally employed for medicinal purposes. It yields Aconite,

Properties and Uses—Although Monkshood in the hands of the intelligent physician is of great service, it should not be used in domestic practice. In improper doses all preparations of aconite act as an energetic acro-narcotic poison. As a sedative and anodyne, it is capable of many beneficial uses in the hands of a skilled person.

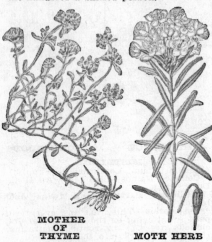

MOTHER OF THYME   MOTH HERB

MOTHER OF THYME

(Thymus Serpyllum—Mint Family)
Common Names—Wild or Creeping Thyme.
Medicinal Part—Herb.
Description—Mother of Thyme is found in thickets, woods and along roadsides. It is creeping, forming broad, flat perennial turfs. The leaves are green and the flowers are purplish or flesh-colored whorls crowded or somewhat spiked at the ends of the flowering branches.
Properties and Uses—Carminative, anti-spasmodic.

MOTH HERB

(Ledum Palustre—Heath Family)
Common Names—Marsh Tea, Swamp Tea, Narrow-leaved Labrador Tea.
Medicinal Part—Leaves.
Description—Moth Herb is a shrub about a foot high, the twigs rusty-tomentose. The leaves are linear, obtuse, dark green and somewhat rugose above with brown wool beneath. The flowers are white and numerous in terminal umbels.
Properties and Uses—Bitter, astringent and vulnerary.

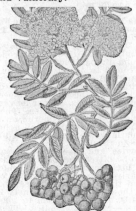

MOUNTAIN ASH

(Pyrus Domesticata—Rose Family)
Common Names—Sorb Apple, Rowan Tree.
Medicinal Part—The fruit.
Description—Mountain Ash is a slender tree or tall shrub, leaves odd pinnate of several (9-17) leaflets; flowers are numerous and white in ample, compound flat cymes terminating the branches of the season. The fruit is berry-like and scarlet red when ripe. The trees are often planted for ornament especially for the clusters of showy fruit in the autumn.
Properties and Uses—Astringent and anti-scorbutic.

MOUNTAIN BALM

(Monarda Didyma—Mint Family)
Common Names—Oswego Tea, Red Bee-Balm.
Medicinal Parts—Leaves and flowers.
Description—The plant is similar in appearance to Wild Bergamot (Monarda fistulosa)—however, the foliage of Mountain Balm is a richer green, and the flowers are a showy scarlet color. Mountain Balm is found in moist woods, stream banks, thickets and roadsides in the Blue Ridge Mountains, Georgia to Alabama, Ontario and New Brunswick.
Properties and Uses—Carminative and aromatic. Used as a beverage and as a tea for flatulence, nausea and vomiting.

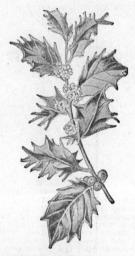

poison those who eat the birds. The leaves are the officinal part. Attention was called to their medicinal virtues by the use which the Indians make of them, viz., a decoction by which they commit suicide.

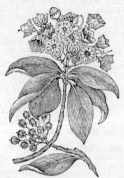

MOUNTAIN HOLLY
(Ilex Aquifolium—Holly Family)
Common Name—European Holly.
Medicinal Part—The leaves.
Description — Mountain Holly is a tree with very glossy and wavy, spiny leaves, umbellate clusters of many flowers. The berries are bright red. Occasionally planted but not hardy.
Properties and Uses—Astringent, emetic and febrifuge.

MOUNTAIN LAUREL
(Kalmia Latifolia, Heath Family.)
Common Names—Sheep Laurel, Spoonwood, Lambkill, Calfkill, Calico Bush, Narrow Leaved Laurel.
Medicinal Part—The leaves.
Description—This handsome plant is a shrub from four to eight feet high, with crooked stems and a rough bark. The leaves are evergreen, ovate, lanceolate, acute at each end, on long petioles, and from two to three inches long. The flowers are white and numerous. The fruit is a day capsule.
Mountain Laurel inhabits the rocky hills, and elevated grounds of most parts of the United States. Its beautiful flowers appear in June and July. The leaves are reputed to be poisonous to sheep and other animals and it is said that birds which have eaten them will

KALMIA
Properties and Uses—The plant, in medicinal doses, is sedative, and somewhat astringent. It is a most efficient agent in simple neuralgia. The preparation should be employed with great care and prudence and its use restricted to external conditions. Externally, stewed with lard, it is serviceable as an ointment for various skin irritations.
Dose—A teaspoonful of the leaves to a pint of boiling water. Take a tablespoonful 2 to 4 times a day, cold. Of the tincture 2 to 5 min.

MOUNTAIN MINT
(Pycnanthemum Flexuosum—Mint Family)
Common Name—Narrow leaved Mountain Mint.
Medicinal Parts — The leaves and flowers.
Description—An upright plant growing about 20 inches high, generally found growing in clumps in oak barrens, meadows, fields and thickets from Florida to Texas, Minnesota and Maine. Leaves narrow, glabrous and entire. Numerous flowers borne on ends of stalks are white, flecked with dots of lavender or else pale lavender, and also similarly marked with a darker shade. The entire plant emits little fragrance until after it is dried or pressed between the fingers, when its pungent odor is strongly exhaled.
Properties and Uses—Tonic and diaphoretic.

MOUNTAIN MINT

(Pycnanthemum incana—Mint Family)

Common Name—Hoary Mountain-mint, Wild Basil.

Medicinal Part—The herb.

Description — Related to last named species but quite different in general appearance. Plant grows in clumps, on hillsides, dry thickets, and open woods, from Florida to Missouri, Ontario and Maine. Small white flowers in compact clusters. Upper leaves have a hoary white frost-like appearance. The entire plant has a refreshing cool minty fragrance.

Medicinal Uses—The herb is reputed to be diuretic, stimulant, anti-spasmodic, carminative, diaphoretic and tonic.

MOUSE EAR

(Gnaphalium Uliginosum.)

Common Names—Mouse Ear, Everlasting.

Medicinal Part—The whole herb.

Description—The root is perennial, and produces upright flowering stems, together with prostrate runners or stolons like the strawberry plant. The leaves and stems bear a silky white wool. The flowers are small collected in the heads, which are assembled in clusters forming a dense treminal group. The prostrate leaves resemble the ears of a mouse.

Properties and Uses—This herb is considered of more value as a diuretic. It is sudorific and mucilaginous.

Dose—A teaspoonful of the herb to a cup of boiling water. Drink cold one or two cupfuls a day, a large mouthful at a time; of the tincture ½ to 1 fl. dr.

* * * *

Most men know when they are ill, but very few when they are well. And yet it is most certain, that 'tis easier to preserve health than to recover it, and to prevent diseases than to cure them. Towards the first, the means are mostly in our power. Little else is required than to bear and forbear; but towards the latter, the means are perplexed and uncertain, and for the knowledge of them the far greatest part of mankind must apply to others.—An Essay of Health and Long Life, by G. Cheyne, M.D., 1725

* * * *

Happy the age to which we moderns give
The name of "Golden" when men chose
    to live
On woodland fruits, and for their
    medicine took
Herbs from the field, and simples from
    the brook.

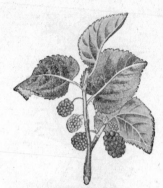

MULBERRY

(Morus Rubra—Nettle Family)

Common Name—Red Mulberry.

Medicinal Part—The bark.

Description—The leaves of the Mulberry are usually large, those on the young shoots deeply lobed, with very oblique and rounded sinuses, the upper surface rough and the lower one soft or variously pubescent. The fruit when fully ripe is almost black. Flowers in the spring.

Properties and Uses—Vermifuge and cathartic.

MULLEIN

(Verbascum Thapsus, Figwort Family.)

Common Names—Velvet Dock, Velvet Plant, Flannel Leaf.

Medicinal Parts—The leaves and flowers.

Description—This biennial plant has a straight, tall, stout, woolly, simple, stem. The leaves are alternate, oblong, acute, and rough on both sides. The flowers are of a golden-yellow color; calyx, five-parted; corolla, five-lobed; stamens, five, and fruit, a capsule or pod. Mullein is common in the United States, but was undoubtedly introduced from Europe. It grows in recent clearings, slovenly fields, and along the side of roads, flowering from June to August. The leaves and flowers are the parts used. They have a faint, rather pleasant odor, and a somewhat bitterish, albuminous taste, and yield their virtues to boiling water.

Properties and Uses—It is demulcent, diuretic, anodyne, and anti-spasmodic. the infusion being useful in coughs, due to colds, diarrhea, etc. It may be boiled in milk, sweetened, and rendered more palatable by aromatics for internal use. A fomentation of the leaves in hot vinegar and water forms an excellent local application for external irritations, as for the itching of piles. A handful of them may be also placed in an old teapot, with hot water,

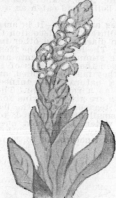

MULLEIN

and the steam be inhaled through the spout, in the relief of nasal congestion or catarrh, throat irritation, etc.

Dose—A teaspoonful of the leaves to a cup of boiling water. Drink cold 1 or 2 cupfuls a day, a large mouthful at a time; of the tincture, ½ to 1 fl. dr.

MYRTLE
(Myrica Cerifera, Bayberry Family)

Common Names—Bayberry, Waxmyrtle, Candleberry, Waxberry.

Medicinal Parts—The bark of the root.

Description—This shrub is branching and partially evergreen, and varies in height from two to a dozen feet. The flowers appear in May, before the leaves are fully expanded. The fruits are small and globular resembling berries, which are at first green, but become nearly white. They consist of a hard stone, inclosing a two-lobed and two-seeded kernel. On the outside of the stone are gunpowder-like grains, and over these is a crust of dry greenish-white wax.

Myrtle is found in woods and fields, from Canada to Florida. The bark of the root is the officinal part, but the wax is also used. Water must be employed to extract the astringent principles of the root-bark, alcohol to extract its stimulating virtues. The period at which the root should be collected is the latter part of fall. Cleanse it thoroughly, and while fresh separate the bark with a hammer or club. Dry the bark thoroughly and keep it in a dry place; then pulverize, and keep the powder in dark and sealed vessels. In order to obtain the wax, boil the berries in water; the wax will soon float on the surface, and may be removed when it becomes cold and hardened.

Properties and Uses — The bark has been successfully used in diarrhea and in **other** cases where astringents were indicated. Powdered, it has been employed as a snuff, with good effect, in nasal congestions or catarrh. It is sometimes applied, in poultice form, to cuts, bruises, scratches, etc., but is better for these when combined with Bloodroot. The wax possesses mild astringent properties.

Dose—I teaspoonful to a cup of boiling water. Drink cold 1 or 2 cupfuls a day; of the tincture, ½ to 1 fl. dr.

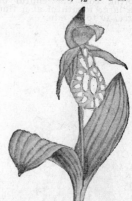

NERVE ROOT
(Cypripedium Pubescens, Orchid Family)

Common Names—American Valerian, Umbel, Ladies' Slipper, Yellow Moccasin Flower, Noah's Ark.

Medicinal Part—The root.

Description — This indigenous plant has a perennial, fibrous, fleshy root from which arise several round leafy stems, from 12 to 18 inches high. The leaves are from 3 to 6 inches long, by 2 or 3 broad, oblong, lanceolate, acuminate, pubescent, alternate, generally the same number on each side. Flowers large and very showy and pale yellow.

This plant grows here in rich woods and meadows, and flowers in May and June. There are several varieties of it, but as they all possess the same medicinal properties, a description of each is not requisite.

Properties and Uses—The fibrous roots are the parts used in medicine, and they should be gathered and carefully cleansed in August or September. The properties and uses are various. The preparations made from these roots are tonic, diaphoretic, and antispasmodic, and have been referred to as gentle nervous stimulants or antispasmodics. The form of the preparation is an alcoholic extract. It is said to be beneficial in cases of ordinary nervous headache, when administered with other remedies, as Catnip, Sweet Balm, etc., in equal parts, taking the tea about every half hour, as indicated.

Dose—A teaspoonful of the root, cut small or granulated to a pint of boiling water. Drink cold one cupful during the day, a large mouthful at a time; of the tincture, 10 to 30 min.

The common Nettle is well known both in America and in Europe, and grows in waste places, beside hedges, and in gardens, flowering from June to September. The leaves and root are the parts used. The prickles of the Common Nettle contain Formic Acid. The young shoots have been boiled and eaten as a remedy for scurvy.

Properties and Uses—It is astringent, tonic and diuretic. In decoction they are valuable in diarrhea and other indicated conditions. The leaves of the fresh Common Nettle stimulate, irritate and raise blisters upon those portions of the skin to which they may be applied, and they have, as a natural consequence, often been used as a rubefacient. The seeds and flowers are given in wine for agues.

Dose—A teaspoonful of the leaves or root, cut small or granulated, to a cup of boiling water. Drink cold, one cupful during the day, a large mouthful at a time; of the tincture, 10 to 20 min.

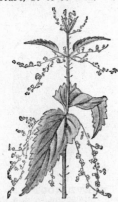

NETTLE
(Urtica Dioica, Nettle Family)

Common Names—Great Stinging Nettles, Great Nettle.

Medicinal Parts—The root and leaves.

Description—This is a perennial, herbaceous, dull-green plant, armed with small prickles, which emit an acrid fluid when pressed. The stem is from two to four feet high; root creeping and branching. The leaves are opposite, cordate, lance-ovate, and conspicuously acuminate. Flowers are small and green.

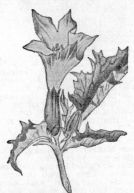

NIGHTSHADE
(Datura Stramonium, Potato Family)

Common Names — Thorn-apple, Stinkweed, Apple-Peru, Jimson Weed.

Medicinal Parts—The leaves and seed.

Description—This plant is a bushy, smooth, fetid, annual plant, two or three feet in height, and in rich soil even more. The root is rather large, of a whitish color, giving off many fibres. The stem is much branched, forked, spreading leafy, of a yellowish-green color. The leaves are large smooth, from the forks of the stem, and are uneven at the base. The flowers are about three inches long, erect, large and white. The fruit is a large, dry, prickly capsule with four valves and numerous black reniform seeds. There is the Datura Tatula, or purple Stramonium, which differs from the above in having a deep purple stem, etc.

Stramonium is a well-known poisonous weed, growing upon waste grounds and road-sides, in all parts of the United States. It is found in very many parts of the world. The whole plant has a fetid, narcotic, odor, which diminishes as it dries. Almost every part of the plant is possessed of medicinal properties, but the officinal parts are the leaves and seeds. The leaves should be gathered when the flowers are in full-bloom, and carefully dried in the shade. They impart their properties to water, alcohol and the fixed oils. The seeds are small, reniform, compressed, roughish, dark or brown or black when ripe, grayish-brown when unripe. They yield what is called Datura.

Properties and Uses—In large doses it is an energetic narcotic poison. The victims of this poison suffer the most intense agonies, and die in maniacal delirium. In medicinal doses it is reported to have been used as a substitute for opium. Although it may have valuable uses in the hands of a skilled herbalist, it is unsuited to domestic use and should not be employed in self-medication.

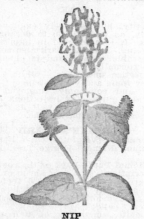

NIP
(Nepeta)
(Nepeta Cataria, Mint Family)
Common Names—Catnip, Catmint.
Parts Used—The whole herb.

Description—Nip is a perennial herb, 3 to 5 feet high with square erect branching stems, covered with fine whitish hairs. Leaves 1 to 2½ inches long, heart-shaped or oblong with pointed apex, upper surface green, under grayish green with whitish hairs, margins finely scalloped. Flowers in spikes, June to September, are whitish dotted with purple, two-lipped, the upper lip notched; the lower with three lobes; the middle lobes broadest and sometimes cleft. Odor, mint-like, bitter, pungent.

Properties—Nip is employed as a mild aromatic and carminative, useful in flatulency and upset stomach. Cats eat it ravenously, being fond of it for its effect.

Dose—A teaspoonful of the herb to a cup of boiling water. Drink cold 1 or 2 cupfuls a day, a large mouthful at a time; ½ to 1 fl. dr. of the tincture.

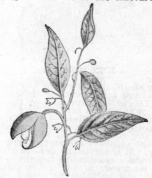

NUTMEG
(Myristica Fragrans)
Common Name—Mace (Arillus of the fruit).
Medicinal Part—Kernels of fruit.
Description—Nutmeg is a tree, native of the Molucca Islands, about 20 feet high, having a grayish brown and somewhat smooth bark. The Nutmeg fruit is oval or nearly round and of a brown and wrinkled aspect.
Properties and Uses—Stimulant and Aromatic.

NUX VOMICA
(Strychnos Nux Vomica)
Common Names—Poison Nut, Ratsbane.
Medicinal Part—The seeds.
Description—This is a moderate-sized tree, with a short and pretty thick trunk.

The wood is white, hard, and bitter. The leaves are opposite, oval, and smooth on both sides. Flowers small, greenish-white, funnel-shaped, and have a disagreeable odor. The fruit is a berry, round, and about the size of a large apple, enclosing five whitish seeds.

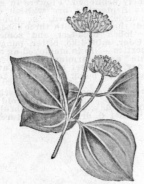

NUX VOMICA

It is an inhabitant of the Coromandel, Ceylon, and other parts of the East Indies. The active principles of the seeds are strychnine and brucia.

Properties and Uses—It is an energetic poison, exerting its influence chiefly upon the cerebro-spinal system. It is supposed to affect the spinal cord principally. If a poisonous dose is given it will produce spasms like tetanus or lockjaw. Its range of service is quite extensive, and valuable for many indications; but as great caution is required in its adminstration, it should only be employed by the educated physician.

OAK
(White, Red and Black, Quercus Alba, Rubra, and Tinctoria, Beech Family)
Medicinal Part—The bark.

Description — These forest-trees vary in size, according to the climate and soil. In diameter they are from 3 to 6 feet; in height, from 60 to 100 feet. They are too well known to require any botanical description.

Quercus is a very extensive and valuable genus, consisting of many species, a large proportion of which grow in the United States. Their usual character is that of astringent, and the three above described are those which have been more particularly employed in medicine.

The bark of the tree is the portion used. White Oak bark is the one chiefly used in medicine. It is a pale brownish color, faintly odorous, very astringent, with a slight bitterness, tough, breaking with a stringy or fibrous fracture, and not readily powdered. It contains a very large proportion of tannic acid. Black Oak bark is also used as an astringent

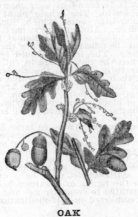

OAK

externally, but is rarely employed internally, as it is liable to derange the bowels. It is also used in tanning and for dyeing. Red Oak bark also contains considerable tannin, and is chiefly applied externally.

Properties and Uses — White Oak is slightly tonic and very astringent. It is useful and commonly employed as a wash and gargle for irritations of the mouth and throat, as well as for the purposes of a vaginal douche.

OLD MAN'S BEARD
(Chionanthus Virginica, Olive Family)
Common Names—Fringe Tree, Poison Ash.
Medicinal Part—Bark of the root.

Description—This is a shrub or small tree, growing from 8 to 25 feet high. The leaves are opposite, oval, oblong, veiny and smooth; flowers are in dense panicles; calyx, very small; corolla snow-white, consisting of four petals; and fruit a fleshy, oval, purple drupe.

This plant is very ornamental, and is much cultivated in gardens, from Pennsylvania to Tennessee. It grows on river-banks and on elevated places, presenting clusters of snow-white flowers in May and June. The bark of the root, which imparts its properties to water or alcohol, is the part used.

Properties and Uses — The bark is aperient and diuretic. By some it is regarded as a tonic with much virtue. It can be used to advantage as a poultice for wounds and external irritations.

Dose—A teaspoonful of the bark of the root, cut small or granulated to a cup of boiling water. Drink cold, one cupful during the day, a large mouthful at a time; of the tincture, 5 to 20 min.

ORACHE
(Chenopodium Vulvaria)

Common Names — Arrach, Stinking Goosefoot, English Mercury, Allgood, Dog Arrach.

Parts Used—The whole plant.

Description—Orache is an annual plant growing on dung hills and waste places, 2 to 3 feet high. It is of a dull glaucous, or greyish green, aspect and invested with a greasy mealiness or bloom which, when touched exhales an odious odor resembling that of stale salt fish. It is attractive to dogs.

Properties — The plant contains trimethylamine, osmazome and nitrate of potash and gives off free ammonia. It is considered of some use in various conditions, but its greatest value is undoubtedly in the form of a poultice mixed with vinegar, honey and salt and as a salve for the usual purposes for which such remedies are commonly employed.

Dose—A teaspoonful of the plant, cut small or granulated to a cup of boiling water. Drink cold one cupful during the day, a large mouthful at a time; of the tincture, 5 to 20 min.

OREGANO
(Origanum Mexicana—Mint Family)

Common names — Mexican Oregano, Mexican Sage.

Parts Used—Leaves and flowering tops.

Description—Oregano is perennial in warm zones, and grown as an annual in cold climates. The plant resembles Origanum vulgare (Wild Marjoram)—however Oregano is more pungent, less leafy and more yellow. Both Oregano and Wild Marjoram are used similarly for flavoring foods—however, Oregano is far more popular among Mexicans, Spanish and Italians.

Oregano is used in pizzas; pasta and spaghetti sauces; chili-con-carne; chili dishes; veal scallopini etc.

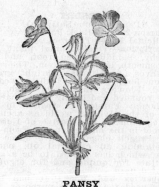

PANSY
(Viola Tricolor—Violet Family)

Common Names—Heartsease, Johnny Jumper, Stepmother.

Medicinal Part—Plant.

Description—Pansy is a low plant with rounded leaves or the upper oval and lowest heart-shaped; petals of various colors and often variegated and under cultivation often very large and showy.

Properties and Uses—Pectoral, mucilaginous, laxative, vulnerary.

PAREIRA BRAVA
(Cissampelos Pareira)

Common Names—Velvet Leaf, Ice Vine.

Medicinal Part—The root.

Description—This plant is a shrub, with a round woody root and smooth stems. Leaves roundish, peltate, subcordate, and smooth above when full-grown. Flowers small, and the fruit a scarlet, round reniform, shrivelled berry.

This is a native of the West India Islands and the Spanish Main. It is sometimes imported under the name of Abuta or Butua Root. It comes in cylindrical pieces, sometimes flattened, and some as thick as a child's arm, and a foot or more in length. The alkaloid obtained from it has been called Cissampelin or Pelosin.

Properties and Uses — Diuretic and aperient. Used by some for irritation of the urinary tract.

Dose—A teaspoonful of the root, cut small or granulated, to a cup of boiling water. Drink cold, one cupful during the day, a large mouthful at a time; of the tincture, 10 to 30 min.

PARSLEY
(Petroselinum Sativum)
Common Name—Rock Parsley.
Medicinal Part—The root.
Description—This biennial plant has a fleshy, spindle-shaped root, and an erect, smooth, branching stem. The radical leaves are biternate, bright green, and on long petioles; leaflets wedge-shaped. Flowers white or greenish, and petals rounded and barely emarginate.

Although Parsley is reared in all parts of the civilized world as a culinary vegetable, it is a native of Europe. The root is the officinal part. From the seeds French chemists have succeeded in obtaining an essential oil, named Apiole, which has proved to be a good substitute for quinia and for ergot in indicated uses.

Properties and Uses—It has been widely used for diuretic purposes, but, as with other products of the fields, it has been largely supplanted by the products of the laboratories of man. The seeds are sometimes used as carminatives. The leaves, bruised, are a good application for contusions.

Dose—A teaspoonful of the root to a cup of boiling water. Drink cold, one or two cupfuls a day, a large mouthful at a time; of the tincture, ⅛ to ½ fl. dr.

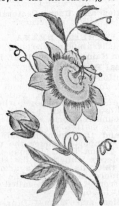

PASSION FLOWER
(Passiflora Incarnata—Passion Flower Family)
Medicinal Part—Plant and flower.
Description—Passion Flower is a woody plant with leaves very deeply cleft or parted into five or seven lance-oblong, entire divisions, pale. The flower is almost white except the purple center and the blue crown banded with whitish in the middle. The plant climbs by simple axillary tendrils.

Properties and Uses—Antispasmodic, sedative.

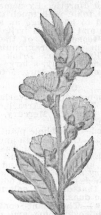

PEACH TREE
(Amygdalus Persica—Rose Family)
Medicinal Part—The leaves and kernels.
Description—Peach is too common to require a detailed description. The peach tree has thin, broad leaves and coarsely serrate leaves and thickfleshed edible fruit and a hard and deeply marked stone.

Properties and Uses—Sedative, bitter, aromatic and laxative.

Peach trees are often sprayed with an arsenic or other poisonous solution. To prevent poisoning purchase these leaves from reliable source. These leaves must not be boiled, merely steeped in hot water. Dose not more than a level teaspoonful to a cup of water.

PENNYROYAL
(Hedeoma Pulegioides, Mint Family)
Common Names—Tickweed, Squawmint, Hedeoma.
Medicinal Part—The herb.
Description—This is an indigenous annual plant, with a fibrous, yellowish root, and an erect, branching stem, from 6 to 12 inches high. The leaves are half an inch or more long, opposite, oblong and on short petioles; floral leaves similar. The flowers are quite small and light blue in color.

This plant should not be confused with the Mentha Pulegioides, or European Pennyroyal. It grows in barren woods and dry fields, and particularly in limestone countries, flowering from June to September and October, rendering the air fragrant to some distance around it. It is said to be very obnoxious to fleas.

Properties and Uses—It is gently stimulant, diaphoretic, and carminative. The warm infusion, used freely, will promote perspiration. It is much used for this last purpose—a large draught being taken at bedtime, the feet being previously bathed in hot water.

Dose—A teaspoonful of the herb to a cup of boiling water. Drink cold one or two cupfuls a day, a large mouthful at a time; of the tincture, ½ to 1 fl. dr.

PEONY
(Paeonia Officinalis)
Medicinal Part—The root.

Description—Peony has many thick, long-spreading, perennial roots, running deep into the ground, with an erect, herbaceous, large green, and branching stem, about 2 or 3 feet high. The leaves are large; leaflets ovate-lanceolate and smooth. The flowers are large, red and solitary; and fruit a many-seeded, fleshy follicle.

This plant is indigenous to Southern Europe, and is cultivated in gardens in the United States and elsewhere on account of the elegance of its large flowers, which appear from May to August. The root is the officinal part. This, with the seeds and flowers, yields its virtues to diluted spirits.

Properties and Uses—It has been credited by some with antispasmodic powers, while others refer to it as purgative and emetic. An infusion of value is made by adding an ounce of the root, in coarse powder to a pint of boiling liquid, composed of one part of good gin and two parts of water.

Dose—A teaspoonful of the root to a cup of boiling water. Drink cold one or two cupfuls a day, a large mouthful at a time; of the tincture, ¼ to 1 fl. dr.

PEPPERGRASS
(Lepidum Apetalum, Mustard Family)
Parts Used—The herb.

Description—Peppergrass is an annual and winter annual. It first forms a rosette of leaves flat on the ground, later the flowering stalk is produced. The plant is much branched and has a bushy appearance; the flowers are very small, white. The seed pods are about 1/10 of an inch wide and somewhat heart-shaped being notched at the top.

Properties and Uses—Peppergrass is recommended as a hair tonic used in combination with Sage, Henna Leaves and Cinchona Bark.

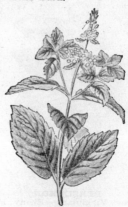

PEPPERMINT
(Mentha Piperita)
Common Names — Lammint, Brandy Mint.

Parts Used—Leaves and flowering tops.

Description—Peppermint is a perennial herb, 1 to 3 feet high, smooth, square stem, erect and branching, leaves dark green, borne on stalk, lance-shaped, sharply toothed, generally smooth on both sides, but sometimes hairy on the veins on lower surface; flowers July to September; blossoms are small purplish; have a tubular 5-toothed calyx and 4-lobed corolla. Peppermint has an aromatic pungent odor and agreeable taste which is at first burning, followed by a cooling sensation.

Properties—Peppermint is an aromatic stimulant with carminative properties. Useful in flatulency, nausea, diarrhea, colic, nervous headache, heartburn, and as a flavoring agent. The oil and menthol are used externally in headache, neuralgia, etc.

Dose—A teaspoonful of the leaves and flowering tops to a cup of boiling water. Drink cold one or two cupfuls a day, a large mouthful at a time; of the tincture; ½ to 1 fl. dr.

A tiny carpeting type of mint, called Corsican Mint (Mentha Requienü) has the purest of all mint fragrances. It is used in the making of "Creme de menthe."

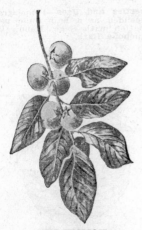

PERSIMMON

(Diospyros Virginiana—Ebony Family)

Common Names—Date Plum, Jove's Fruit, Lotus Tree, Seeded Plum, Winter Plum.

Medicinal Part—Bark.

Description—Persimmon trees grow from twenty to sixty feet high with very hard blackish wood. The calyx is four parted and the corolla pale yellow, four cleft. The fruit is plum-like, green and very puckery until after frost when it is sweet and yellow and eatable.

Properties and Uses—Astringent, febrifuge and anti-periodic.

PERUVIAN BARK

(Cinchona)

Common Names—Foso Bark, Jesuits' Bark, Red Bark, Crown Bark.

Medicinal Part—The bark.

Description — The bark is obtained from the Cinchona Calisaya, Cinchona Condaminea, Cinchona Succirubra and Cinchona Lancifolia. These trees are all evergreen or shrubs. Their generic character is to have opposite entire leaves, flowers white, or usually roseate or purplish, and very fragrant; calyx a turbinated tube; corolla salver-shaped; stamens, five; anthers, linear; style simple; stigma, bifid. The fruit a capsule, ovate or oblong, filled with numerous winged seeds. About thirteen varieties of cinchona are known to commerce, but the above are the most important. Of these species the former three yield respectively the pale yellow and red cinchona barks, and the fourth is one of the sources of quinine.

Cinchona is a very old discovery, and takes its names from the wife of the Spanish viceroy, County de Cinchon, who was cured of fever by it at Lima, about the year 1638. For some time after its introduction into Europe, the Jesuits, who received the bark from their brethren in Peru, alone used it, and kept to themselves the secret of its origin; and their use of it was so successful that it received the name which till clings to it of "Jesuits' Bark." The bark richest in the antiperiodic alkaloids is the Cinchona Calisaya. The geographical range of the cinchonas appears to be exclusively confined to the Andes. within the boundaries of Peru, Bolivia, Ecuador and New Granada. Thirteen species furnish the barks of commerce, and all of them were found growing from one to ten thousand feet above the level of the sea. The four species we have named at the head of this article are, however, the only ones recognized by the United States Pharmacopoeia, and are favorites everywhere. Since the seventeenth century these barks have been the study of men versed in medical and chemical science, and they and the preparations made from them rank among the most important articles of the Materia Medica. It contains numerous active principals, but the most important, and one chiefly used, is quinine.

Properties and Uses—Peruvian Bark is tonic, antiperiodic, astringent to a moderate extent, and eminently febrifuge. It is freely used as a mouth wash and gargle and given internally as a remedy for malaria. The properties and uses of this bark have become well known in recent years. When taken internally it imparts a sensation of warmth to the stomach, which gradually spreads over the body.

Quinine is a white flocculent powder, inodorous, and has a very bitter taste. It is very sparingly soluble in warm water, still less so in cold water. It is readily soluble in hot alcohol, and tolerably so in ether. It is always best to administer quinine instead of the bark, unless some of the effects of the other principles are desired.

Dose—Steep a teaspoonful of the bark into a cup of boiling water for half hour. Drink a half cupful upon retiring at night, hot or cold. Or take a mouthful 3 times a day. One or two cupfuls may be taken; of the tincture, ¼ to ½ fl. dr.

* * * *

Nature, Time and Patience, are the Three Great Physicians.

—an old proverb

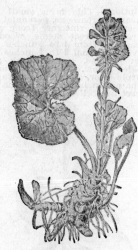

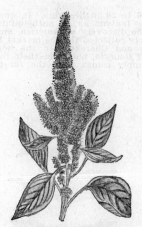

PILE WORT
(Amaranthus Hypochondriacus,
Amaranth Family)

Common Names — Prince's Feather,
Red Cock's Comb, Amaranth, Lady
Bleeding.

Medicinal Part — The leaves.

Description — This is an annual herb,
with a great stout upright stem, from
3 to 4 feet high. The leaves are oblong,
lanceolate, mucronate, green with a red
purplish spot, clustered flowers, five
stamens.

This plant is a native of the middle
states, where it is cultivated in gardens
as an ornamental plant, but contains
more medicinal virtues in its wild state.
It flowers in August. The leaves impart their virtues to water.

Properties and Uses — Pilewort is astringent and as such may be employed
for diarrhea, etc. It is useful as a local
application to mouth and throat irritations and as a wash for external purposes.

Dose — One teaspoonful to a cup of
boiling water. Drink cold 1 or 2 cupfuls
a day; of the tincture, ½ to 1 fl. dr.

PINK ROOT
(Spigellia Marilandica, Logania Family)

Common Names — Carolina Pink, Worm
Grass.

Medicinal Part — The root.

Description — This herbaceous, indigenous plant has a perennial, very fibrous,
yellow root, which sends up several
erect, smooth stems of purplish color,

PEST ROOT
(Petasites Officinalis — Thistle Family)

Common Names — Butter-bur, Butterfly
Dock.

Medicinal Part — Root and leaves.

Description — Pest Root herb has a
very scaly scape from six to fifteen
inches high. The leaves are orbicular or
hastate-reniform, often twelve inches
broad when mature, rounded or pointed
at the apex. White tomentose beneath
and green and glabrous above. The
heads are in a dense green raceme. The
flowers are pink, purple and fragrant.

Properties and Uses — Tonic, Stimulant,
diuretic.

PETTY SPURGE
(Euphorbia Peplus — Spurge Family)

Medicinal Part — The root.

Description — Petty Spurge is found
growing in waste places. It has an erect
stem, leaves petioled, entire, round-
obovate, the upper floral ones ovate;
umbel first three-rayed, afterwards two-
forked; pod two-crested on each lobe.

Properties and Uses — Cathartic and
diuretic.

* * * *

"He that takes medicine and neglects
to diet, wastes the skill of his doctors."
— old Chinese proverb

from 6 to 20 inches high. It was used by the Indians as an anthelmintic before the discovery of America, and was formerly collected for the market by the Creeks and Cherokees in the northern part of Georgia, but since their removal the supply comes from the far Southwest.

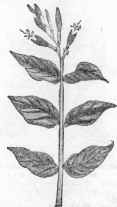

PINK ROOT

It inhabits the Southern States, and is seldom found north of the Potomac. The leaves are opposite, sessile, ovate, lanceolate, acute or acuminate, entire and smooth. Flowers few in number and club-shaped. Fruit a double capsule.

Properties and Uses—It is an active vermifuge in cases of round-worm especially among children. It should not be given alone, however, as it is very apt to produce various unpleasant symptoms, increased action of the heart, dizziness, etc.

Dose—It gives best results when mixed as follows:

One teaspoonful Pink Root, 1 teaspoonful Senna Leaves, I teaspoonful Anise Seed, 1 teaspoonful Male Fern, 1 teaspoonful Turtlebloom.

One teaspoonful of above mixture to a cup of boiling water. Drink one cupful as often as indicated. Children, a tablespoonful.

PIPSISSEWA
(Chimaphila Umbellata, Wintergreen Family)

Common Names—Princess Pine, False Wintergreen, Ground Holly.

Medicinal Part—The whole plant.

Description— This is a small evergreen, nearly herbaceous, perennial herb, with a creeping rhizome, from which spring several erect stems, woody at their base, and from 4 to 8 inches high. The leaves are from 2 to 3 inches long, on short petioles, and of dark green color, paler below. The flowers are of light purple color, and exhale a fragrant odor. The pollen is white, and the fruit is an erect five-celled capsule.

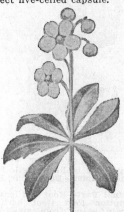

PRINCE'S PINE

This plant is indigenous to the north temperate regions of both hemispheres, and is met with in dry, shady woods, flowering from May to August. The leaves have no odor when dried, but when fresh and rubbed they are rather fragrant. Boiling water or alcohol extracts their virtues. They contain resin, gum, lignin and saline substances.

Properties and Uses—It is diuretic and is favored by some for its apparently beneficial influence on the urinary tract, it being preferable to other herbs on account of being less obnoxious to the stomach.

Dose—A teaspoonful of the plant to a cup of boiling water. Drink cold one or two cupfuls a day, a large mouthful at a time; of the tincture, ½ to 1 fl. dr.

PITCHER PLANT
(Sarracenia Purpurea)

Common Names — Huntsman's Cup, Eve's Cup, Fly Trap.

Parts Used—The whole plant.

Description—This is a most interesting plant. The leaves are all radical winged down the innerside, open at the top with an arching hood, each leaf resembling a pitcher; the basal leaves or pitchers are partially filled with water.

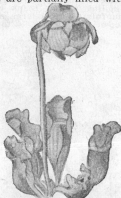

PITCHER PLANT

Just below the rim of the pitchers on the inside is a sticky substance to attract and trap insects, which become food for the plant after they decompose. Scape tall, naked, bearing a single large red nodding flower.

Properties — Pitcher plant has been used by some for its tonic and beneficial action on the stomach.

Dose—A teaspoonful of the plant to a cup of boiling water. Drink cold, one cupful during the day, a large mouthful at a time. Tincture, 5 to 20 min.

PLANTAIN
(Plantago Lanceolate)

Common Names—Ribwort, Soldiers Herb.

Medicinal Part—The leaves.

Description—Plantain is one of the most common flowering weeds about dooryards everywhere.

The leaves all radiate from the base; they are lanceolate, sharply pointed and set on long, troughed stems; they are dark green in color and are strongly ribbed lengthwise.

The flower stem is stiff and smooth and attains heights of 6 to 18 inches. The head is short and studded with tiny, four-parted, dull white flowers, with long slender stamens. There are often perfect, staminate and pistillate flowers on the same plant. It is now as abundant in all parts of our range as it is in its native European home.

Properties and Uses—The fresh leaves are a mild astringent and useful for cuts and scratches and for dressing wounds, when mashed to a pulp and applied. The same is also highly recommended to give quick relief for the external rectal irritation of piles.

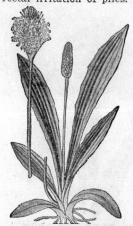

LANCE LEAF PLANTAIN

Plantain is an old English remedy at one time widely used internally.

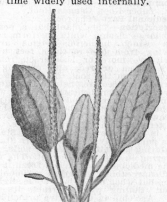

Greater Plantain—Plantago Major is identical with above except that the leaves are broader and larger and the flowering spike 3 to 5 inches longer. It is of equal value medicinally.

Dose—A teaspoonful of the leaves to a cup of boiling water. Drink cold one or two cupfuls a day, a large mouthful at a time; of the tincture, ½ to 1 fl. dr.

tion and expectoration in conditions in which such action is indicated. In full doses it is emetic and cathartic.

Dose—A teaspoonful of the root to a cup of boiling water. Drink cold one or two cupfuls a day, a large mouthful at a time; of the tincture, ½ to 1 fl. dr.

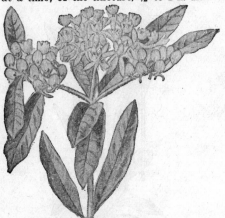

PLEURISY ROOT
(Asclepias Tuberosa, Milkweed Family)

Common Names—Butterfly Weed, Wind Root, Tuber Root, Canada Root.

Medicinal Part—The root.

Description—This plant has a perennial, large, fleshy, white fusiform root, from which numerous stems arise, growing from one to three feet high, which are more or less erect, round, hairy, green or red, and growing in bunches from the root. The leaves are alternate, lanceolate, hairy, dark green above and paler beneath. The flowers are numerous, erect and of a beautifully bright orange color. The fruit is a long, narrow, green follicle. Seeds are ovate, and terminate in long silken hairs.

It is a native of the United States, more particularly of the Southern States, inhabiting gravelly and sandy soils, and flowering in July and August. The root is the medicinal part. When fresh it has a disagreeable, slightly acrimonious taste, but when dried the taste is slightly bitter. Boiling water extracts its virtues. Asclepin is the active principle.

Properties and Uses—Butterfly Weed is much used in decoction or infusion, for the purpose of promoting perspira-

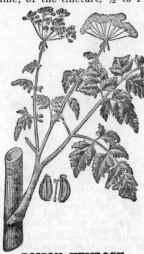

POISON HEMLOCK
(Conium Maculatum—Parsley Family)

Common Names—Poison Root, Spotted Hemlock, Cicuta, Spotted Cowbane, Poison Snakeweed.

Medicinal Part—Leaves and seed.

Description—A smooth branching herb found in waste grounds. The stems are spotted, about three feet high, very compound leaves with lanceolate and pinnatifid leaflets, ill-scented when bruised.

Properties and Uses—A virulent poison suitable for use only by the skilled physician.

POISON IVY
(Rhus Toxicodendron—Cashew Family)

Common Names—Poison Oak, Poison Oak Sumach, Poison Vine.

Description—The poison ivy's range reaches from as far North as Nova Scotia as far south as Florida and Texas, and as far west as Utah and British Columbia. It is often confused with the beautiful Virginia Creeper. Poison Ivy is a prodigal climber, inclined to run over everything in sight. Even the oak is sometimes smothered when the ivy reaches its topmost branches. It begins to blossom in May and June, its flowers being small, fragrant and yellowish green and arranged in densely clustered spikes. Toward fall these develop into smooth, white, wax-like berries that often hold fast the winter through. The three leaves are shining green, short-stemmed and oval pointed.

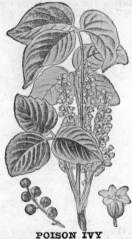

POISON IVY

The poison of the poison ivy is a powerful, nonvolatile oil which penetrates the pores of the human skin and develops hosts of tiny itching blisters, followed by a burning swelling of the affected parts.

POISON IVY RECIPE

Huron Smith, author of Ethnobotany of the Forest Potawatomi Indians wrote in regard to Jewel Weed, or Wild Touch-me-not (Impatiens biflora): "This is accounted a valuable Medicine among the Forest Potawatomi who use the fresh juice of the plant to wash nettle stings or poison ivy infections. The writer knows that it instantly alleviates the sting of Stinging Nettle, and has it from the Indians that it will alleviate the itching of Poison Ivy."

Another source states: "An Indian gathered and put some on W.P.A. workers for ivy poisoning, as they were working in bush land. He squeezed the juice on affected parts, and it healed right up. He also claims it is a cure for other surface caused minor skin troubles."

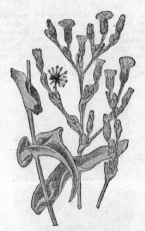

POISON LETTUCE
(Lactuca Virosa—Chicory Family)

Common Names—Acrid Lettuce, Prickly Lettuce.

Medicinal Part—The leaves.

Description—Poison Lettuce is a biennial, green and glaucous. The stem is stiff, leafy, from two to seven feet high. The leaves are oblong or oblong-lanceolate. The lower leaves are much larger than the upper ones. The heads are from six to twelve flowered, very numerous in an open panicle.

Properties and Uses—Narcotic and poisonous.

POKE
(Phytolacca Decandra. Pokeweed Family)

Common Names—Pigeon Berry, Garget, Scoke, Coakum, Inkberry.

Medicinal Parts—The root, leaves and berries.

Description—This indigenous plant has a perennial root of large size, frequently exceeding a man's leg in diameter, fleshy, fibrous, easily cut or broken, and covered with a thin brownish bark. The stems are annual, about an inch in diameter, round, smooth, when young green, and grow from five to nine feet in height. The leaves are scattered, petiolate, smooth on both sides, and about five inches long and three broad. The flowers are numerous, small, and greenish-white in color, and the berries are round, dark purple, and in long clusters.

99

This plant is common in many parts of the country, growing in dry fields, hillsides and roadsides, and flowering in July and August. It is also found in Europe and northern parts of Africa. The leaves should be gathered just previous to the ripening of the berries. The berries are collected when fully matured. Phytolaccin is its active principle.

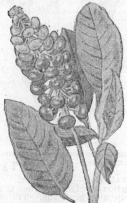

POKEBERRY
Properties and Uses—Poke is cathartic, alterative, and slightly narcotic. While it also is a slow-acting emetic, its use for that purpose is not favored. However, few, if any, of the alteratives have superior power to Poke, if it is properly gathered and prepared for medicinal uses.

Dose—A tablespoonful of the root, leaves or berries cut small to a pint of boiling water. Take one teaspoonful at a time as required; of the tincture, 2 to 5 min.

POMEGRANATE
(Punica Granatum)
Medicinal Parts—The rind of the fruit and bark of the root.

Description—This is a small tree or shrub. The leaves are opposite, entire, smooth and 2 or 3 inches long. The flowers are large, red, two or three, and nearly sessile. Calyx five-cleft, corolla consists of five much-crumpled petals. The fruit is a large pericarp, quite pleasant in flavor, and quite watery.

The Pomegranate is Asiatic, but has been naturalized in the West Indies and the Southern States.

Properties and Uses—The flowers and bark and rind are astringent, and are an ancient remedy for tapeworm. It is astringent and has been employed as a gargle for throat irritations. Also used for diarrhea and as a vaginal douche.

Dose—A teaspoonful of the bark of the root, cut small or granulated to a cup of boiling water. Drink cold one cupful during the day, a large mouthful at a time; of the tincture, 5 to 40 min.

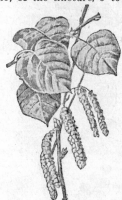

POPLAR
(Populus Tremuloides)
Common Names—White poplar, American Aspen.

Parts Used—Leaves, buds and bark.

Description—This is a rather small tree with thin foliage 30 to 40 feet high; trunk diameter 20 inches, tapering to the very top of the tree; branches slender, alternating and scattered. Bark horizontally marked, smooth on younger trees and gray or rusty green with a whitish bloom and dark patches below the branches. Older trees sepia brown and rough toward the base. Leaves broad heart-shaped, dull, whitish, dark green with white veins, roundly fine toothed. Grows everywhere in the U. S.

Properties—The bark and leaves long have been used in some countries for medicinal purposes, because of their balsamic and soothing qualities. Externally as a wash for cuts, scratches, burns, fetid perspiration. The buds of this species and Populus Candicans are commonly called Balm Gilead.

Dose—A teaspoonful of the leaves, buds or bark to a cup of boiling water. Drink cold one or two cupfuls a day, a large mouthful at a time; of the tincture, ½ to 1 fl. dr.

When used externally as a wash, a teaspoonful of borax should be added to the cupful of tea.

POPULUS CANDICANS
(Balm Gilead)

Description—These buds as well as those of other species of Populus which are covered with a resinous exudation which has a peculiar, agreeable, balsamic odor and a bitterish balsamic somewhat pungent taste.

Properties—The buds boiled in olive oil or lard make an excellent salve. Internally they are valuable in coughs resulting from colds.

Dose—The buds must be soaked in alcohol to dissolve the resin before they can be used as a tea. A teaspoonful of the buds to a cup of boiling water. Drink cold one cupful during the day, a large mouthful at a time; of the tincture, 5 to 20 min.

PRICKLY ASH
(Xanthoxylum Fraxineum, Rue Family)
Common Names—Yellow-wood, Toothache-bush.

Medicinal Parts—The bark and berries.

Description — This indigenous shrub has a stem ten or twelve feet high, with alternate branches, which are armed with strong conical prickles. The leaves are alternate and pinnate, leaflets ovate and acute. The flowers are small, greenish, and appear before the leaves. The fruit is an oval capsule, varying from green to red in color.

It is a native of North America, growing from Canada to Virginia, and west to the Mississippi, in woods, thickets and on river banks, and flowering in April and May. The medicinal parts render their virtues to water and alcohol. Xanthoxyline is its active principle.

Properties and Uses—Prickly Ash bark is stimulant, diaphoretic, and sometimes used for flatulence and diarrhea. The berries, which contain a volatile oil, are aromatic.

Dose—A teaspoonful of the bark, cut small or granulated, to a cup of boiling water. Drink cold, one cupful during the day, a large mouthful at a time; of the tincture, 5 to 20 min.

The Aralia Spinosa, or Southern Prickly Ash, differs from Xanthoxylum, both in botanical character and medicinal virtues.

PRIDE WEED
(Erigeron Canadense, Aster Family)
Common Names — Colt's Tail, Horse Weed, Canada Fleabane, Butter Weed, Bitter Weed.

Medicinal Part—The whole plant.

Description—This is an indigenous annual herb, with a high bristly hairy stem, from 6 inches to nine feet high. The leaves are lanceolate; flowers small, white and very numerous.

Pride Weed is common to the Northern and Middle States, grows in fields and meadows, by roadsides, and flowers from June to September. It should be gathered when in bloom and carefully dried. It has a feeble odor, somewhat astringent taste, and yields its virtues to alcohol or water.

Properties and Uses—It is tonic, aromatic, and astringent. Useful in indicated conditions, such as diarrhea.

Dose—Steep a level teaspoonful of the plant cut into small pieces into a cup of boiling water for half hour. When cold drink 1 or 2 cupfuls a day, a good mouthful at a time. Of the tincture, 10 to 40 min.

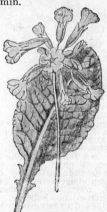

PRIMROSE
(Primula Veris)
Common Names—Butter Rose, English Cowslip.

Parts Used—Flowers and herb.

Description—Primrose is a perennial downy herb native of England, growing 6 to 9 inches high; leaves are radical, oval, oblong, wrinkled. Flowers in umbels on slender pedicles, rising from the root stock above the leaves, yellow corolla and calyx bell-shaped.

Properties—The flowers are said to be useful in ordinary headache. The whole plant has a somewhat soothing and quieting influence.

Dose—A teaspoonful of the flowers and herbs, cut small or granulated to a cup of boiling water. Drink cold, one cupful during the day, a large mouthful at a time; of the tincture, 5 to 20 min.

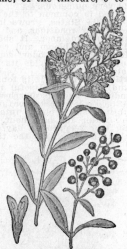

PRIVET
(Ligustrum Vulgare, Olive Family)
Common Names—Privy, Prim.

Medicinal Part—The leaves.

Description—This is a smooth shrub, growing 5 to 6 feet high. The leaves are dark green, 1 or 2 inches in length, about half as wide, entire, smooth, lance-olate, and on short petioles. The flowers are small, white, and numerous, and fruit a spherical black berry.

It is supposed to have been introduced into America from England, but it is indigenous to Missouri and found growing in wild woods and thickets from New England to Virginia and Ohio. It is also cultivated in American gardens. The leaves are used for medicinal purposes. They have but little odor, and an agreeable bitterish and astringent taste. They yield their vitrues to water or alcohol. The berries are reputed cathartic, and the bark is said to be as effectual as the leaves, as it contains sugar, mannite, starch, bitter resin, bitter extractive, albumen, salts and a peculiar substance called Ligustrin.

Properties and Uses—The leaves are astringent. A decoction of them may be employed internally in indicated conditions. These leaves also may be used as a mouth wash and gargle or as a vaginal douche.

Dose—A teaspoonful of the leaves to a cup of boiling water. Drink cold one or two cupfuls a day, a large mouthful at a time; of the tincture, ½ to 1 fl. dr.

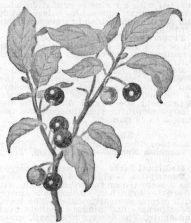

PURGING BUCKTHORN
(Rhamnus Frangula)
Common Names—Buckthorn, Arrow Wood, Alder Dogwood, Bird Cherry.

Medicinal Parts—Bark of young trunks and large branches.

Description—Purging Buckthorn is a shrub introduced from Europe, 5 to 8 feet high, with spreading, thornless branches, the young twigs very fine, hairy. The small leaves light olive green, obovate, very obscurely round-toothed or toothless, smooth about 2 inches long. Flowers green in tiny stemless clusters, perfect, with 5 petals. Blooms May to June. Fruit black, ¼ inch in diameter with three seeds. Grows in swamps in the Northeastern and Northern parts of the United States.

Properties and Uses—The bark should be at least one year old before using. It is purgative, its action said to be similar to that of rhubarb. Useful in costiveness and constipation. An ointment made of the fresh bark is excellent for skin irritations.

Dose—A teaspoonful of the bark, cut small of granulated, to a cup of boiling water. Drink cold, one cupful during the day, a large mouthful at a time; of the tincture, 5 to 20 min.

PYROLA
(Round Leaved Pyrola Rotundifolia)
Common Names — Shin-leaf, Canker-Lettuce, Pear-Leaf Wintergreen.

Medicinal Part—The herb.

Description—This is a low, perennial, evergreen herb. The leaves are radical, ovate, nearly two inches in diameter, smooth, shining and thick. The petioles are much longer than the leaf. The flowers are many, large, fragrant, white and drooping. The fruit is a five-celled, many-seeded capsule.

This plant is common in damp and shady woods in various parts of the United States, flowering in June and July. The whole plant is used, and imparts its medicinal properties to water.

Properties and Uses—It is astringent and is used, among other purposes, as a vaginal douche. The herb is applied with profit as a poultice, to bruises, bites of insects, etc. The decoction will be found beneficial as a gargle for throat and mouth irritation, and as a wash for the eyes.

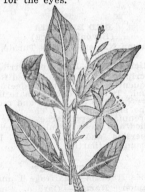

QUASSIA
(Picraenia Excelsa)
Common Names—Bitter Root, Bitter Ash.

Medicinal Part—The wood.

Description—This is a tree growing from 50 to 100 feet high, with an erect stem, 3 or more feet in diameter at the base. The bark is grayish and smooth. The leaves are alternate, unequally pinnate; leaflets opposite, oblong, acuminate and unequal to the base. Flowers are small, pale or yellowish green. Fruit three drupes, about the size of a pea. The Quassia Amara or Bitter Quassia is a shrub, or moderately sized branching tree, having a grayish bark.

Quassia Amara inhabits Surinam, Guiana, Colombia, Panama and the West Indies. It flowers in November and December. The bark, wood and root, which are intensely bitter, are used to the greatest advantage in some conditions.

Properties and Uses—Quassia is a well known bitter tonic. Cups made of the wood have been used for many years by persons requiring a strong tonic. Any liquid standing in one of these vessels a few moments will become impregnated by its peculiar medicinal qualities. Wherever a bitter tonic is required, Quassia is an excellent remedy.

Dose—A teaspoonful of the wood cut small or granulated, to a cup of boiling water. Drink cold, one cupful during the day, a large mouthful at a time; of the tincture, 2 to 5 min.

QUEEN OF THE MEADOW
(Eupatorium Purpureum, Aster Family)
Common Names—Gravel-Root, Joe-Pie, Trumpet Weed, Purple Boneset.

Medicinal Part—The root.

Description — This is a herbaceous plant, with a perennial woody root, with many long dark-brown fibres, sending up one or more solid green, sometimes purplish stems, 5 or 6 feet in height. The leaves are oblong, ovate or lanceolate, coarsely serrate, and from three to six in a whorl. The flowers are tubular, purple, often varying to whitish.

Queen of the Meadow grows in low places, dry woods or meadows, in the Northern, Western and Middle States of the Union, and flowers in August and September. The root is the officinal part. It has a smell resembling old hay, and a slightly bitter, aromatic taste, which is faintly astringent but not unpleasant. It yields it properties to water by decoction or spirits.

Properties and Uses—In decoctions, the flowers are diuretic and tonic. The roots are astringent and useful as such, as in diarrhea.

Dose—A teaspoonful of the root to a cup of boiling water. Drink cold one or two cupfuls a day, a large mouthful at a time. Of the tincture, ½ to 1 fl. dr.

RAGGED CUP
(Silphium Perforiatum, Aster Family)
Common Names—Indian Cup-plant, Indian Gum.

Medicinal Part—The root.

Description—This plant has a perennial, horizontal, pitted rhizome, and a large smooth herbaceous stem, from 4 to 7 feet high. The leaves are opposite, ovate, from 8 to 14 inches long by 4 to 7 wide. The flowers are yellowish and the fruit a broadly ovate winged achenium.

This plant is common to the Western States, and is found growing in rich bottoms, bearing numerous yellow flowers, which are perfected in August. It has a large, long and crooked root, which is the part used medicinally, and which readily imparts its properties to alcohol or water. It will yield a bitterish gum, somewhat similar to frankincense, which is frequently used to sweeten the breath.

Properties and Uses—It is tonic, diaphoretic and alterative. A strong infusion of the root, made by long steeping, or an extract, is said to give good results.

Dose—A teaspoonful of the root, cut small or granulated, to a cup of boiling water. Drink cold, one cupful during the day, a large mouthful at a time; of the tincture, 5 to 20 min.

Silphium Gummiferum, or Rosin-weed and Silphium Laciniatum, or Compass-weed, are used for coughs resulting from colds.

RATTLE SNAKE PLANTAIN
(Goodyera Pubescens, Orchid Family)

Common Names—Net Leaf Plantain, Scrofula Weed, Adder's Violet, etc.

Medicinal Part—The leaves.

Description—The scape or stem of this plant is from 8 to 12 inches high, springing from a perennial root. The leaves are radical, ovate and dark green. The flowers are white, numerous and pubescent.

This herb grows in various parts of the United States, in rich woods and under evergreens, and is more common southward than northward, although there is a variety (Goodyera Repens) which is plentiful in colder regions of America. It bears yellowish-white flowers in July and August. The leaves are the parts employed, and yield their virtues to boiling water.

Properties and Uses—The fresh leaves are steeped in milk and applied as a poultice to bruises, bites of insects, skin irritations. The leaves also may be used whole if preferred.

* * * *

"For one believeth that he may eat all things; another, who is weak eateth herbs."   —St. Paul to the Romans

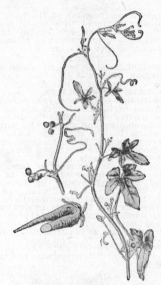

RED BRYONIA
(Bryonia Dioica)

Common Names—Devil's Turnip, Wild Hops, Wild Vine.

Medicinal Part—Root and berries.

Description—The common Red Bryony is frequently found in the hedgerows in England. It has cordate-palmate leaves, axillary bunches of flowers and red berries the size of a pea. The root stock is perennial, very large, white and branched and has a repulsive smell.

Properties and Uses—Acrid, bitter, emetic and cathartic.

RED CURRANT
(Ribes Rubrum—Saxifrage Family)

Common Names — Garden Currant, Wineberry, Raisin Tree, Garnet Berry.

Medicinal Part—The fruit.

Description—Red currant is a low shrub with straggling or reclining stems, somewhat heart-shaped moderately three-five lobed leaves; edible berries red, or white.

Properties and Uses—Refrigerant and febrifuge.

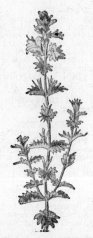

Description—This is a shrubby and strongly hispid plant, about 4 feet high. Leaves, pinnate; leaflets, oblong-ovate; flowers, white; corolla, cup-shaped, and fruit a red berry, of a rich delicious flavor.

The Red Raspberry grows wild, and is common to Canada and the Northern and Middle United States. It grows in hedges and thickets, and upon neglected fields. It flowers in May and its fruit ripens from June to August. The leaves and bark of the root are the parts used medicinally. They impart their properties to water, giving to the infusion an odor and flavor somewhat similar to black tea.

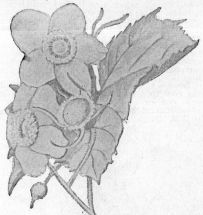

RASPBERRY

Properties and Uses—It is very useful as an astringent. An infusion or decoction of the leaves has been found an excellent remedy in diarrhea. The decoction of the leaves combined with cream will suppress nausea and vomiting.

Dose—A teaspoonful of the bark of the root or the leaves, cut small or granulated, to a cup of boiling water. Drink cold, one or two cupfuls a day, a large mouthful at a time; of the tincture, ½ to 1 fl. dr.

RED EYE BRIGHT
(Euphrasia Officinalis)
Common Name—Eye Bright.
Medicinal Part—The leaves.

Description—This is an elegant little annual plant, with a square, downy, leafy stem, from one to five inches in height. The leaves are entirely opposite, ovate or cordate, and downy; the flowers very abundant, inodorous, with a brilliant variety of colors. The fruit is an oblong pod, filled with numerous seeds.

This plant is indigenous to Europe and America, bearing red or white flowers in July. The leaves are commonly employed; they are inodorous, but of a bitter astringent taste. Water extracts their virtues.

Properties and Uses — Slightly tonic and astringent. Useful in form of infusion or poultice, in nasal congestion or catarrh; also in coughs, hoarseness, earache and headache associated with colds.

Dose—Steep a heaping teaspoonful of the leaves into a cup of boiling water for half hour. When cold drink 1 or 2 cupfuls a day; a good mouthful at a time; of the tincture, ½ to 1 fl. dr.

RED RASPBERRY
(Rubus Strigosus, Rose Family)
Common Name—Wild Red Raspberry.
Medicinal Parts—The bark of the root and leaves.

RED ROOT
(Ceanothus Americanus, Buckthorn Family)
Common Names — New Jersey Tea, Wild Snowball.

Medicinal Part—The bark of the root.

Description—This plant has a large root with a red or brownish bark, tolerably thick, and body of dark-red color. The stems are from 2 to 4 feet high, slender, with many reddish, round, smooth branches. The leaves are ovate or oblong-ovate, serrate, acuminate, rather smooth above and cordate at the base. The flowers are minute and white and fruit a dry capsule.

This plant is very abundant in the United States, especially in the Western portions thereof. It grows in dry woodlands, bowers, etc., and flowers from June to August. The leaves are sometimes used as a substitute for Chinese Tea, which, when dried, they much resemble. The root, which is officinal, contains a large amount of Prussic acid. Ceanothine is the name that has been given to its active principle.

Properties and Uses—Red Root is astringent, expectorant, and has been credited with various uses. Among other purposes, it has been used as a gargle in mouth and throat irritations.

Dose—A teaspoonful of the bark of the root to a cup of boiling water. Drink cold one or two cupfuls a day, a large mouthful at a time; of the tincture, ½ to 1 fl. dr.

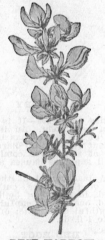

REST HARROW
(Ononis Spinosa)
Common Names—Petty Whin, Cammock, Stay Plough.

Medicinal Part—Root.

Description—Rest Harrow has a five-cleft bell-shaped calyx, the standard of the corolla large and striated, the keel beaked, the pod turgid and few seeded. The lower leaves have three leaflets, the upper are simple. The flowers are axillary and rose-colored, or very rarely white. The plant is half shrubby, with spiny stems, viscid and its smell unpleasant.

Properties and Uses—Diuretic, detergent and aperient.

RHATANY
(Krameria Triandria)
Medicinal Part—The root.

Description—The root of this plant is horizontal, very long, with a thick bark. The stem is round and procumbent, branches two or three feet long; when young, white and silky; when old, dark and naked. The leaves are alternate, sessile, oblong and obovate, hoary and entire. The flowers are red on short stalks. Calyx has four sepals, and corolla four petals. The fruit is a dry hairy drupe.

Rhatany flowers all the year round, and grows upon the sandy, dry and gravelly hills of Peru. The root is the officinal part, and is dug up in large quantities after the rains. It was made officinal in 1780 by Ruiz, but long before that the natives had used it as a strong astringent for various diseases, afflictions, maladies and complaints. In Portugal, to which the Peruvians send the bulk of the roots gathered, it is used to adulterate red wines. The best method of extracting the medicinal qualities of the root is to put it powdered in a displacer and pass water through. This will bring a brick-red aqueous solution, which will embrace all the medicinal virtues. There is a false Rhatany, the source of which is unknown.

Properties and Uses—It is a strong astringent, and slightly tonic. It is beneficial wherever active astringents are required, and may be used to advantage, if properly prepared, for all conditions which call for the application of a decided astringent.

Dose—A teaspoonful of the root, cut small or granulated, to a cup of boiling water. Drink cold, one cupful during the day, a large mouthful at a time; of the tincture, 5 to 20 min.

RHUBARB
(Rheum Palmatum)
Common Names—Chinese or Turkey Rhubarb.
Medicinal Part—The root.

Description—Rhubarb is a large compact perennial herb, resembling our garden rhubarb; stems 4 to 6 inches thick on mature plants, many branches 10 to 15 inches long, 3 to 6 inches thick, dark brown coat from withered acreas and leaf bases, inside fleshy, semi-pulpy, juice yellow; leaves very large, 2 to 4 feet long and wide petioles 12 to 18 inches long, palmately veined, 7 lobed; flowering stems 5 to 10 feet high; flowers in clusters; greenish white, fruit crimson red. The root or rhizome is sub-cylindrical, conical, irregular, 2 to 6 inches long, 2 to 3 inches thick.

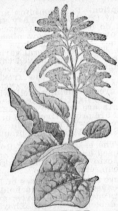

RHUBARB

There are several varieties met with in commerce termed the Russian, Chinese, English and French Rhubarb, among which the Russian is considered the best. The names are given not that they are produced in indicated countries, but of the channels by which they are thrown upon the market. Rhubarb has a peculiar aromatic odor, bitter, faintly astringent taste, and when chewed tinges the saliva yellow.

Properties and Uses—Rhubarb is cathartic, astringent and tonic. It is much used as a laxative for infants, its mildness and tonic qualities making it peculiarly applicable. It is a valuable medicine.

Dose—A teaspoonful of the root, cut small or granulated, to a cup of boiling water. Drink cold, one cupful during the day, a large mouthful at a time; of the tincture, 5 to 20 min.

ROCK ROSE
(Helianthemum Canadense, Rock Rose Family)

Common Names—Frost Plant, Frost Wort.

Medicinal Part—The herb.

Description—Rock Rose is a perennial herb, with a simple, ascending downy stem, about a foot high. The leaves are alternate, from one-half to one inch long, about one-fourth as wide; oblong, acute, lanceolate, erect and entire. The flowers are large and bright yellow, some with petals, and some without petals. The flowers open in sunshine and cast their petals next day.

It is indigenous to all parts of the United States, growing in dry, sandy soils, and blossoming from May to July. The leaves and stems are covered with a white down, hence its name. The whole plant is official, having a bitterish, astringent, slightly aromatic taste, and yields its properties to hot water. Prof. Eaton, in his work on botany, records this curious fact of the plant: "In November and December of 1816 I saw hundreds of these plants send out broad, thin, curved ice crystals, about an inch in breadth from near the roots. These were melted away by day, and renewed every morning for more than twenty-five days in succession."

Properties and Uses—It is used in form of decoction, syrup or fluid extract, but had better be used in combination with other remedies. In combination with Corydalis Formosa and Stillingia it forms a most valuable remedy. It is tonic and astringent. It can be used with advantage in diarrhea, as a gargle in throat irritations, and as an eye wash. The Helianthemum Corybosum, or Frost Weed, growing in the pine barrens and sterile lands of the Southern and Middle States, possesses similar qualities, and may be employed if the former Frost Weed is not to be had.

Dose—Steep a teaspoonful of the granulated herb into a cup of boiling water for half hour. Strain. Take a tablespoonful 3 to 6 times a day; of the tincture, 5 to 10 min.

ROMAN MOTHERWORT
(Leonurus Cardiaca, Mint Family)

Common Names—Lion's Tail, Throwwort.

Medicinal Parts—The tops and leaves.

Description—This perennial plant has stems from 2 to 5 feet in height. The leaves are opposite, dark green, rough and downy. The flowers are purplish or whitish-red; calyx, rigid and bristly;

corolla, purplish; anthers in pairs, and fruit an oblong achenium.

Motherwort is an exotic plant, but extensively introduced into the United States, growing in fields and pastures, and flowering from May to September. It has a peculiar, aromatic, not disagreeable odor and a slightly aromatic bitter taste. It yields its properties to water and alcohol.

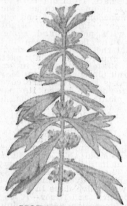

MOTHERWORT

Properties and Uses—It apparently is a valuable remedy for many purposes, and deserves greater attention than it receives. It has been used as a vaginal douche for simple vaginitis.

Dose—A teaspoonful of the tops and leaves to a cup of boiling water. Drink cold 1 or 2 cupfuls a day, a large mouthful at a time; of the tincture, ½ to 1 fl. dr.

ROSEMARY
(Rosemarinus Officinalis)
Medicinal Part—The tops.

Description—Rosemary is an erect perennial, evergreen shrub, 2 to 4 feet high, with numerous branches of an ash color, and densely leafy. The leaves are sessile, opposite, and linear, over an inch in length, dark green and shining above, and downy. The flowers are few, bright blue or white. Calyx purplish.

Rosemary is a native of the countries surrounding the Mediterranean, and is cultivated in nearly every garden for its fragrance and beauty. It flowers in April and May. The parts used in medicine are the flowering tops.

Properties and Uses—It is gently stimulant. The oil is principally used as a perfume for ointments, liniments and embrocations.

Dose—A teaspoonful of the tops, cut small or granulated, to a cup of boiling water. Drink cold, one cupful during the day, a large mouthful at a time; of the tincture, 5 to 20 min.

ROSE-SCENTED GERANIUM
(Pelargonium graveolens

Part Used—The leaves.

Description—Pelargoniums are native of Cape of Good Hope. They are perennial, but do not tolerate freeze or frost. Field grown plants grow about 3 feet high. They prefer hot days and cool evenings. There are several variations of graveolens. The small leaved variety has the strongest aroma. Old leaves have a stronger scent than the fresh young leaves. Leaves are deeply veined and grayish green, turning yellowish with age. Flowers light lavender flecked with red. Plants are easy to propagate from slips, and are productive for 5 or 6 years. They are grown mainly in southern France, Spain, Algeria and Reunion.

Uses—The essential oil of Rose geranium is used as an adulterant or substitute for otto of roses in making perfumes, soap, etc.

There are a variety of uses of Rose geranium leaves in the household. Fresh butter wrapped in the leaves, gives the butter a delectable scent. They may be used to flavor apple pie, jellies and custards. Layer cake is delicious with a few leaves of Rose geranium placed in the bottom of pans.

A favorite old-fashioned sachet is made of one part Rose Geranium and one part each of Lemon Verbena and Lavender.

There are many other varieties of scented Geraniums, a few of the most popular are:

P. Crispum—a refreshing lemon-scented variety used for finger bowls—often called Finger-bowl Geranium.

P. Limonium—balm scented. Adds a pleasant flavor when added to Chinese tea.

P. Odoratissimum—apple-like fragrance. Adds a delicate aroma to jellies.

P. Tomentosum—peppermint scented.

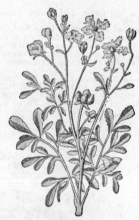

RUE
(Ruta Graveolens)
Common Names—German Rue, Garden Rue.

Medicinal Part—The herb.

Description—This plant is a native of Southern Europe, but is cultivated in many gardens in the United States. It grows 2 to 3 feet high and has a woody stem. The flowers are yellow. The fruit a capsule, 4-5 lobed; seeds black, numerous; leaflets ½ to 1 inch long, ¼ inch wide, crenate, thick, pellucid-punctate.

Properties and Uses—Rue is a bitter, aromatic stimulant very valuable for gas pains or colic.

Dose—A teaspoonful of the herb, cut small or granulated, to a cup of boiling water. Drink cold one cupful during the day, a large mouthful at a time; of the tincture, 5 to 20 min.

SACRED BARK
(Rhamnus Purshiana, Buckthorn Family)
Common Names—Chittembark, Cascara.

Part Used—The bark.

Description — This indigenous tree grows on the sides and bottom of the Rocky Mountains; it is 15 to 20 feet high. The thin dark green leaves are elliptical, fine saw-toothed, rounded or slightly heart-shaped at the base, blunt at the apex or with a short, sharp point, veins prominent, somewhat hairy on undersides. The flowers are produced in umbels or clusters, small greenish and are followed by black ovoid 3 seeded

berries of an insipid taste. It is very difficult to distinguish this from other similar species of Rhamnus. When dried the outer surface of the bark is reddish brown, wrinkled and usually covered with light grayish lichen; the inner surface is smooth and marked with very fine lines, taste very bitter.

Properties—Sacred Bark is an old Indian remedy. It is purgative, and seems to excite peristalsis of the bowels. It gives best results when combined with other herb simples. The bark should be at least one year old before using; it improves with age. The Indians held this bark sacred and modern physicians have found it one of the very best remedies for constipation.

Dose—A teaspoonful of the bark, cut small or granulated, to a cup of boiling water. Drink cold one cupful during the day, a large mouthful at a time; of the tincture 5 to 20 min.

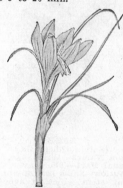

SAFFRON
(Carthamus Tinctorus.)
Common Names—Safflower, **Bastard** Saffron, American Saffron.

Medicinal Part—The flowers.

Description—This annual plant has a smooth, straight stem, from one to two feet high, and branching at the top. The leaves are alternate, ovate-lanceolate, sessile, smooth and shining. The flowers are numerous, long, slender and orange-colored. Corolla five-cleft.

This plant is cultivated in England and America, although it is a native of Egypt and the countries surrounding the Mediterranean. The orange-red florets are the officinal parts. The cultivated Safflower is usually sold in the shops, and contains two coloring matters; the first of which is yellow and soluble in water; the second a beautiful red, and readily soluble in alkaline solutions only.

Properties and Uses—Saffron has been and still is employed to some extent for medicinal purposes in some countries, because of its apparently soothing qualities, but saffron tea now is only occasionally used.

Dose—A teaspoonful of the flowers, cut small or granulated, to a cup of boiling water. Drink cold one cupful during the day, a large mouthful at a time; of the tincture, 5 to 20 min.

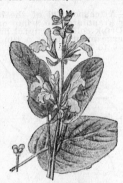

SAGE
(Salvia Officinalis.)
Common Names—Wild Sage.
Medicinal Part—The leaves.
Description—Sage is a plant with a pubescent stem, erect branches, hoary with down, leafy at the base, about a foot or foot and a half long. The leaves are opposite, entire, petioled, ovate-lanceolate, the lowermost white, with wool beneath. The flowers are blue and in whorls.

Sage is a native of southern Europe, and has been naturalized for very many years in this country as a garden plant. The leaves and tops should be carefully gathered and dried during its flowering season, which is in June and July. They have a peculiar, strong, aromatic camphorous odor, and a sharp, warm, slightly bitter taste, which properties are owing to its volatile oil, which may be obtained by distilling the plant with water. It imparts its virtues to boiling water in infusion, but more especially to alcohol.

Properties and Uses—It is feebly tonic and once was highly valued as a medicinal agent. Though it sometimes is used even now for its beneficial influence on digestion, its chief modern uses are a condiment.

Dose—A teaspoonful of the leaves to a cup of boiling water. Drink cold one to two cupfuls a day, a large mouthful at a time; of the tincture, 20 to 60 min.

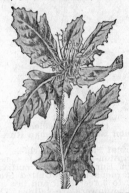

ST. BENEDICT THISTLE
(Carduus Benedictus)
Common Names — Blessed Thistle, Spotted Thistle, Cardin.
Part Used—Leaves and flowering tops.
Description—Blessed Thistle is an annual herb growing about 2 feet high with coarse erect stem, branched and rather wooly; leaves 2 to 3 inches long, oblong, lance-shaped, thin more or less hairy, margins wavy lobed and spiny. The yellow flower heads, which appear from May to August are situated at the ends of the branches almost hidden by the upper leaves. The flowers are surrounded by scales of a leathery texture tipped with long yellowish red spines.

Properties—Blessed Thistle is tonic and diaphoretic. Taken cold in a mild dose as prescribed below it is a mild tonic; taken hot it produces copious perspiration; taken double or triple strength it becomes an emetic.

Dose—A teaspoonful of the leaves and flowering top, cut small or granulated, to a cup of boiling water. Drink cold, one cupful during the day, a large mouthful at a time; of the tincture, 5 to 20 min.

ST. IGNATIUS' BEAN
(Ignatius Amara)

Description—The Ignatius Amara is a branching tree with long, taper, smooth, scrambling branches. The leaves are veiny, smooth, and a span long. The flowers are long, nodding and white, and smell like jessamine. The fruit is small and pear-shaped, and the seeds number about twenty, are angular, and are imbedded in a soft pulp.

The tree is indigenous to the Philippine Islands, and the seeds thereof are the St. Ignatius' Bean of the drug-shops. The bean yields its properties best to alcohol, but will also yield them to water. It contains about one-third more strychina than nux-vomica, but is seldom used for the production of strychina on account of its extreme scarcity.

Properties and Uses—Very similar to nux-vomica seeds, but perhaps more energetic. It is employed in various conditions with partial good effect, but is a dangerous article, however well prepared, and should be used only upon the advice of a physician. It should not be employed in domestic practice as it is too powerful.

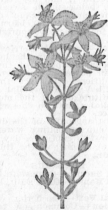

ST. JOHNSWORT
(Hypericum Perforatum, St. John's Wort Family)

Common Name—John's Wort.
Medicinal Parts—The tops and flowers.
Description—This a beautiful shrub, and is a great ornament to our meadows. It has a hard and woody root, which abides in the ground many years, shooting anew every year. The stalks run up about two feet high, spreading many branches, having deep-green, ovate, obtuse, and composite leaves, which are full of small holes, which are plainly seen when the leaf is held up to the light. At the tops of the stalks and branches stand yellow flowers of five leaves apiece, with many yellow threads in the middle, which, being bruised, yield a reddish juice, like blood, after which come small, round heads, wherein is contained small blackish seed, smelling like resin. The fruit is a three-celled capsule.

This plant grows abundantly in this country and Europe, and proves exceedingly annoying to farmers. It flowers from June to August. It has a peculiar terebinthine odor, and a balsamic, bitterish taste. It yields its properties to water, alcohol and ether.

Properties and Uses—It is astringent, and has been credited by former generations with peculiar soothing effects. Externally, in fomentation, or used as an ointment, it is serviceable for bruises, scratches, bites of insects, and skin irritation.

Dose—A teaspoonful of the tops and flowers, cut small or granulated, to a cup of boiling water. Drink cold one cupful during the day, a large mouthful at a time; of the tincture, 10 to 20 min.

ST. JOSEPHWORT
(Ocymum Basilicum)

Common Name—Sweet Basil.
Part Used—The herb.
Description—This is an annual plant native of India and Persia and cultivated here and in Europe. Leaves ovate, slightly serrate, smooth extending from the stem. The flowers vary in colors, white, pink and red.

Properties and Uses—This herb is aromatic, with the usual qualities and uses of that class of plant.

Dose—One teaspoonful to a cup of boiling water. Drink 1 or 2 cupfuls a day.

SANICLE
(Sanicula Marilandica, Parsley Family.)

Common Names—Black Snake Root, Pool Root, American Sanicle.
Medicinal Part—The root.
Description—Sanicle is an indigenous, perennial herb, with a smooth furrowed stem, from one to three feet high. The leaves are digitate, mostly radical, and on petioles from six to twelve inches long. Cauline leaves few, and nearly sessile. The flowers are mostly barren

white, sometimes yellowish, fertile ones sessile.

It is common to the United States and Canada, and is found in low woods and thickets, flowering in June. The fibrous root is aromatic in taste and odor. It imparts its virtues to water and alcohol.

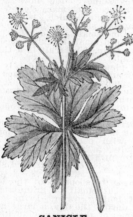

SANICLE

Properties and Uses—Domestically, it is used with advantage in throat irritation and is very beneficially employed in various other conditions.

Dose—A teaspoonful of the root, cut small or granulated, to a cup of boiling water. Drink cold, one cupful during the day, a large mouthful at a time. Of the tincture, 15 to 30 min.

SASSAFRAS
(Laurus Sassafras, Laurel Family)
Common Names—Saxafrax.
Medicinal Part—The bark of the root.
Description—This is a small tree, varying in height from ten to forty feet. The bark is rough and grayish, that of the twigs smooth and green. The leaves are alternate, petiolate, bright green, very variable in form, smooth above and downy beneath. The flowers appear before the leaves, are small, greenish-yellow; fruit an oval, succulent drupe.

Indigenous to North America and common to the woods from Canada to Florida, and flowering in the latter part of April or early in May. The bark has an aromatic, agreeable taste, and similar odor. It yields its properties to hot water by infusion and to alcohol.

Properties and Uses—It is a warm aromatic, stimulant, alterative, diaphoretic and diuretic. It is much used in alterative compounds as a flavoring adjuvant. In domestic practice it enjoys a wide field of application and use, especially as a so-called spring tonic.

Dose—A teaspoonful of the bark of the root, cut small or granulated, to a cup of boiling water. Drink cold one cupful during the day, a large mouthful at a time; of the tincture, 15 to 30 min.

SAW PALMETTO
(Serenoa Serrulata.)
Common Names — Dwarf Palmetto, Fan Palm.
Medicinal Part—The dried berries.
Description—This plant or shrub grows near the Atlantic ocean, in Georgia and Florida, on a strip of coast hundreds of miles in length, and from one to five miles wide. The edge of the leaf has the appearance of a saw, hence its name. The Saw Palmetto fruit or berries are very abundant, and about the size and shape of olives, and grow in bunches. They are dark purple or nearly black in color, ripen from October to December, and are very sweet and juicy, being much sweeter than sugar cane, and richer in nutrition. People who live near it learn to love the fruit, for it is very nourishing and satisfying.

Properties—Palmetto Berries are of great service in cold in the head, irritated mucous membrane of the throat, nose and air passages, and in numerous other conditions. In fact they have been credited with peculiar virtues. They constitute one of the most valuable remedial agents in the whole materia medica.

Dose—A teaspoonful of the dried berries to a cup of boiling water. Drink cold one or two cupfuls a day, a large mouthful at a time; of the tincture ½ to 1 fl. dr.

SCABIOUS
(Scabiosa Succisa—Composite Family)
Common Names—Devil's Bit, Primrose Scabious.
Medicinal Part—The herb.
Description — Common on roadsides, meadows, and cultivated ground in England. Slender little-branched plant, with hairy stem, few leaves, oblong and entire. Flowers globular and deep purplish-blue.
Properties and Uses—The plant is still used in England for its diaphoretic, demulcent and febrifuge properties.

Several other varieties are also still used as medicinals in Europe.

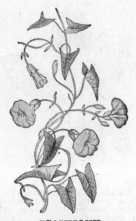

SCAMMONY
(Convolvulus Scammonia—Convolvulus Family)
Common Name—Bindweed.
Medicinal Part—The root.
Description—Scammony is found in low grounds, twining freely and spreading by running rootstocks; leaves arrow-shaped.
Properties and Uses—Cathartic, diuretic and herpatic; flowers yellow.

SCULLCAP
(Scutellaria, Lateriflora, Mint Family)
Common Names—Side-flowering Scullcap, Mad Dogweed, Blue Pimpernell and Hood-wort.
Medicinal Part—The whole plant.
Description—Scullcap has a small, fibrous, yellow, perennial root, with an erect and very branching stem, from one to three feet in height. The leaves are on petioles about an inch long, opposite, thin subcordate on the stem, ovate on branches, acuminate, acute and coarsely serrate. The flowers are small, and of a pale-blue color. It is an indigenous herb, growing in damp places, meadows, ditches, and by the side of ponds from Connecticut south to Florida and Texas, flowering in July and August. The whole plant is medicinal, and should be gathered while in flower, dried in the shade, and kept in well-closed tin vessels. Chemically it contains an essential oil, a yellowish-green fixed oil, chlorophyll, a volatile matter, albumen, an astringent principle, lignin, chloride of soda, salts of iron, silica, etc.

Properties and Uses—This is another of the botanicals once in rather common use which have been crowded from the medicinal picture in modern times. Formerly seems to have been employed by some as a nervine or tonic.

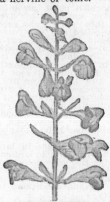

SCULLCAP

Dose—Place one teaspoonful of the granulated leaves into a cup of boiling water. Drink one or two cupfuls during the day, or use from half to one teaspoonful of the fluid extract three times a day.

SEA WRACK
(Fucus Vesiculosus)
Common Names—Bladder Wrack, Gulf-wrack.
Part Used—The dried plant.
Description—Sea Wrack grows on muddy rocks in the Atlantic ocean and gulf and often floats to the shore; it is 40 inches long and about ½ inch broad, flattened, branched, with a midrib; air-vessels in pairs, blackish, seaweed odor, saline, mucilaginous taste.
Properties—It is considered alterative, and has been employed as such in some cases of reducible overweight.
Dose—A teaspoonful of the dried plant to a cup of boiling water. Drink cold one or two cupfuls a day, a large mouthful at a time; of the tincture ½ to 1 fl. dr.

SENEKA
(Polygala Senega, Milkwort Family)
Common Names—Seneca Snake Root, Senega.
Medicinal Part—The root.
Description—This indigenous plant has

a perennial, firm, hard, branching root, with a thick bark, and sends up several annual stems, which are erect, smooth, from eight to fourteen inches high, occasionally tinged with red. The leaves are alternate, nearly sessile, lanceolate, with a sharpish point, smooth; flowers white; calyx consists of five sepals, corolla of three petals, and capsules are small, two-celled and two-valved.

It is found in various parts of the United States, in rocky woods and on hill-sides, flowering in July. It is more abundant in the West and South than in the East. The officinal root varies in size from two to four or five lines in diameter, crooked, and a carinate line extends the whole length of it. Its chemical constituents are polygalic, virgineic, pectic, and tannic acids, coloring matter, an oil, cerin, gum, albumen, salts of alumina, silica, magnesia, and iron.

Properties and Uses—In large doses emetic and cathartic; in ordinary doses it stimulates the secretions, acting particularly as an expectorant. It is a good expectorant and as such has been employed in various conditions indicating that quality.

Dose—A teaspoonful of the root, cut small or granulated, to a cup of boiling water. Drink cold, one cupful during the day, a large mouthful at a time; of the tincture 5 to 10 min.

SEVEN BARKS
(Hydrangea Arborescens)
Medicinal Part—The root.
Description — Hydrangea grows in shady places in the woods and on the banks of streams throughout our middle and southern states. It is a shrub 4 to 8 feet high with ovate or almost heart-shaped leaves from 3 to 6 inches long, generally acuminate, serrately toothed. The flat clusters of white, tiny, pistilate flowers often contain a few large sterile flowers around the margin. They appear in June and July, fruit a 2-horned capsule, containing many seeds. A peculiar characteristic of this shrub, from which it has derived its name, is the peeling off of the stem bark, which comes off in seven successive layers of thin different colored bark.

Properties—Seven Barks is a mild and soothing diuretic and has been preferred by some for such uses. It is reputed to be an old Cherokee Indian remedy.

Dose—A teaspoonful of the root, cut small or granulated, to a cup of boiling water. Drink cold one cupful a day, a large mouthful at a time; of the tincture, 5 to 20 min.

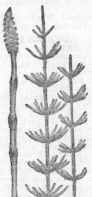

SHAG BARK HICKORY
(Carya Amara—Walnut Family)
Common Names—Shagbark Walnut, Ackroot, Shagbark Tree.
Medicinal Part—Bark.
Description—Barks of the old trunks of the Shag Bark Hickory are very shaggy, separating in rough wide strips. The nut is white and the meat highly flavored.
Properties and Uses—Cathartic.

SHAVE GRASS
(Equisetum Hiemale)
Common Name—Horsetail Grass.
Medicinal Part—The plant.
Description—This is a perennial plant rising from creeping root stocks, the

numerous stems are furrowed, many-jointed; fruitication in terminal cone-like spikes. These spikes are the first to appear in the spring and die after a few weeks, after which the clump of stems appear. These are the parts used in medicine. The plant grows in sand and gravel along road sides and railroad tracks and in wet places.

Properties—This is said to have some diuretic action and has been employed in various combinations.

Dose—A teaspoonful of the plant to a cup of boiling water. Drink cold one or two cupfuls a day, a large mouthful at a time; of the tincture, ½ to 1 fl. dr.

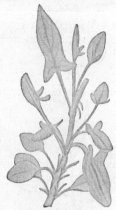

SHEEP SORREL
(Rumex Acetosella.)

Common Names — Sourgrass, Red Sorrel.

Part Used—The herb.

Description—Sheep Sorrel is a perennial, with shallow running root stalk, yellowish in color. The leaves are arrow shaped and have a decidedly sour taste.

Properties and Uses—Sheep Sorrel when used green in salads is very beneficial. It contains acid potassium, oxalate and tartaric acid. It is refrigerant and diuretic but not very active after drying.

Dose—A teaspoonful of the herb to a cup of boiling water. Drink cold 1 or 2 cupfuls a day, a large mouthful at a time; ½ to 1 fl. of the tincture.

SHEPHERD'S PURSE
(Capsella Bursa Pastoris, Mustard Family)

Common Names—Shepherd's Heart.
Medicinal Part—The whole herb.

Description—This is one of the most common of wayside weeds. The name Capsella signifies a little box, in allusion to the seed pods. It is a Cruciferous plant, made familiar by the diminutive pouches or flattened pods, at the end of its branching stems.

Properties and Uses—Has been used at times as a stimulant diuretic and also as an anti-scorbutic.

Dose—A teaspoonful of the herb to a cup of boiling water. Drink cold 1 or 2 cupfuls a day, a large mouthful at a time; of the tincture, ½ to 1 fl. dr.

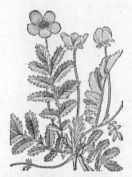

SILVER WEED
(Potentilla Anserina)

Common Names — Silver Cinquefoil, Cramp Weed, Goose Tansy, Moor Grass.
Medicinal Part—The whole herb.

Description—Silver weed is a common and very handsome species found in dry, barren ground throughout our range, but most abundantly near the coast. It is from 5 to 12 inches high. The little, yellow flowers are clustered at the ends of the branches. The stems and the undersides of the divided and deeply cut leaves are covered with fine while silvery wool, contrasting sharply with the dark green of the upper surfaces. This species bloom from May until September.

Properties and Uses—Silver Weed Tea has been used for various astringent purposes, as in diarrhea, etc. The root has been used as a red dye.

115

Dose—A teaspoonful of the herb to a cup of boiling water. Drink cold, one or two cupfuls a day, a large mouthful at a time; of the tincture ½ fl. dr.

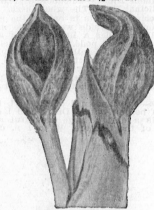

SKUNK CABBAGE
(Symplocarpus Foetidus, Arum Family.)

Common Names—Skunk Weed, Pole Cat Weed, Meadow Cabbage, Swamp Cabbage.

Medicinal Parts—The roots and seeds.

Description—This plant has been a troublesome one for botanists to classify; but the term Symplocarpus is now generally preferred. It is perennial, having a large, abrupt root or tuber, with numerous crowded, fleshy fibres, which extend some distance into the ground. The spathe appears before the leaves, is ovate, spotted, and striped, purple and yellowish-green, the edges folded inward, and at length coalescing. The flowers are numerous, of a dull purple within the spathe, on a short, oval spadix. Calyx consists of four fleshy, wedge-shaped petals; corolla, none; stamens 4, seeds round and fleshy, and about as large as a pea.

Skunk Cabbage is a native of the United States, growing in moist grounds, flowering in March and April, and maturing its fruit in August and September, forming a roughened, globular mass, two or three inches in diameter, and shedding its bullet-like fruit one-third to one-half inch in diameter, which are filled with a singular solid, fleshy embryo. The parts used are the seeds and roots, which have an extremely disagreeable odor. Water or alcohol ex-tracts their virtues. Chemically it contains a fixed oil, wax, starch, volatile oil and fat, salts of lime, silica, iron and manganese.

Properties and Uses—Internally it is a stimulant, exerting expectorant anti-spasmodic, with slightly narcotic influences. It has been used in the spasms of asthma, whooping-cough, nasal catarrh, and bronchial irritation.

Externally in the form of an ointment it has a soothing effect.

Dose—A teaspoonful of the root, cut small or granulated, to a cup of boiling water. Drink cold one cupful during the day, a large mouthful at a time; of the tincture 5 to 20 min.

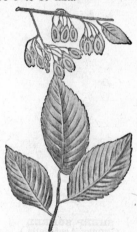

SLIPPERY ELM
(Ulmus Fulva)

Common Names—Indian Elm, Moose Elm, Rock Elm, Sweet Elm.

Parts Used—Inner bark.

Description—A commonly slim and characteristically rough tree, rough in bark and leaf, 40-50 and rarely 70 feet high, with a trunk diameter of 1-4 feet. Bark dark brown, deeply furrowed perpendicularly, very rough-scaly, the under layers ruddy brown, the innermost layer next to the wood buff white, aromatic, and very mucilaginous, used medicinally for its demulcent quality. The twigs rough, grayish, hairy.

The leaves are extremely rough above, deep yellowish olive green, lighter and sometimes a rusty-downy beneath. Flowering in March and April. Fruit nearly round in outline, winged, without hairy fringe, ripening in spring, at intervals of 2-4 years.

Properties—Slippery Elm is demulcent, emollient. Useful internally for diarrhoea, coughs due to colds, etc. Externally as a poultice for skin irritation and in rectal and vaginal suppositories.

Dose—A teaspoonful of the inner bark to a cup of boiling water. Drink cold one or two cupfuls a day, a large mouthful at a time.

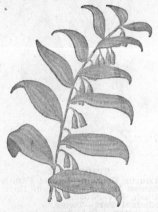

SOLOMON'S SEAL
(Convallaria Multiflora)
Medicinal Part—The root.

Description—The stem of this plant is smooth, from one to four feet high, and growing from a perennial root. The leaves are alternate, lanceolate, smooth, and glossy above, paler and pubescent beneath; flowers greenish-white, the Convallaria Racemosa, the root of which possesses similar qualities to that of Solomon's Seal.

Both plants are to be found throughout the United States and Canada. They flower from May to August. The root, which is the part used, is inodorous, and has a sweetish, mucilaginous taste, which is followed by a slight sense of bitterness.

Properties and Uses—The root seems to be tonic, mucilaginous, and astringent. It also is said to be emetic. Once rather freely used as an external application for bruises, etc., it does not now enjoy much if any favor.

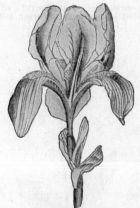

SPANISH IRIS
(Iris Florentina—Iris Family)
Common Names—Orris Root.

Medicinal Part—Root.

Description—Spanish Iris has stems from two to three feet high, with broad leaves and white flowers with blue veins, the obovate outer divisions 2½ to 3 inches long with yellow beard. The flowers are faintly scented. Its violet-scented root stalk yields orris root.

Properties and Uses—Used mostly as a sachet for its violet-like odor.

SPEEDWELL
(Veronica Officinalis)
Common Names—Veronica, Paul's Betony, Ground-hele, Fluellin, Low Speedwell.

Medicinal Part—The leaves and flowering tops.

Description—The little perennial is found growing from Nova Scotia to Michigan and south to North Carolina and Tennessee. It creeps over the ground by means of rather woody stems rooting at the joints and sends up branches from 3 to 10 inches in height. It is hairy all over. The leaves are opposite, on short stalks, greyish green and soft, hairy, oblong, or oval shape, ½ to 1 inch diameter, margins saw-toothed; flowers pale blue in spikes, from May to July. Seed capsule is triangular, compressed and contains numerous flat seeds.

Properties—Veronica is tonic, alterative and diuretic, and has been used with apparent benefit for expectorant and diaphoretic purposes.

Dose—Steep a teaspoonful of the granulated leaves and flowering tops in-

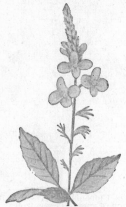

VERONICA

to a cup of boiling water for half an hour. Strain. Take a tablespoonful 3 to 6 times a day. Of the tincture, 10 to 20 min.

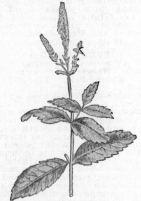

SPEARMINT
(Mentha Viridis—Mint Family)
Common Name—Mint.
Medicinal Part—The herb.
Description—Spearmint may be found on roadsides, spreading rapidly by run-

ning rootstock. The plant is green, nearly smooth with oblong or lance-ovate, wrinkled, veiny, sessile leaves and spikes narrow, dense and leafless. The small flowers are purplish-bluish or almost white in summer.

Properties and Uses—Carminative, antispasmodic, stimulant, aromatic and diuretic.

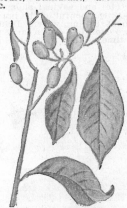

SPICEBUSH
(Laurus Benzoin—Laurel Family)
Common Names—Benjamin Bush, Fever Bush, Feverwood.
Medicinal Part—Twigs.
Description — Spicebush is a shrub found growing in rich woods. It is from six to fifteen feet high, almost smooth. The leaves are thin, obovate-oblong, acute at the base and from three to five inches long. Flowers in the spring preceding the leaves.

Properties and Uses—Aromatic, vermifuge and febrifuge.

SPIKENARD
(Aralia Racemosa)
Common Names—Spignet, Wild Licorice, Nard, Oldman's Root.
Part Used—The root.
Description—Spikenard is quite an imposing plant with its long, curving, zig-zag stem, its numerous light green, deeply ribbed leaves and its feathery terminal flower clusters. The white flowers are tiny but perfect, with 6 parted perianth, six slender stamens and a short, thick style. The root stalk is thick and fleshy with prominent stem scars and furnished with numerous long, thick roots.

118

Properties and Uses—Spikenard is a mild stimulant, alterative, and expectorant. While it is employed to some extent as a pectoral, its value is uncertain.

Dose—1 or 2 teaspoonfuls of the root to a cup of boiling water. Drink cold one or two cupfuls a day. Tincture, 1 to 2 fl. dr.

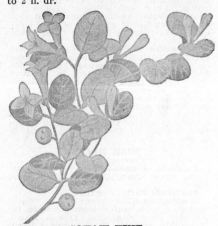

SQUAW VINE
(Mitchella Repens, Madder Family)
Common Names—Partridge Berry, One Berry, Checkerberry, Winter Clover, Deerberry, Hive Vine.
Medicinal Part—The vine.
Description — This indigenous evergreen herb has a perennial root, from which arises a smooth and creeping stem. The leaves are ovate, slightly cordate, opposite, flat and dark-green; flowers are white, often tinged with red, in pairs, very fragrant, and have united ovaries. Calyx four-parted; corolla funnel-shaped; stamens four, inserted on the corolla. The fruit is a dry berry-like double drupe.

Squaw Vine is indigenous to the United States. It grows both in dry woods and swampy places, and flowers in June and July. The berry is bright scarlet and edible, but nearly tasteless. The leaves, which look something like clover remain green throughout the winter. The whole plant is used, readily imparting its virtues to alcohol or boiling water.
Properties and Uses — The use of Squaw Vine goes back to the Indian, hence its name. It has been likened in

diuretic, tonic and alternative effect to the Pipsissewa.

Dose—A teaspoonful of the vine to a cup of boiling water. Drink cold one or two cupfuls a day, a large mouthful at a time; of the tincture, ¼ to ½ fl. dr.

SQUAW WEED
(Senecio Aureus, Aster Family)
Common Names—Life Root, Ragwort, False Valerian, Golden Senecio, Female Regulator, Coughweed, Cocash Weed.
Medicinal Parts—The root and herb.
Description—Squaw Weed has an erect, smoothish stem, one or two feet high. Radical leaves are simple and rounded, mostly cordate and long petioled, lower cauline leaves lyrate, upper ones few, dentate and sessile. Flowers golden yellow.

The plant is perennial and indigenous, growing on low marshy grounds, and on the banks of creeks. The northern and western parts of Europe are where it is mostly found, and the flowers culminate in May and June. There are several varieties of this plant, but as all possess the same medicinal properties, it is unnecessary to specify them. The whole herb is used of all the varieties.
Properties and Uses—It once enjoyed high repute as a so-called female tonic or regulator but has lost much of its standing in modern times.

SQUILLS
(Urginea Maritima)
Common Names—Sea Onion, Scilla.
Part Used—The bulb, outer scales and center rejected.
Description—Squills is a perennial herb, roots fibrous from base of large bulb; leaves appear long after flower, 1 to 2 feet long, shiny deep green leathery similar to our common onion; flowers white on succulent stem 1 to 3 feet high in close spike, no calyx, peduncle purplish, fruit dry capsule, one-half inch long, 3 lobed, yellow, seeds 6 in each cell one-fourth inch long, flattened purplish brown. Bulb pear-shaped when fresh, 3 to 6 inches long and broad; consists of fleshy scales onion like. Collected in August.
Properties—Squills somewhat resembles Digitalis in physiological action and is an irritant poison in over doses causing death by heart paralysis. If properly used it is valuable in certain conditions suggested by its properties, but it is only for the physician or trained herbalist. A fine rat poison.

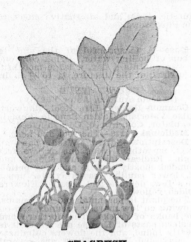

tree growing in China, Japan and Tartary. The fruit consists of from five to ten brownish ligneous capsules, four or five lines long, united together in the form of a star, each containing a brown, shining seed. It is much used in France to flavor liquors; and the volatile oil, upon which its aromatic properties depend, and of which it is said to yield about 2.3 per cent, is imported into this country from the East Indies, and sold as common oil of anise, to which, however, it is thought by some to be much superior.

Properties and Uses—Stimulant and carminative; used in causes of flatulency, and to remove nausea. Sometimes added to other medicines to improve their flavor or to correct disagreeable effects. Should not be confused with botanicals closely resembling Star Anise but wholly unfit for medicinal use.

Dose—A teaspoonful of this to a cup of boiling water. Drink cold, 1 to 2 cupfuls a day. Of the tincture, ¼ to ½ fl. dr.

STAR ROOT
(Aletris Farinosa, Lily Family.)

Common Names—Star Grass, Ague Root, Crow Corn, Unicorn Root, Colic Root.

Medicinal Part—The root.

Description—This plant has a perennial root, with radical leaves, sessile, lying flat on the ground, ribbed, broad, lanceolate, smooth, the large ones being about four inches long. The flower-stem is from one to three feet high, erect and simple, bearing bell-shaped flowers, which as they grow old have a wrinkled, mealy appearance. The fruit is a triangular capsule.

It is indigenous to North America, growing in low grounds, sandy soils, and at the edges of woods. Its flowers are white, and appear from May to August. The root is the part used. Alcohol is the best solvent.

Properties and Uses—Its root, when thoroughly dried, is a valuable bitter tonic, and in decoction or tincture is of great utility in flatulent colic, etc.

Dose—A teaspoonful of the root, cut small or granulated, to a cup of boiling water. Drink cold, one cupful during the day, a large mouthful at a time; of the tincture, 5 to 10 min.

* * * *

Big Elk, a Pequot Indian, who died at the age of 105, attributed his longevity to "herb concoctions he made himself, and to right eating, thinking and acting, and a sincere faith in the Great Spirit God."

STAGBUSH
(Viburnum Prunifolium)

Common Names—Black Haw, Sweet Viburnum, Sheepberry, Sloe.

Part Used—The dried bark of the root.

Description—This is an erect bushy shrub, sometimes gaining the height of a tree, 10 to 28 feet high, with a trunk diameter of 10 inches. Dark gray brown, rough with short narrow, rounded ridges broken laterally into small sections. The deep green leaves are broadly elliptical or obovate, finely and sharply toothed, the undersurface smooth, 1 to 3 inches long, the stem sometimes slightly margined. Flowers very small and white with 3 to 5 lobes, in clusters 2 to 4 inches broad. Bloom from May to June. Fruit ovid, dark cadet blue, on red stems, edible but insipidly sweet. Grows in the northern and central parts of the U. S.

Properties and Uses—This botanical has been quite freely used as a stimulant diuretic in some conditions.

Dose—A teaspoonful of the bark of root to a cup of boiling water. Drink cold one or two cupfuls a day, a large mouthful at a time; of the tincture, 2 fl. dr.

STAR ANISE
(Illicium Verum, Magnoliaceae Family)

Common Name—Star Anise.

Medicinal Part—Seed.

Description—The Star Aniseed is the fruit of Illicium Anisatum, an evergreen

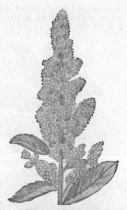

STEEPLEBUSH
(Spiraea Tomentosa)

Common Name—Meadow Sweet.

Part Used—The root and leaves.

Description—Steeplebush is a shrub 2 to 3 feet high, leaves alternate, lanceolate, toothed, dark green above, rusty white beneath; flowers in spikes small, purplish pink turning to a rusty color in the fall.

Properties—Steeplebush is useful as an astringent, tonic in diarrhoea, etc.

Dose—A teaspoonful of the root or leaves, cut small or granulated, to a cup of boiling water. Drink cold 1 cupful during the day, a large mouthful at a time; of the tincture, 5 to 20 min.

STICKLEWORT
(Agrimonia Eupatoria, Rose Family)

Common Names—Cockleburr or Agrimony.

Medicinal Part—The root and leaves.

Description—Sticklewort has a reddish, tapering and creeping root, with brown stems covered with soft, silky hairs; two or three feet high; leaves alternate, sessile, interruptedly pinnate. The stipule of the upper leaves large, rounded, dentate, or palmate. The flowers grow at the top of the stem, are yellow, small and very numerous, one above another in long spikes, after which come rough heads hanging downwards, which will stick to garments or anything that rubs against them.

This perennial plant is found in Europe, Canada and the United States, along roadsides, and in fields and woods, flowering in July or August. Both the flowers and roots are fragrant, but harsh and astringent to the taste, and yield their properties to water or alcohol.

Properties and Uses—It is a mild astringent. Useful in all conditions calling for such a remedy. It is exceedingly useful in coughs resulting from cold.

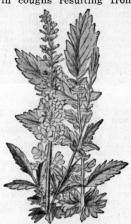

STICKLEWORT

As a gargle for throat and mouth irritation, it is very serviceable. The Indians of North America and the Canadians are reported to have employed the root with advantage in many ailments.

Dose—A teaspoonful of the root or leaves, cut small, steeped into a cup of boiling water. Drink a cupful every day, a few mouthfuls at a time. Of the tincture, ¼ to ½ fl. dr.

STILLINGIA
(Stillingia Sylvatica, Spurge Family)

Common Names—Queen's Root, Queen's Delight, Yaw Root and Silver Leaf.

Medicinal Part—The root.

Description—This perennial herb has a glabrous, somewhat angled stem from two to four feet high, which when broken gives a milky sap. The leaves are sessile, somewhat leathery, and tapering at the base. The flowers are yellow, and arranged on a terminal spike. Fruit, a three-grained capsule.

Stillingia grows in sandy soils, and is a native of the southern part of the United States. The root is the part used.

It should be used as soon after being gathered as possible, as age impairs its properties. The latter yield to water, but are better extracted by diluted alcohol. Its properties appear to be owing to a very acrid oil, known as the Oil of Stillingia.

Properties and Uses—In large doses Stillingia vomits and purges, but it is not in much favor today for those purposes, though there is some evidence of its alterative effect in smaller doses. The oil, unless well incorporated with some mucilaginous or saccharine substance, should never be used internally.

Dose—A teaspoonful of the root, cut small or granulated, to a cup of boiling water. Drink cold, one cupful during the day, a large mouthful at a time; of the tincture, 5 to 20 min.

STONE ROOT

(Collinsonia Canadensis, Mint Family)
Common Names — Hardrock, Horseweed, Heal-all, Richweed, Oxbalm, Knob Root, Wild Citronella.

Medicinal Part—The plant.

Description—This plant has a knobby root and a four-sided stem, from one to four feet in height. The leaves are thin, broadly ovate, acuminate, coarsely serrate, from six to eight inches long, and from two to four broad. Flowers large, corolla greenish-yellow; stamens two, and very long; seeds four, of which two or three are sterile.

This plant grows in moist woods from Canada to Carolina, and flowers from July until September. The whole plant has a strong odor and a pungent and spicy taste. The odor of the fresh root is slightly disagreeable. The whole plant is generally used, and has its value. The chief virtues of the plant are, however, concentrated in the root, which should always be used when fresh. Its active principle is Collinsonin, which name is derived from its discoverer, Peter Collinson.

Properties and Uses—It is used with good effect in a variety of conditions. It is a very fair stimulant, and a gentle tonic and diuretic. The largest dose is five grains; the average dose two grains. The infusion or decoction of the plant may be moderately used without additional remedies; but in about every case a skillful combination of the latter with other standard preparations is necessary to insure best results. Stone Root is used externally—the leaves particularly—in fomentation and poultice, for bruises, wounds, blows, sprains, cuts, etc.

Dose—A teaspoonful of the root, cut small or granulated, to a cup of boiling water. Drink cold one cupful during the day, a large mouthful at a time; of the tincture, 5 to 20 min.

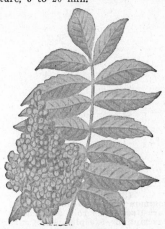

SUMACH

(Rhus Glabrum, Sumac Family)
Common Names—Smooth Sumach, Scarlet Sumach.

Medicinal Part—The bark and fruit.

Description—Sumach is a shrub, from six to fifteen feet high, consisting of many straggling branches, covered with a pale-gray bark, having occasionally a reddish tint. The leaves are alternate, consist of from six to fifteen leaflets, which are lanceolate, acuminate, acutely serrate, shining and green above, whitish beneath, becoming red in the fall. The flowers are greenish red, and fruit a small red drupe, hanging in clusters, with a crimson down, extremely sour to the taste, which is due to malate of lime.

Sumach grows in the thickets and waste grounds of Canada and the United States. It flowers in June and July, but matures its fruit in September and October. The bark and berries are officinal. The berries should be gathered before the rains have washed away the acid properties which reside in their external, downy efflorescence. Both the bark and the berries yield their active influence to water. Great care is to be taken in the selection of several species of Rhus, as many of them are highly poisonous.

Properties and Uses—The berries are rather widely used in medicine for their astringent effect. A gargle prepared from them has given good results in throat irritation.

Dose—A teaspoonful of the bark to a cup of boiling water. Drink cold one or two cupfuls a day, a large mouthful at a time; of the tincture, ¼ to ½ fl. dr.

SUMMER SAVORY
(Satureja Hortensis, Mint Family)
Common Names—Bean Herb, Bohnenkraut.

Medicinal Part—The leaves.

Description—This annual plant has a branching, bushy stem, about eighteen inches in height, woody at the base, frequently changing to purple. The leaves are numerous, small entire, and acute at the end. The flowers are pink-colored. Calyx tubular, corolla bilabiate, stamens diverging.

It is a native of the south of France. It is extensively cultivated for culinary purposes in Europe and America, and flowers in July and August. The leaves are the part employed. They have an aromatic odor and taste analogous to those of thyme.

Properties and Uses—It is a stimulant, carminative. A warm infusion is beneficial in wind colic.

Dose—A teaspoonful of the leaves to a cup of boiling water. Drink cold one or two cupfuls a day, a large mouthful at a time. Of the tincture, ½ to 1 fl. dr. Satureja Montana, or Winter Savory, possesses similar qualities.

SUNDEW
(Drosera Rotundifolia)
Part Used—The whole herb.

Description—This plant is found in moist sandy or peaty soil in Canada and United States. The leaves are round on long stems extending from the root. They are thickly covered with hairy glands that exude drops of a clear glutinous fluid that have the appearance of dew drops which deceive insects alighting on the leaves. Having caught a victim the leaf slowly folds up and digests it.

Properties—Sundew has been esteemed by the Eclectic School of Medicine for relief of the spasm of whooping cough and employed for other pectoral purposes, but its virtues are not conceded by other schools of medicine.

Dose—A teaspoonful of the herb, cut small to a pint of boiling water. Take 1 teaspoonful at a time as required; of the tincture, 2 to 5 min.

SUMBUL
(Ferula Sumbul)
Common Name—Musk Root.

Part Used—The root.

Description—Sumbul is a native of Central and Western Asia. The dried root is ¼ to 4 inches thick, dusky brown, annulate, longitudinally wrinkled or with smooth, silver grey periderm, interior light brown, spongy, porous with numerous brownish yellow resin reservoirs, odor musk like, taste bitter.

Properties—Sumbul has been credited with a soothing influence over the nervous system in ordinary cases and employed by some for that quality.

Dose—A teaspoonful of the root to a pint of boiling water. Drink cold a mouthful 2 or 3 times a day. Tincture 2 to 5 min.

SWAMP BEGGAR'S TICK
(Bidens Connata)
Common Names—Cockhold Herb, Beggar's Tick, Harvest Lice, Spanish Needles.

Medicinal Parts—The herb.

Description—This herb has a smooth stem, from one to three feet high. The leaves are lanceolate, opposite, serrate, acuminate, and decurrent on the petiole. Flowers, terminal; florets, yellow; and fruit, a wedge-formed achenium.

Properties and Uses—Root and seeds are employed domestically as an emmenagogue to some extent, as well as for the purposes of an expectorant in throat irritation.

Dose—A teaspoonful of the root, cut small or granulated, to a cup of boiling water. Drink cold, one cupful during the day, a large mouthful at a time; of the tincture, 5 to 20 min.

Bidens Bipinnata, or Spanish Needles, and Bidens Frondosa, or Beggar Tick, can be employed, medically, the same.

SWEET CICELY
(Osmorrhiza longistylis—Ammiaceae Family)
Common Names—Anise root, Sweet Anise, Sweet Jarvil.

Part Used—The root.

Description—Found in rich woods and thickets from Alabama to Kansas, South Dakota, Ontario, south to South Carolina. Root has a sweet anise-like fragrance. Plant grows about 20″ high: foliage is glabrous or finely pubescent: leaf segments mainly ovate or oblong-ovate. Flowers white and inconspicuous. Seeds long, narrow and adhere to clothing, fur, etc.

Properties—Aromatic, carminative, expectorant, stomachic.

SWEET FERN
(Comptonia Asplenifolia)

Common Name—Spleenwort Bush.

Part Used—The entire plant.

Description—This shrub grows 1 to 3 feet high, slender, erect and spreading branches, bark reddish brown, leaves thin narrow, hairy when young; are linear oblong 3 to 6 inches long and ¼ inch to one inch wide, deeply divided into many lobes, the margins of which are sometimes sparingly toothed. The male flowers are produced in cylindrical catkins in clusters at the end of the branches and are about 1 inch in length. The female flowers are born in egg shaped catkins. The whole plant has a spicy, aromatic odor.

Properties—Sweet Fern is useful for its tonic and astringent properties, as in diarrhoea.

Dose—A teaspoonful of the plant to a cup of boiling water. Drink cold 1 or 2 cupfuls a day, a large mouthful at a time; of the tincture, ½ to 1 fl. dr.

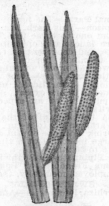

SWEET FLAG
(Acorus Calamus—Arum Family)

Common Names—Myrtle Flag, Sweet Grass, Sweet Cane, Sweet Root, Sweet Rush.

Medicinal Part—Root.

Description—A perennial herb, resembling the blue flag. It is not an Iris, however, and may be distinguished from it by its corm and the aromatic taste of its leaves. It grows on the borders of ponds and marshes throughout the United States.

Properties and Uses—It is a mild aromatic and employed as a household rem-

edy for upset stomach, sour stomach, and associated conditions. In some countries it seems to be employed for various purposes.

Dose—A teaspoonful of the root to a cup of boiling water. Drink cold one or two cupfuls a day, a large mouthful at a time; of the tincture, ½ to 1 fl. dr.

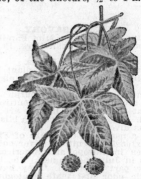

SWEET GUM
(Liquidambar Styraciflua, Witch Hazel Family)

Common Names—Red Gum, Star-leaved Gum.

Medicinal Part—The bark and concrete juice.

Description—The Sweet Gum tree grows to the height of from fifty to sixty feet. Its bark is gray and deeply furrowed, and there are corky ridges on the branches; the leaves are palmate, rounded, smooth and shining, fragrant when bruised, and turn a deep red in the fall. Fruit, a kind of strobile.

This tree is very abundant in the Southern and Middle States, and can be found in the moist woods of nearly all parts of the Union. From incisions made in the tree a gum exudes which is resinous and adhesive, and somewhat like white turpentine in appearance.

Properties and Uses—As a household remedy for coughs resulting from colds it enjoys much favor. It is also very useful when made into an ointment.

Dose—A teaspoonful of the bark, cut small or granulated, to a cup of boiling water. Drink cold, one cupful during the day, a large mouthful at a time; of the tincture, ¼ to ½ fl. dr.

* * * *

Man should observe kind nature's laws, and from them learn result and cause.

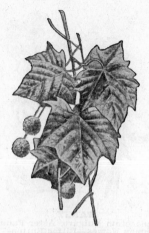

SYCAMORE
(Acer Pseudo-Platinus—Soapberry Family)
Medicinal Part—Bark.

Description—A fine tree with spreading branches, ample five-lobed leaves, whitish and rather downy beneath on long reddish petioles, the lobes toothed, elongated. The flowers are clusters and greenish; wings of the pubescent fruit moderately spreading.

Properties and Uses—Astringent, opthalmicum and vulnerary.

TACAMAHAC
(Populus Balsamifera)
Common Name—Balsam Poplar.
Medicinal Part—The buds.

Description—This tree, also called Tachamahac Poplar, attains the height of from fifty to seventy feet, with a trunk about eighteen inches in diameter. The branches are smooth, round and deep brown. The leaves are ovate, gradually tapering and pointed, deep-green above, and smooth on both sides.

This tree is found in Siberia, and in the northern parts of the United States and Canada. In America it is in blossom in April. The leaf-buds are the officinal part. They should be collected in the spring, in order that the fragrant, resinous matter with which they are covered may be properly separated in boiling water, for upon this their virtues depend. They have an agreeable, incense-like odor, and an unpleasant,

bitterish taste. The balsamic juice is collected in Canada in shells, and sent to Europe under the name of Tacamahaca. Alcohol, or spirits, is the proper solvent. The Populus Balsamifera is generally confounded with the Populus Candicans, from whose buds we get the virtues known as the Balm of Gilead; but it is much the superior tree for medical purposes.

Properties and Uses—The buds have been employed internally as a stimulating expectorant but now seem to be used chiefly for external purposes as counter-irritants in the form of ointments and plasters.

Dose—A teaspoonful of the buds to a cup of boiling water. Drink cold one or two cupfuls a day, a large mouthful at a time; of the tincture, ½ to 1 fl. dr.

TAG ALDER
(Alnus Rubra, Birch Family)
Common Names—Common Alder, Smooth Alder, Red Alder.

Description—This is a well known shrub, growing in clumps, and forming thickets on the borders of ponds and rivers and in swamps. The stems are numerous, and from six to fifteen feet high. The layers are obovate, acuminate, smooth and green, from two to four inches long.

The Alnus Rubra is indigenous to Europe and America, and blossoms in March and April. The bark is the part used medicinally.

Properties and Uses—The bark is commonly known to be alterative and emetic, and is preferred by some for those purposes, but it is inferior to Rock Rose or Stillingia, of which there are many varieties, some of which have and some of which have not been classified.

Dose—One teaspoonful to a cup of boiling water. Drink cold 1 or 2 cups a day; of the tincture, ½ to 1 fl. dr.

TALL RAGWEED
(Ambrosia Trifida—Ambrosia Family)
Common Names—Great or Giant Ragweed, Horse-cane.
Part Used—Leaves.

Description—A very tall weed sometimes growing from 6 to 9 feet high. Found on river banks, cultivated ground, and waste places from Florida to Texas, Colorado to Canada. Coarse hispidulous or hirsute leaves and stem. Upper small leaves are lancelote, lower leaves 3 or 5 lobed. Small flowers yellowish green.

Properties—The leaves are reputed to be stimulating, astringent and antiseptic.

TALL NASTURTIUM

Common Names—Water Cress.

Medicinal Parts—Leaves and roots.

Description—Tall Nasturtium grows in running water. The branching stems are 1 to 2 feet long and generally extend with leaves above the water. The leaves are somewhat fleshy, elliptic and in pairs of 3 to 7. The flowers are white and small.

Properties and Uses—Water cress is a literal storehouse of natural vitamins, minerals and trace elements.

Dose—A teaspoonful of the leaves of roots to a cup of boiling water. Drink cold, one or two cupfuls a day, a large mouthful at a time; of the tincture, ½ to 1 fl. dr.

TAMARIND
(Tamarindus Indica—Legume Family)

Part Used—Pulp of fruit.

Description and Uses—A native tree of Africa, now found over a large part of the tropical world where it is grown for its fruit and as a shade tree. Tamarind is a large handsome, spreading, symmetrical tree with small pinnate leaves that fold up at night-time. The fruit of Tamarind is a thin shell pod containing a cinnamon brown sweetish acidulated pulp that is used in many ways. Tamarind has refrigerant and gentle laxative properties. It is widely used to make refreshing cooling drinks, containing both citric and tartaric acid. They form an important ingredient in Indian Cookery, especially in curries, and in preserving or pickling of fish. Tamarinds were an important article of diet on old-time sailing ships, as the acid and sugar content of the fruit helped offset the starchy diet of seamen.

An old "Bajan" friend informed me that at one time, great quantities of Tamarinds in molasses, were shipped from Barbados to Leghorn Italy, and used as a laxative medicine.

Tamarind pulp is highly nutritious, rich in Vitamin B, and in calcium, riboflavin, and other food values. Natives in the tropics use the tender fresh leaves of Tamarind as poultices and as fomentations.

The pulverized seeds are also used to make a very strong cement for wood. The leaves yield a yellow dye, and the trunk of the tree yields beautiful red timber.

The wood is very hard and is used to make tools, furniture, etc.

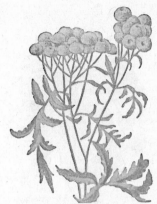

TANSY
(Tanacetum Vulgare, Aster Family)

Common Names—Bitter Buttons, Parsley Fern.

Medicinal Part—The herb.

Description—Tansy has a perennial creeping root, and an erect herbaceous stem, one to three feet high. The leaves are smoothish, dark green; flowers, golden yellow; fruit, an achenium.

Indigenous to Europe, but has been introduced into this country and cultivated by many; but grows also spontaneously in old grounds, along roads, flowering in the latter part of summer. Drying impairs much of the activity of the plant. It contains volatile oil, wax, stearine, chlorophyll, bitter resin, yellow coloring matter, tannin with gallic acid, bitter extractive gum, and tanacetic acid, which is crystallizable, and precipitates lime, baryta and oxide of lead.

Properties and Uses—Tansy has been said to add to the medicinal virtues of aromatic bitters the qualities of an irritant narcotic. While it may be capable of beneficial use in the hands of a skilled person, it should be greatly diluted, 1 teaspoonful to a pint of water.

THUJA
(Thuja Occidentalis, Pine Family)

Common Names—Arbor-Vitae, Yellow Cedar.

Parts Used—Branchlets and leaves.

Description—The Arbor Vitae or Thuja is a handsome ornamental evergreen, much cultivated for hedge rows and windbreaks, grows 20 to 40 feet high with a trunk diameter of 2 to 4 feet. The trunk often buttressed at the base, and sometimes distorted and twisted; branches short, the lower ones horizontal, the upper closely crowded with foliage and forming a dense conical head. Bark light brown, shredded, separating into long narrow strips. The leaves are bright green in overlapping scales, 4 rows on the two-edged small twigs, the middle row flat with a tiny slightly raised tubercle on each scale; with an aromatic odor when crushed. Cones small, when very young pale green, about ½ inch long; when old, light reddish brown with 6 to 12 pointless, thin oblong scales.

Properties and Uses—The leaves and twigs of Thuja are useful as a counter-irritant in the relief of muscular aches and pains, and for the usual purposes of such a remedy. Boiled with lard they form an excellent salve.

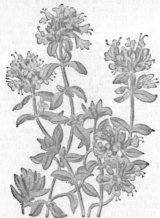

THYME
(Thymus Vulgaris)
Common Name—Garden Thyme.
Medicinal Part—The herb.

Description—Thyme is a small undershrub, with numerous erect stems, procumbent at base, and from six to ten inches in height. The leaves are oblong, ovate, lanceolate and numerous. The flowers are bluish purple, small, and arranged on leafy, whorled spikes.

A native of Europe, but introduced into this country, and extensively cultivated in gardens for culinary purposes. It blossoms in the summer, when it should be collected and carefully dried.

It has a strong, pungent, spicy taste and odor, both of which are retained by careful drying. The herb yields its properties to boiling water and alcohol.

Properties and Uses—Thyme seems to enjoy rather common use in throat and bronchial irritation, and also to be domestically employed for the spasms of Whooping Cough by some. The warm infusion is useful in flatulence, colic, and to promote perspiration. The leaves are used externally in fomentation.

Dose—A teaspoonful of the herb to a cup of boiling water. Drink cold one or two cupfuls a day, a large mouthful at a time; of the tincture, ½ to 1 fl. dr.

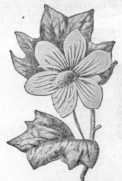

TULIP TREE
(Liriodendron Tulipifera—Magnolia Family)
Common Names—Lyre Tree, Canoewood, Lime Tree.
Medicinal Part—Bark.

Description—Tulip tree is a magnificent tree sometimes attaining the height of 190 feet. It is found growing in rich soil. The yellow with greenish and orange flowers blossom in the late spring. The leaves have two short side lobes and the end appears as if cut off.

Properties and Uses—Bitters, aromatic, stimulant, febrifuge and vermifuge.

TURKEY CORN
(Corydalis Formosa, Poppy Family)
Common Names—Wild Turkey Pea, Stagger Weed, Choice Dielytra.
Medicinal Part—The root.

Description—This indigenous perennial plant has a tuberous root, and a stem from six to ten inches in height. The leaves are radical, rising from ten to fifteen inches high, and somewhat triternate. The scape is naked, eight to twelve inches high, and bearing from six to ten reddish purple nodding flowers. The fruit is a pod-shaped, many-seeded capsule.

This beautiful little plant flowers very early in the spring, and the root should only be gathered while the plant is in flower. It grows in rich soil, on hills, among rocks, and old decayed timber, and is found westward and south of New York to North Carolina. The alkaloid, Corydalia, is the active principle.

Properties and Uses—Tonic, diuretic and alterative. Its tonic properties are similar to Gentian, Columbo and other pure bitters. Its beneficial action as an alterative renders it one of the best botanical drugs.

Dose—A teaspoonful of the root, cut small or granulated, to a cup of boiling water. Drink cold one cupful during the day, a large mouthful at a time; of the tincture, 5 to 20 min.

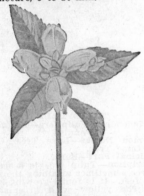

TURTLEBLOOM
(Chelone Glabra, Figwort Family)
Common Names—Snake Head, Salt Rheum Weed, Balmony, Turtle Head, Shell-flower.
Medicinal Part—The leaves.
Description—This is a perennial, smooth, herbaceous plant, with simple erect stem about two or three feet high. The leaves are opposite, sessile, oblong-lanceolate, acuminate, serrate and of a dark shining green color. The fruit is a capsule.

This valuable medical plant is found in the United States, in damp soils,

flowering in August and September. The flowers are ornamental, and vary in color, but inodorous, and impart their virtues to water and alcohol.

Properties and Uses—It is tonic and aperient and believed by some to have a beneficial effect on the liver. In small doses it is a good tonic in and during convalescence. An ointment made from the fresh leaves is valuable for the itching and irritation of piles.

Dose—One teaspoonful to a cup of boiling water. Drink cold 1 or 2 cupfuls a day. Tincture, ½ to 1 fl. dr.

TWIN LEAF
(Jeffersonia Diphylla, Barberry Family)
Common Names—Rheumatism Root, Ground Squirrel Pea, Yellow Root.
Medicinal Part—The root.
Description—This plant is perennial, and has a horizontal rhizoma or fleshy root, with matted fibrous radicles. The stem is simple, naked, one-flowered, and from eight to fourteen inches in height. The leaves are in pairs, broader than long, ending in an obtuse point, smooth and petioled; flowers, large and white; fruit, an obovate capsule.

This plant is found from New York to Maryland and Virginia, and in many parts of the Western States. It grows chiefly in limestone soil, but also is found in woods and near rivers, irrespective of limestone, and flowers in April and May. The root is the part used, and its virtues are extracted by water or alcohol. A chemical analysis of this plant showed it to contain tannic acid, gum, starch, pectin, fatty resin, bitter matter, similar to polygalic acid, carbonate and sulphate of potassa, lime, iron, magnesia, silica, etc.

Properties and Uses—In small doses it seems to be expectorant and tonic, and in large doses, emetic. As a gargle it is useful in throat irritations.

Dose—A teaspoonful of the root, cut small or granulated, to a cup of boiling water. Drink cold one cupful during the day, a large mouthful at a time; of the tincture, 5 to 20 min.

VANILLA
(Vanilla Aromatica)
Medicinal Part—The fruit or pods.
Description—Vanilla Aromatica is a shrubby, climbing, aerial parasite, growing in the clefts of rocks, or attaching itself to the trunks of trees. It suspends itself to contiguous objects, and is truly an aerial plant. The stem is round, about as thick as the finger, from twenty to thirty feet in length, and often thicker at the summit than at the base.

The leaves are alternate, oblong, entire, on short petioles, green fleshy, and pointed by a species of bean, yellow or buff color, of an agreeable aromatic odor; the beans must be dried with care or they will lose their properties.

Vanilla grows in Mexico and other parts of tropical South America. There are several species which are supposed to furnish the vanilla of commerce. It yields its virtues to water or alcohol.

Properties and Uses—Vanilla has been employed for its stimulating action, but its use today is as a flavoring agent.

VIRGINIA SNAKE ROOT
(Serpentaria Aristolochia)

Common Names—Red River Snake Root, Texas Snake Root, Sangrel, Sangree Root, Birthwort, Serpentaria.

Medicinal Part—The dried rhizone and roots.

Description—Virginia Snake Root is a perennial plant with one or more slender erect, zigzag jointed stems, about one foot high, purple toward the base; leaves cordate, ovate, 2 to 3 in. long, pale green, entire, flowers June to July, few purple, due to calyx which is tubular inflated at both ends and bent like letter S. The rhizone has numerous stem scars and bears a dense tress of thin branching roots about 3 in. long with camphorous odor and bitter aromatic taste.

Properties—Virginia Snake Root belongs to the aromatic bitters and in proper dosage promotes appetite and digestion in indicated conditions. In large doses, however, it is irritant, causing vomiting, vertigo, purging, etc.

Dose—Steep a teaspoonful of the granulated roots into a cup of boiling water for half an hour. Strain. Take a tablespoonful 3 to 6 times a day. Of the tincture 5 to 20 min.

WAFER ASH
(Ptela Trifoliata, Rue Family)

Common Names—Wing Seed, Shrubby Trefoil, Swamp Dogwood, Hop Tree.

Medicinal Part—The bark and the root.

Description—This is a shrub from six to eight feet in height, with the leaves trifoliate, and marked with pellucid dots; the leaflets are sessile, ovate, shortly acuminate, downy beneath when young. The flowers are polygamous, greenish-white, nearly half an inch in diameter, and of disagreeable odor. Stamens, mostly four; style short, and fruit a two-celled samara.

Wafer Ash or Ptela, is a shrub common to America, growing most abundantly west of the Alleghanies, in sandy, moist places and edges of woods, and also in rocky places. It flowers in June. The bark of the root is officinal, and yields its virtues to boiling water. Alcohol, however, is its best solvent. Ptelein is its active principle.

Properties and Uses—It is especially tonic and unirritating. It is said to be very useful as a promoter of appetite. It may be tolerated by the stomach when other tonics are rejected.

Dose—A teaspoonful of the bark of the root cut small to a cup of boiling water. Drink cold one cupful during the day, a large mouthful at a time; of the tincture 5 to 20 min.

WAHOO
(Euonymus, Atropurpureus)
Staff Tree Family

Common Names—Spindle Tree, Burning Bush, Indian Arrow Wood, Euonymus.

Medicinal Part—The bark of the root.

Description—Wahoo is a small shrub or bush, with smooth branches and from five to ten feet high. The leaves are from two to five inches in length, lanceolate, acute, and finely serrated. Flowers dark purple, and the fruit a crimson, five celled capsule. There is another variety known as Euonymus Americanus, which is equally useful medicinally, and this and the foregoing are both known by the name of Wahoo better than by any other title.

These plants grow in many sections of the United States, in woods and thickets, and in river bottoms, flowering in June. The bark of the root has a bitter and unpleasant taste in its natural state, and yields its qualities to water and alcohol.

Properties and Uses—Wahoo has been employed for its peculiar cathartic effect, but is not recommended for home use.

WALTHERIA AMERICANA

(Sterculia or Chocolate Family)

Part Used—The leaves and bark of root.

Description—This bush is found in the Florida peninsula, Keys, West Indies, Mexico and in most of the islands of tropical Pacific. The bush grows to about 5 feet high—lower branches are woody. The branches and leaves are densely tomentose to softly villous with stellate hairs. Leaves are ½ to 3 inches long, opposite, ovate-oblong and broadcast at the base. The sweet scented small yellow flowers grow in dense axillary clusters.

Properties and Uses — Mucilaginous, demulcent emollient and febrifuge.

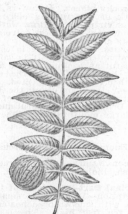

WALNUT, BLACK
(Juglans Nigra—Walnut Family)
Common Name—European Walnut.
Medicinal Part—The bark.
Description—Black Walnut is a large tree with dark, rough branches; stalks and shoots not clammy, minutely downy. The leaflets are smoothish, ovate-lanceolate and serrate. The fruit is spherical.
Properties and Uses—Astringent.

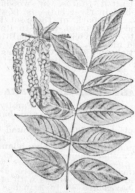

WALNUT (WHITE)
(Juglans Cinerea, Walnut Family)
Common Names—Butternut, Oil Nut.
Medicinal Parts—The inner bark of the root, and leaves.

Description—This indigenous tree attains a height of from thirty to fifty feet, with a trunk about four feet in diameter; the branches are wide-spreading, and covered with a smooth gray bark. The leaves are alternate, twelve to twenty inches long, and consist of seven or eight pairs of leaflets, which are oblong-lanceolate, and finally serrate. Male and female flowers distinct upon the same tree. Fruit is dark colored hard nut, kernel oily, pleasant flavored and edible.
Properties and Uses—Butternut is a mild cathartic whose action has been likened to that of Rhubarb. It appears to have been used as a laxative during our Revolutionary War.
Dose—A teaspoonful of the inner bark of the root, cut small or granulated to a cup of boiling water. Drink cold one cupful a day, a large mouthful at a time; of the tincture, 5 to 20 min.

WATER ERYNGO
(Eryngium Aquaticum, Carrot Family
Common Names—Button Snake Root, Rattlesnake's Master, Rattlesnake Weed, Cornsnake Root.
Medicinal Part—The root.
Description—This indigenous, perennial herb has a simple stem from one to five feet high. The root is a tuber, the leaves are one or two feet long, half an inch to an inch wide, and taper-pointed. The flowers are white or pale, and inconspicuous.
This plant is indigenous, growing in swamps and low, wet lands from Virginia to Texas, especially on prairie lands, blossoming in August. The root is the officinal part. Water or alcohol extracts its properties.
Properties and Uses—It is diuretic, stimulant, diaphoretic, expectorant, and, in large doses, emetic. Very useful, when chewed, to promote the flow of saliva and then to aid digestion. A good substitute for Senega.
Dose—A heaping teaspoonful of the root to a pint of boiling water. Take a tablespoonful 2 to 4 times a day, cold. Of the tincture, 10 to 20 min.

WATER PEPPER
(Polygonum Punctatum, Buckwheat Family)
Common Names—Smartweed, Water Smartweed.
Medicinal Part—The whole herb.
Description—This is an annual plant, with smooth stem, branches often decumbent at the base, of reddish or greenish brown color, and growing from one to two feet high. The leaves are

alternate, lanceolate, petiolate, with pellucid dots, wavy, and scabrous on the margin. The flowers are small, greenish-white, greenish-pink, and are disposed in loose, slender, drooping, but finally erect spikes.

It is a well known plant, growing in England and America, in ditches, low lands, among rubbish, and about brooks, and water courses. It flowers in August and September. The whole plant is medicinal. It has a bitter, pungent, acrid taste, and imparts its virtues to alcohol and water. It should be collected and made into a tincture while fresh. When it is eight months old it is almost worthless. The English variety of the plant possesses the same properties.

Properties and Uses—It is a stimulant, diuretic, diaphoretic, etc. The infusion in cold water has been found serviceable in common colds and coughs.

It is used as a wash in skin irritation. The fresh leaves bruised with the leaves of Plantain, and moistened with oil of Turpentine, and applied to the skin, will speedily vesicate. The infusion in cold water forms an excellent local application. The decoction or infusion in hot water is not so active as when prepared in cold or warm water.

Dose—A teaspoonful of the herb, cut small or granulated, to a cup of boiling water. Drink cold, one cupful during the day, a large mouthful at a time. Of the tincture, 30 to 60 min.

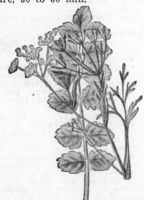

WATER PIMPERNEL
(Pimpinella-Saxifraga)
Common Names—Burnet, Pimpinella.
Parts Used—The root and herb.

Description—This plant reaches a height of 1 to 3 feet, nearly smooth with numerous lance-oblong coarsely toothed leaflets, often heart-shaped at base and hairy. The perfectly white flowers appear in September and October.

Properties—Pimpernel is useful as a stomachic, diuretic and diaphoretic.

Dose—A teaspoonful of the root or herb, cut small or granulated to a cup of boiling water. Drink cold, one cupful during the day, a large mouthful at a time; of the tincture, 5 to 20 min.

WHITE HOLLY
(Ilex Opaca)
Common Name—American Holly.
Parts Used—Leaves and bark.

Description—A native shrub or tree 15 to 40 feet high with a slender brown gray, rather smooth bark, 10 to 20 inches in diameter and spreading slender branches, horizontal or drooping; foliage olive or bronzy green. Leaves evergreen, leathery, elliptical, deep olive or yellow olive green, spiny, 2 to 3 inches long. Flowers white in loose clusters at the bases of the leaves or branchlets, with 4 to 5 oval or obovate petals. Fruit scarlet, not glossy, berrylike about 2-3 inch in diameter, short stemmed, persisting through the winter.

Properties and Uses—Leaves and bark are purgative, diuretic and emetic, and hence useful in promoting proper elimination of the waste products of the body—a most important function.

WHITE MELILOT
(Melilotus Alba—Pea Family
Common Names—Sweet White Clover, Bokhara Clover, Sweet Lucerne, Sweet Melilot.
Parts Used—Flowers.

Description—A tall weed from Europe, now found over a large part of the U.S. and southern Canada, especially along roadsides, meadows, cultivated grounds and waste places. Small trifoliate leaflets are narrow or oblong. Tiny white flowers are borne on slender racemes. Seedpods are tiny oval or roundish. The entire plant has a sweet vanilla-like scent when dried, containing considerable coumarin.

Medicinal Uses—Expectorant and diuretic. Used to flavor tobacco, cheese, and other products.

Used also in sachets, and potpourri mixtures.

A yellow flowering species (Melilotus officinalis) is used in the same way as White Melilot.

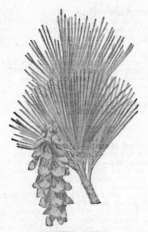

WHITE PINE
(Pinus Strobus)

Common Names—Deal Pine, Soft Pine.

Part Used—Inner bark and sprigs.

Description—This is a handsome, plumy foliaged, straight-stemmed evergreen tree, 50 to 75 feet high and occasionally 180 feet high; trunk diameter 2 to 5 feet, bark perpendicularly seamed, dark gray, brown, rough. The needles soft, slender, delicate, three-sided, 3 to 4 inches long, light or dark bluish brown, the inner side with a strong line of white bloom; the sheaths deciduous, always in clusters of five. The cones 4 to 6 inches long, narrow, cylindrical, the scales broad-wedge shaped, without spines or prickles.

Properties and Uses—The bark and sprigs are very useful as an expectorant, to modify quality and quantity of the mucous secretions, and to favor its removal, in common colds and coughs. It should be mixed, however, with wild cherry, sassafras and spikenard.

Dose—One teaspoonful to a cup of boiling water. Drink a large mouthful as often as necessary; of the tincture, ½ to 1 fl. dr.

A strong tea of the Boneset will help break up an ordinary Cold quickly. Just make and sweeten to taste.

WHITE SANDAL
(Santalum Album)

Common Names—White, Red, Yellow Sandalwood, White Saunders.

Medicinal Part—The wood and oil.

Description—The several varieties of Sandal are of the same medicinal value and all furnish Oil of Sandal of good quality. Sandal is a small tree 20 to 30 feet high, bark greyish brown, leaves oval, smooth, glaucous, flower small, numerous cymes, odorless, color variable violet pink, red and yellow. The heartwood of White Sandal is yellow; the outside or sap wood is white. The heart wood only should be used.

PROPERTIES—The oil, extract and infusion or tea are astringent, stimulant, diuretic, expectorant. Apparently much like Copaiba and Cubebs in action the oil is employed for the somewhat peculiar urinary action for which remedies of that class are commonly used and popularly known. Extensively used in perfumery. The wood is used in making temple incense and by art-cabinet makers.

Dose—Steep a heaping teaspoonful of the wood, cut into small pieces, into a cup of boiling water for half an hour. When cold drink one or two cupfuls a day, a good mouthful at a time. Of the tincture 20 to 40.

WHITE WEED
(Leucanthemum Vulgare, Aster Family)

Common Names—Ox Eye Daisy, White Daisy.

Medicinal Parts—The leaves and flowers.

Description—This is a perennial herb, having an erect, branching, and furrowed stem, from one to two feet high. The leaves are few, alternate, lanceolate-serrate, the lower ones petiolate; the upper ones small, sublate, and sessile.

The plant was introduced into the United States from Europe, and is a very troublesome weed to farmers in nearly every section. It bears white flowers in June and July. The leaves are odorous and somewhat acid; the flowers are bitterish; they impart their virtues to water.

Properties and Uses—While it seems to have some medicinal uses and has been mentioned as an external application for some purposes, it is chiefly employed as an insect powder for fleas, etc. The fresh leaves or flowers will destroy or drive away fleas.

Dose—Steep a heaping teaspoonful of this herb into a cup of boiling water for half an hour. When cold drink 1 or 2 cupfuls a day; a good mouthful at a time. Of the tincture, ½ to 1 fl. dr.

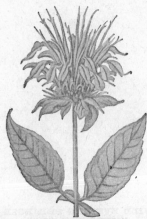

WILD BERGAMOT
(Monarda Fistulosa—Mint Family)
Common Names—Wild Burgamot.
Medicinal Part—Leaves.

Description—A soft, downy or smooth-ish herb, leaves petioled, the floral ones often whitish and the calyx hairy in the throat, the corolla rose-color, purple or white. Found growing in dry soil.

Properties and Uses—Aromatic, bitter, nervine, stomachic.

WILD BULL NETTLE
(Solanum Carolinense)
Common Names—Bull Nettle, Band Brier, Horse Nettle, Sand Brier.
Medicinal Part—The root and dried berries and leaves.

Description—Bull Nettle is a native perennial common on dry fields and sandy or gravelly banks of rivers and lakes. It is rough, hairy, about 1 foot high, with ovate-oblong or sinuate-lobed leaves; yellowish prickles, and pale blue or white flowers about 1 inch wide.

Properties and Uses—The root of Bull Nettle is the most used. It seems to be somewhat anodyne and capable of beneficial use as an adjunct to the bromides, or in combination with other medicinal agents, but is of limited virtue when used alone.

Dose—Steep a teaspoonful of the root into a cup of boiling water for half an hour. Drink a half cupful at night upon retiring, hot or cold—or take a mouthful 3 times a day. One or two cupfuls may be taken. Tincture, ½ to 1 fl. dr.

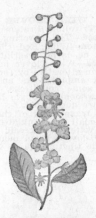

WILD CHERRY
(Prunus Serotina)
Common Names—Choke Cherry, Rum Cherry.
Medicinal Part—The inner bark.

Description—Wild Cherry grows in woods and open places. Its range extends from Nova Scotia to Florida and westward from Texas to South Dakota. The trunk is straight, bark rough black, young branches smooth and reddish brown, fine grained and hard. The leaves are thick and oval, 2 to 5 inches long; smooth and shining, bright green above and somewhat hairy on the veins beneath, toothed. The clusters of white flowers borne at the ends of leafy branches, are somewhat drooping. The cherries ripen in August and September, are globular, very dark purple or black, about the size of a pea and have a sweet astringent taste that puckers the mouth. The outside layer of the bark should be removed, the green layer is then stripped off and carefully dried. Young thin bark is the best.

Properties—Wild Cherry Bark appears to have the stomachic action of the simple bitters and also to be of value in cough syrups. For the latter purpose it is an old-time home remedy.

Dose—A teaspoonful of the inner bark to a cup of boiling water. Drink cold one or two cupfuls a day, a large mouthful at a time; of the tincture, ½ to 1 fl. dr.

133

WILD CLOVER
(Trifolium Pratense)

Parts Used—The flowering tops.

Description—Wild Red Clover is so common it needs no description.

Properties—Wild Clover has been regarded as an alterative by former generations and employed as an anti-spasmodic in some conditions, as in the spasm of whooping cough, but its virtues now are questioned.

Dose—A teaspoonful of the flowering tops, cut small or granulated, to a cup of boiling water. Drink cold one cupful during the day, a large mouthful at a time; of the tincture, 20 to 40 min.

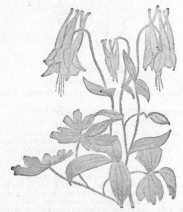

WILD COLUMBINE
(Aquilegia Vulgaris)

Common Name—Rocky Mt. Columbine.

Part Used—The entire plant.

Description—Columbine is a perennial herbaceous plant, indigenous to the U. S. and cultivated in gardens for its ornamental flowers. The root, leaves and flowers have a disagreeable odor and a bitterish acrid taste. The seeds are small black, shining.

Properties and Uses—Once regarded as a diuretic and diaphoretic but in recent years it has not been much used in medicine.

Dose—Steep a teaspoonful of the granulated plant into a cup of boiling water for half hour, strain. Take a tablespoonful 3 to 6 times a day. Of the tincture, 5 to 10 min.

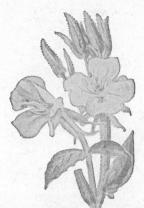

WILD EVENING PRIMROSE
(Oenothera Biennis)

Common Names — Tree Primrose, Scurvish, Scabbish, Kings Cureall, Nightwillow Herb.

Parts Used—The entire plant.

Description—This is a coarse annual or biennial weed. Its flowers do not open until evening. Stem erect, stout, 1 to 5 feet high, hairy and leafy. Leaves 1 to 6 inches long, lance-shaped, pointed at top, wavy toothed margin, narrowing at base. The spikes of yellow flowers bloom from June to October. The seed capsules are oblong and hairy, about an inch in length.

Properties—This plant has a somewhat astringent and mucilaginous taste. It has been used for coughs resulting from colds. An ointment made therefrom has been found beneficial in skin irritations.

Dose—A teaspoonful of the plant, cut small or granulated, to a cup of boiling water. Drink cold, one cupful during the day, a large mouthful at a time; of the tincture, 5 to 20 min.

WILD GERANIUM
(Geranium Maculatum, Geranium Family)

Common Names—Dove's Foot, Crow Foot, Wild Alum Root, Spotted Geranium. Cranesbill.

Medicinal Part—The root.

Description—This plant has a perennial, horizontal, thick, rough, and knotty root, with many small fibres. The stems are grayish-green, erect, blossoms large, and generally purple, mostly in pairs. The Doves Foot, or Cranebill, which grows in England, is a different plant, bearing many small bright-red, flowers of five leaves apiece, though it possesses medicinal properties similar to the American varieties.

Geranium is a native of the United States, growing in nearly all parts of it, in low grounds, open woods, etc., blossoming from April to June. The root is the officinal part. Its virtues are yielded to water and alcohol.

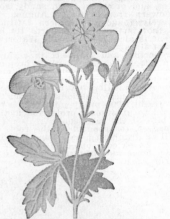

WILD ALUM ROOT

Properties and Uses—It is a strong astringent, used in diarrhoea; in infusion, with milk. Both internally and externally it may be used wherever astringents are indicated. This makes it a very popular domestic remedy, particularly for children and persons with delicate stomachs, as it is agreeable to the taste and without upsetting effect. Also employed as a gargle for throat irritation.

Dose—Steep a teaspoonful of the root, cut into small pieces, into a cup of boiling water for half an hour. When cold drink 1 or 2 cupfuls a day; a good mouthful at a time. Of the tincture, ½ to 1 fl. dr.

* * * *

"Wild Alum root is powerfully astringent, without bitterness or unpleasant taste, and is useful in diarrhoea, and other diseases where a medicine of this kind is required. Boiled in water, and mixed with sugar and milk, it is easily administered to children."

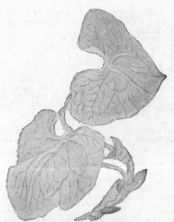

WILD GINGER
(Asarum Canadense)

Common Names—Canada Snake Root, Indian Ginger, Vermont Snake Root.

Medicinal Part—The root.

Description—The beautiful little plant may be found flowering in rich woods during April and May from Maine to Michigan, and southwards. It has two large heart-shaped leaves on long petioles from the base; deep green above and light below, soft woolly and handsomely veined. The flower is small, of a dull red color, on a weak short stem that barely raises it from the ground and often leaves it concealed by the dead leaves that carpet the woods.

Properties and Uses—Wild Ginger is an aromatic and useful in flatulency. It also has been employed as a local irritant or errhine.

Dose—A teaspoonful of the granulated root to a pint of boiling water. Take two tablespoonfuls at a time as often as required; of the tincture, 2 to 5 min.

WILD HYSSOP
(Pycnanthemum Virginicum)

Common Names—Prairie Hyssop, Virginia Thyme, Mountain Mint.

Medicinal Part—The plant.

Description—This pubescent plant has a simple stem, growing from one to two feet high. The leaves are sessile, entire, and linear; flowers are white, and fruit an achenium.

It is found in low grounds, dry hills, and plains from Ohio and Illinois, extending southward, and flowering in July and August. The whole plant is used, and has the taste and odor peculiar to the mint family.

Properties and Uses—It is carminative and, when taken hot, diaphoretic. In warm infusion it is good for gas colic and the cold infusion is a good tonic and stimulant during convalescence.

Dose—A teaspoonful of the plant to a cup of boiling water. Drink warm or cold one or two cupfuls a day, a large mouthful at a time; of the tincture, ½ to 1 fl. dr.

WILD INDIGO
(Baptistia Tinctoria, Pea Family)

Common Names—Rattle Bush, Horse fly Weed, Yellow Indigo.

Medicinal Part—The bark of the root and leaves.

Description—The blackish and woody root of this perennial plant sends up a stem which is very much branched, round, smooth, and from two to three feet high. The leaves are small and alternate, leaflets rounded at their extremity; calyx four-cleft, and fruit a short, bluish-black legume.

This small shrub grows in dry places in many parts of the United States, and bears bright yellow flowers in July and August. The fruit is of a bluish-black color in the form of an oblong pod, and contains indigo, tannin, an acid, and baptisia. Any portion of the plant, when dried, yields a blue dye, which is however, not equal in value to indigo. If the shoots are used after they acquire a green color they will cause drastic purgation. Alcohol or water will take up the active properties of this plant. Medicinally, both the root and the leaves are valuable, and deserve to be better known than they are at present as remedial agents. The virtues of the root reside chiefly in the bark.

Properties and Uses—Internally it is purgative and emetic in strong doses, while externally it may be applied to bruises, small cuts and scratches, etc. May be used as a decoction or in fomentation.

Dose—A teaspoonful of the bark of the root or the leaves, cut small, to a pint of boiling water. Take one teaspoonful at a time as required; of the tincture 2 to 5 min.

WILD JALAP
(Convolvulus Panduratus, Morning Glory Family.)

Common Names — Man-in-the-earth, Man-in-the-ground, Wild Potato, Mechameck.

Medicinal Part—The root.

Description—This has a perennial very large tapering root, from which arise several long, round, slender, purplish stems, from four to eight feet high. The leaves are cordate at base, alternate, and acuminate, and about two or three inches long. Flowers large and white, opening in the forenoon; fruit an oblong, two-celled capsule.

Wild Jalap belongs to the United States, and grows in light, sandy, soils. It flowers from June to August, but is rarely found in northern latitudes. The root is the officinal part. Its best solvent is alcohol or spirits. Water will extract its active properties.

Properties and Uses—It is regarded as a strong cathartic that promotes copious and watery stools. Often given in combination with other botanicals to moderate its action. Overdoses are to be avoided because of serious reactions that may result. The milky juice of the root is said to give some protection against the bite of the rattlesnake.

Dose—A teaspoonful of the root, cut small or granulated, to a cup of boiling water. Drink cold, one cupful during the day, a large mouthful at a time; of the tincture, 5 to 20 min.

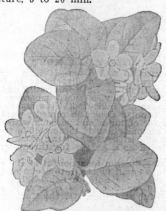

WILD MAY FLOWER
(Epigaea Repens)

Common Names—Gravel Plant, Trailing Arbutus, Ground Laurel.

Parts Used—The whole plant, especially leaves.

Description—This is a small trailing plant, with woody stems, from six to eighteen inches, which appear early in the spring. It is found in woods and sides of hills with northern exposure.

Properties and Uses—Mayflower has been compared with Uva Ursi as the two drugs seem to have substantially the same active principles, and is said to have been used by some as a substitute for Uva Ursi.

Dose—Steep a heaping teaspoonful of the whole plant, cut into small pieces, into a cup of boiling water for half hour. When cold drink 1 or 2 cupfuls a day, a good mouthful at a time. Of the tincture, ½ to 1 fl. dr.

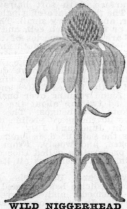

WILD NIGGERHEAD
(Brauneria Angustifolia)

Common Names—Echinacea, Purple Cone Flower, Sampson Root, Kansas Niggerhead.

Part Used—The root.

Description—Echinacea is a native herbaceous perennial belonging to the Aster family, grows 2 to 3 feet high. Stem stout bristly hairy, leaves thick rough-hairy, broadly lanceshaped or linear lanceshaped entire, 3 to 8 inches long, narrowed at the end and strongly, three nerved. The flower heads appear from July to October. The color varies from whitish rose to pale purple.

Properties and Uses—Echinacea has been credited with medicinal virtues by some but its merits are uncertain. It may be used to promote perspiration.

Dose—Steep a teaspoonful of the granulated root into a cup of boiling water for half hour. Strain. Take a tablespoonful 3 to 6 times a day. Of the tincture, 5 to 10 min.

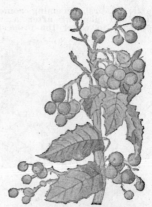

WILD OREGON GRAPE
(Berberis Aquifolium)

Common Names — Rocky Mountain Grape, Oregon Grape, Trailing Mahonia, California Barberry.

Parts Used—Rhizome and roots.

Description—Oregon Grape is a low trailing glabrous shrub, leaves petiolate, pinnate, leaflets 3 to 7, ovate acute, cordate at base, sessile, thick, dentate with spine-bearing teeth; flowers April to May, yellow racemes, fruit globular berry, blue, resembling the Whortle Berry. Rhizome irregular, knotty, wood yellowish, hard, tough, bark brownish; taste bitter.

Properties and Uses—Oregon Grape is alterative, diuretic, tonic, laxative. Very useful in some skin conditions and irritation.

Dose—Steep a teaspoonful of the granulated root into a cup of boiling water, strain. Take a tablespoonful 3 to 6 times a day. Of the tincture, 5 to 10 min.

WILD SOAPWORT
(Saponaria)

Common Names—Bouncing Bet, Dog Cloves.

Parts Used—The root and leaves.

Description—Soapwort is a perennial herbaceous plant, growing wild in this country, probably introduced from Europe. It is one to two feet high, smooth stem, leaves lanceolate, flowers in clusters varying in color from white to pink and purplish white. They appear from July to August. The leaves and root are inodorous and of a bitterish taste, at first becoming somewhat sweetish and pungent after a while. They impart to water the property of

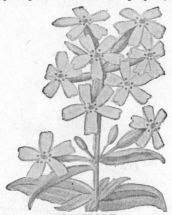

SOAPWORT

forming a lather, when agitated, like a solution of soap. The active principle is Saponin. As a substitute for soap in shampoo compounds it is excellent.

WILD STRAWBERRY
(Fragaria Virginia)

Parts Used—The herb.

Description—Wild Strawberry is so well known in the United States it requires no description.

Properties—Strawberry herb is astringent and tonic and valuable as a tonic for convalescents and especially for children.

Dose—A teaspoonful of the herb to a cup of boiling water. Drink cold 1 or 2 cupfuls a day, a large mouthful at a time; of the tincture, ½ to 1 fl. dr.

WILD VIOLETS

Parts Used—The flowers and leaves.

Description—Violets are too well known to require a description.

Properties and Uses—Violets are alterative and expectorant. Useful in throat and bronchial irritation.

Dose—Steep a teaspoonful of the leaves or flowers into a cup of boiling water for half hour, strain. Take a tablespoonful 3 to 6 times a day. Of the tincture, 5 to 10 min.

WILD YAM
(Dioscorea Villosa, Yam Family)

Common Names—Colic Root, Rheumatism Root.

Medicinal Part—The root.

Description—This is a delicate twining vine, with a perennial root. From this root proceeds a smooth, woolly, reddish-brown stem, the sixth of an inch in diameter, and from five to fifteen or eighteen feet long. The leaves average from two to four inches in length and about three-quarters of their length in width. They are glabrous on the upper surface, with soft hairs on the lower. The flowers are of a pale-greenish color, and are very small. The seeds are one or two in each cell, and flat.

There are several species of the Yam Root which grow in the South, and which the natives eat as we do potatoes, but these are not medicinally like the Dioscorea Villosa, which I have described above, and which is a slender vine growing wild in the United States and Canada, and found running over bushes and fences, and twining about the growths in thickets and hedges. The farther south we go the more prolific it is. It flowers in June and July. The root, which is the part used, is long, branched, crooked, and woody. From this is made a preparation called Dioscorein, or Dioscorin, which contains all its active qualities.

Properties and Uses—The Eclectic School of Medicine has regarded this as an anti-spasmodic and employed it in biliary colic. In large doses it seems to be diuretic and to act as an expectorant, but its medicinal virtues are questioned by other schools of medicine.

Dose—A teaspoonful of the root, cut small or granulated, to a cup of boiling water. Drink cold, one cupful during the day, a large mouthful at a time; of the tincture, 5 to 20 min.

WILLOW
(Salix Nigra—Willow Family)

Common Names—Black Willow, Pussywillow, Catkins Willow.

Medicinal Part—Bark.

Description—Willow is to be found growing along river banks, attaining a height of from fifteen to fifty feet. The bark is rough while the narrow-lanceolate leaves are taper pointed. There are from three to six stamens and short-ovate pods.

Properties and Uses—Bitter, astringent, detergent and anti-periodic.

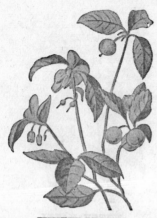

Wintergreen differs from Pippsissewa in that it has a distinct wintergreen aroma and flavor and the flowers are generally below the leaves, whereas the Pippissewa bears its flowers several inches above the leaves. The leaves also differ in their shape.

Properties and Uses—Wintergreen is diuretic and is believed by some to have a peculiarly beneficial action in indicated condition. Small doses stimulate the stomach, large doses have the opposite effect and cause vomiting. It is an old-time remedy.

Dose—A teaspoonful of the plant, cut small cr granulated, to a cup of boiling water. Drink cold, one cupful during the day, a large mouthful at a time; of the tincture, 5 to 20 min.

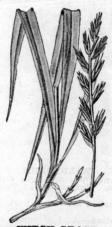

WINTERGREEN
(Gaultheria Procumbens)
Common Names — Periwinkle, Spice Berry, Deerberry, Teaberry.

Medicinal Part—The whole plant.

Description—Wintergreen is a low-growing, broad-leaved, evergreen plant with a creeping stem. The shoots from the stem grow to a height of 4 to 5 inches and bear solitary white flowers, which are followed by red berries. These berries are edible and are widely known as teaberries or checkerberries. Wintergreen is a common plant in woods and clearings from eastern Canada southward to the Gulf States, but its collection is somewhat difficult. Both the dry herb and the oil form marketable products.

Like other woodland plants, wintergreen thrives only in partial shade, and plantings should be made in a grove or under a specially constructed shade, such as is used for Golden Seal or Ginseng. A fairly good growth may be expected in soil which is thoroughly mixed with leaf mold to a depth of 4 inches or more. Wild plants may be used for propagation. Divisions of these may be set in the fall or spring, about 6 inches apart each way, in permanent beds.

Wintergreen is usually gathered in October or at the end of the growing season. The plants are carefully dried and packed in bags or boxes for marketing. For the production of the volatile oil the plants are soaked in water for about 24 hours and then distilled with steam.

WITCH GRASS
(Agropyron Repens)
Common Names—Quick Grass, Dog Grass, Couch Grass, Triticum, Durfa Grass.

Medicinal Part—The rootstock.

Description—Witch Grass is a perennial plant, rather coarse, 1 to 3 feet high and when in flower much resembles rye or beardless wheat. The pale yellow, smooth rootstock is long, tough and jointed, creeping along underneath the ground and pushing in every direction. It should be collected in spring carefully cleaned and dried.

Properties and Uses—Witch Grass is diuretic, aperient, demulcent. Useful in conditions in which it is desired to pro-

139

mote or increase the flow of urine. Large and frequent doses are considered a good tonic or "spring medicine." May be used freely.

Dose—Steep a heaping teaspoonful of the rootstock, cut into small pieces, into a cup of boiling water for half an hour. When cold drink 1 or 2 cupfuls a day; a good mouthful at a time. Tincture, 1 to 4 fl. dr.

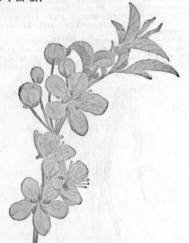

WILD PLUM
(Prunus Spinosa—Rose Family)

Common Names—Sloe Tree, Black Thorn.

Medicinal Part—The bark and the fruit.

Description—A low and spreading, thorny, European tree appearing in this country chiefly in the double-flowered variety. The flowers are borne singly or in pairs (rarely in threes), very small as compared with the garden Plum. The leaves are small and mostly obovate and obtuse (or in some forms very blunt-pointed), finely and doubly serrate, rugose and more or less hairy beneath. The fruit is small and round and purple and is scarcely edible.

Properties and Uses—Bark, antispasmodic and sedative; berries, acidulous and astringent.

"He causeth the grass to grow for the cattle, and herb for the service of man." (Psalm 104, 14.)

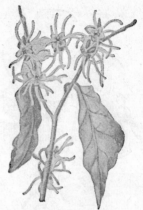

WITCH HAZEL
(Hamamelis Virginica, Witch Hazel Family)

Common Names—Winterbloom, Snapping Hazelnut, Spotted Alders.

Medicinal Parts—The bark and leaves.

Description—Witch Hazel is an indigenous shrub consisting of several crooked branching stems, from the same root, from four to six inches in diameter and ten to twelve feet high, covered with a smooth gray bark. The leaves are on short petioles, alternate, oval or obovate; flowers yellow; calyx small, petals four, and the fruit a nutlike capsule or pod.

It grows in damp woods, in nearly all parts of the United States, flowering from September to November, when the leaves are falling and maturing its seeds the next summer. The bark and leaves are the parts used in medicine. They possess a degree of fragrance, and when chewed are at first somewhat bitter, very sensibly astringent, and leave a pungent, sweetish taste, which remains for a considerable time. Water extracts their virtues. The shoots are used as divining rods to discover water and metals under ground by certain adepts in the occult arts.

Properties and Uses—It is an old-time remedy that still is in popular use. The Indians used it in the form of poultice, in external irritations, bruises, etc.

The tea may be advantageously used as a mouth wash for conditions of irritation and as a vaginal douche for simple vaginitis.

An ointment made with lard, and a decoction of white-oak bark, apple-tree bark, and witch-hazel, is a very valuable remedy for the itching and irritation of piles.

Dose—A teaspoonful of the bark or leaves, cut small or granulated, to a cup of boiling water. Drink cold, one cupful during the day, a large mouthful at a time; of the tincture, 5 to 20 min.

WOOD ANEMONE
(Anemone Quinquefolia)

Common Name—Wind Flower.
Medicinal Part—The whole herb.
Description—This is an exceedingly delicate looking plant, common in our woods. The slender stem is from 4 to 8 inches high. The solitary flower is white inside and purplish on the outer surface.
Properties and Uses—It has been extensively used by Eclectic physicians but its virtues are said to depend upon its effect as a local irritant.

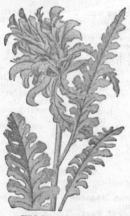

WOOD BETONY
(Betonica Officinalis—Mint Family)

Common Names—Betony, Lousewort.
Medicinal Part—Leaves.
Description—A European plant occasionally seen in old gardens growing from six inches to two feet high with pediate and oblong-cordate, obtuse, crenate leaves and red-purple corolla three-quarters inch long. The flowers are borne in spicate whorls.
Properties and Uses—Aperient and cordial.

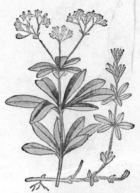

WOODRUFF
(Asperula Odorata)

Common Names — Sweet Woodruff, Master of the Wood.
Medicinal Part—The whole herb.
Description—Woodruff is a favorite little plant, growing commonly in our woods and gardens, with a pleasant smell, which like the good deeds of the worthiest persons, delights by its fragrance most after it has been dried. This herb is of the Rubiaceous order, and gets its botanical name from the Latin asper, rough, in alusion to the rough leaves possessed by its species.

It may be readily recognized by its small white flowers set on a slender stalk with narrow leaves growing round it in successive whorls, just as in the Cleaver (Goosegrass) which belongs to the same order.

Properties and Uses—A fragrant and exhiliarating tea may be made from the leaves and blossoms of the Sweet Woodruff. "When it is desired," says Mrs. Jones, "to preserve the leaves merely for their scent, the stems should be cut through just below and above a joint, and the leaves pressed in such a way as not to destroy their star-like arrangement. The dried herb may be kept amongst the linen, like lavender to preserve it from insects."

It is also of value as an aid to digestion. A small handful of the dried herb if placed into a gallon of wine or liquor of any kind for 4 to 6 hours, imparts to it a very fine flavor.

Dose—A teaspoonful of the herb to a cup of boiling water. Drink cold one or two cupfuls a day, a large mouthful at a time; of the tincture, ½ to 1 fl. dr.

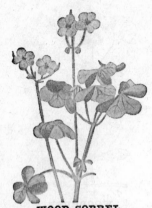

WOOD SORREL
(Oxalis Acetoselia, Wood Sorrel
Family)
Common Names—Shamrock, Trefoil.
Medicinal Part—The whole herb.
Description—This is a small perennial herb, with a creeping and scaly-toothed root stock. The leaves are numerous, radical and on long, weak, hairy stalks; leaflets broadly obcordate, and of yellowish green color. Flowers white, yellowish at the base and scentless. Fruit a five-lobed, oblong capsule.

It is indigenous to Europe and this country, growing in woody and shady places, and flowering from April to June. It is inodorous, and has a pleasantly acid taste. The acidity is due to oxalic acid, which, in combination with potassa, forms the binoxalate of that alkalai. The "Salts of Sorrel," formerly used so much to remove inkspots and iron marks from linen, is merely this salt separated from the plant.

Properties and Uses—Cooling and diuretic and employed to some extent by Eclectic physicians, but care is to be observed in its use.

Dose—A teaspoonful of the herb, cut small or granulated, to a cup of boiling water. Drink cold, one cupful during the day, a large mouthful at a time; of the tincture, 10 to 30 min.

Rumex Acetosa, or Garden Sorrel, Rumex Acetosella or Sheep Sorrel, and Rumex Vesicarius possess similar qualities.

* * * *

He 'scapes the best, who, nature to repair,
Draws physic from the fields, in draughts
of vital air.

WORM ROOT TREE
(Melia Azedarach)
Common Names—Pride of China, Pride of India, Bead tree.
Medicinal Part—The bark of the root.
Description—This is an elegant tree, which attains the height of thirty or forty feet, with a trunk about a foot and half in diameter. The bark is rough; leaves bipinnate, flowers lilac color; calyx five parted; corolla has five petals; stamens deep violet, anthers yellow. The fruit is a five-celled bony nut.

It is a native of China, but cultivated in the warm climates of Europe and America. It does not grow to any extent north of Virginia, and flowers early in the spring. Its name of Bead Tree is derived from the use to which its hard nuts are put in Roman Catholic countries, viz., for making rosaries. The recent bark of the root is the most active part for medicinal purposes. It has a disagreeably bitter taste, and a very unpleasant odor, and imparts its properties to boiling water.

Properties and Uses—The bark is anthelmintic, and in large doses narcotic and emetic.

The fruit is somewhat saccharine, and is an excellent remedy to expel worms. Its pulp is used as an ointment for destroying lice and other extozoa.

Standley's "Trees and Shrubs of Mexico," states: "In the southern U.S. there is a belief that if horses eat the fruits they will be protected against attacks of bots. It is said also, that the berries packed with dried fruit will prevent the attacks of insects, and if laid among clothes, they will keep away moths. A decoction of the fruits sprinkled over growing plants, is reported to guard them from injury by cutworms and other insects."

WORMSEED
(Chenopodium Anthelminticum, Goosefoot Family)
Common Names—Jerusalem Oak, Chenopodium.
Medicinal Part—The seeds.
Description—This plant has a perennial branched root, with an erect, herbaceous stem, from one to three feet high. The leaves are alternate, oblong-lanceolate, of yellowish green color, and marked beneath with small resinous particles. The numerous flowers are of the same color as the leaves. Seeds solitary and lenticular.

This plant grows in waste places in almost all parts of the United States, flowering from July to September, and ripening its seeds throughout the fall, at which time they should be collected. The whole plant has a disagreeable odor, and the seeds partake of the same odor.

Properties and Uses—Its chief use seems to be as an anthelmintic. Excellent to expel the lumbrici from children. The oil is the best form of administration, which may be given in doses of 4 to 8 drops on sugar. The infusion with milk is also given often in wineglassful doses.

Dose—A teaspoonful of the seeds mixed with honey to be given twice a day and to be followed with a good laxative.

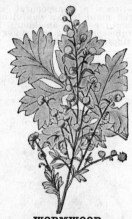

WORMWOOD
(Artemisia Absinthium, Aster Family.)
Common Name—Absinth.
Medicinal Parts—The tops and leaves.

Description—This is a perennial plant, with a woody root, branched at the crown, and having numerous fibres below. The whole herb is covered with close silk hoariness; the stems are numerous, bushy, and from 1 to 2 feet in height. Their lower part exists for some years, from which young shoots spring forth every year, decaying in cold weather. The leaves are alternate, broadish and blunted, the lower ones on long petioles, upper ones on shorter, broader, and somewhat winged ones.

Wormwood grows nearly all over the world, from the United States to Siberia. It flowers from June to September. The tops and leaves are the part used. The dried herb, with the flowers, has a whitish gray appearance, a strong, aromatic odor, and is extremely bitter to the taste. Alcohol or water takes up its active principles. It yields what is known to druggists as absinthine.

Properties and Uses—It is anthelmintic, tonic and narcotic. It is used for many conditions, among which may be enumerated want of appetite, diarrhoea, etc. It is also used externally in country places as a fomentation for sprains, bruises and local irritations. Taken too often, or in large quantities, it will irritate the stomach, and dangerously increase the action of the heart and arteries. For this reason, it should be greatly diluted: 1 teaspoonful to a pint of water.

Dose—A teaspoonful of the tops and leaves, cut small or granulated, to a cup of boiling water. Drink cold, one cupful during the day, a large mouthful at a time; of the tincture, 5 to 30 min.

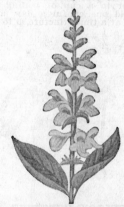

WOUND WORT
(Prunella Vulgaris, Mint Family)
Common Names — Hercules Wound Wort, Panay, All Heal, Brownwort, Sickle Wort, Blue Curls, Self Heal.
Medicinal Part—The whole herb.

Description—This plant is 1 to 3 feet high with a downy, bristly stem and purple two-lipped flowers in terminal spikes.

This plant is found in the United States and England and other parts of Europe. In the United States it flowers usually until the end of summer, but in some parts of Europe it flowers from May to December.

Properties and Uses—Wound Wort is pungent and bitter and slightly diuretic.

143

It once was used as a gargle for throat irritation and for other purposes.

Dose—A teaspoonful of the herb is placed in a pint of good brandy or whiskey for a few days. Two tablespoonfuls of this is taken during the day or when needed.

YELLOW BEAR'S FOOT
(Polymnia Uvedalia, Aster Family)
Common Names — Yellow Leafcup, Uvedalia, Bearsfoot.
Part Used—Root.
Description—This is a large, native, perennial, 3 to 6 feet high, growing in ravines and edges of woods from New York to Michigan, south to Florida and Texas.
Properties and Uses—By some this plant is credited with considerable value in certain malarial conditions.
Dose—One teaspoonful of the granulated root to a cup of boiling water. Drink cold one cupful a day, a large mouthful at a time; tincture, 3 to 5 min.

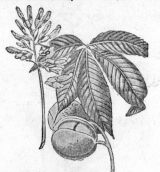

YELLOW CHESTNUT
(Æsculus Flava—Soapberry Family)
Common Name—Sweet Buckeye.
Medicinal Part—Bark.
Description—A tree of the slopes of the Alleghenies west of Iowa and Texas commonly from 75 to 90 feet high. The leaves are dark, green, pointed at either end and short stemmed. The flowers are in terminal spikes, yellow and blossoming in June.
Properties and Uses—Astringent and febrifuge.

YELLOW CHIRETTA
(Swertia Chirayita)
Medicinal Part—The dried plant.
Description—Chiretta is an annual plant of Northern India, with smooth

stem about 3 feet high, yellowish, with numerous opposite ascending branches. Wood yellowish, thin, yellowish pitch. Leaves opposite, sessile, ovate-lanceolate, entire, 5 nerved about 2½ in. long, flowers small, panicled. Fruit a one-celled ovoid, acute capsule containing numerous seeds. Should be collected when in flower.
Properties and Uses—Chiretta belongs to the clan of pure bitters, and as such it has tonic properties. It also is believed by some to exert a favorable influence on the bile and to relieve constipation.
Dose—Steep a teaspoonful of the granulated plant into a cupful of boiling water for half an hour. Strain. Take a tablespoonful 3 to 6 times a day. Of the tincture, 5 to 10 min.

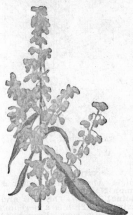

YELLOW DOCK
(Rumex Crispus, Buckwheat Family)
Common Names—Curled Dock, Narrow Dock, Sour Dock, Rumex.
Medicinal Part—The root.
Description—There are four varieties of Dock which may be used in medicine; the Rumex Aquaticus (Great Water Dock); Rumex Britannica (Water Dock); Rumex Abtusifolius (Blunt Leaved Dock); and the Rumex Crispus or Yellow Dock. They all possess similar medicinal qualities, but the Yellow Dock is the only one entitled to extensive consideration. It has a deep spindle-shaped yellow root, with a stem 2 or 3 feet high. The leaves are lanceolate, acute, and of a light green color. The flowers

are numerous, pale green, drooping and interspersed with leaves below. The fruit is a nut contracted at each end.

The Docks are natives of Europe, excepting the blunt-leaved, which is indigenous, but they have all been introduced into the United States. Yellow Dock grows in cultivated grounds, waste grounds, about rubbish, etc., flowering in June and July. The root has scarcely any odor, but an astringent bitter taste, and yields its virtues to water and alcohol.

Properties and Uses—Yellow Dock is an alterative, tonic and astringent that has come down from the ancients. For some conditions it has no equal, especially if properly compounded with appropriate adjutants and corrigents. The fresh root bruised in cream, lard or butter, forms a good ointment for various purposes.

Yellow Dock root is a very rich source of digestible plant iron—the mineral so important for men, animals, and plants. It was a favorite ingredient of herbal formulaes of old-time doctors, Indian medicine men, and early settlers.

YELLOW JESSAMINE
(Gelseminum Sempervirens, Logania Family)

Common Names—Gelsemin, Wild Jessamine, Woodbine.

Medicinal Part—The root.

Description—This plant has a twining, smooth, glabrous stem, with opposite, perennial, lanceolate, entire leaves, which are dark green above and pale beneath. The flowers are yellow and have an agreeable odor. Calyx is very small, with five sepals, corolla funnel-shaped, stamens five, pistils two, and the fruit a two-celled capsule.

Yellow Jessamine abounds throughout the southern states, growing luxuriantly, and climbing from tree to tree, forming an agreeable shade. It is cultivated as an ornamental vine, and flowers from March to May. The root yields its virtues to water and alcohol. Gelsemin is its active principle. It also contains a fixed oil, acrid resin, yellow coloring matter, a heavy volatile oil, a crystalline substance, and salts of potassa, lime, magnesia, iron and silica.

Properties and Uses—This herb has been used for many purposes by former generations and still seems to be credited with a sedative or soothing influence in such conditions as facial neuralgia. It may have such strong reaction, however, including effect upon the vision, that it should not be used as a home remedy.

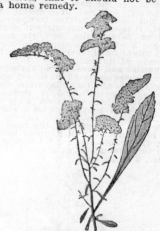

YELLOW GOLDENROD
(Solidago Nemoralis—Composite Family)

Common Name—Oldfield Golden Rod.

Medicinal Part—The leaves and flowers.

Description — A slender, ashy-gray plant from six inches to two feet high, finely and densely pubescent. The leaves are thick, roughish, the upper ones gradually smaller. The yellow flower heads are usually one-sided panicles.

Properties and Uses—Carminative and diaphoretic.

YELLOW PARILLA
(Menispermum Canadense, Moonseed Family)

Common Names—Vine-Maple, Moonseed.

Medicinal Part—The root.

Description—This plant has a perennial, horizontal, very long woody root of a beautiful yellow color. The stem is round and climbing, and about a foot in length. The leaves are roundish, cordate, peltate, smooth, glaucous green above, paler below, entire, and 4 to 5 inches in diameter. The flowers are in clusters, and are small and yellow. The fruit, a drupe, is about the third of an inch in diameter, and one-seeded.

145

Yellow Parilla grows in moist woods and hedges, and near streams, from Canada to Carolina, and west to the Mississippi. It flowers in July. The root, which is the part used, has a bitter, lasting, but not unpleasant acrid taste, and yields its virtues to water and alcohol. It is called, not without justice, American Sarsaparilla, and its active principle, known as menispermin, shows that it might have received a name less expressive of its merits.

Properties and Uses—Some authors of herbalist dispensatories have set down Yellow Parilla as "tonic, laxative, alterative and diuretic," and it seems to possess all of these qualities. It is said to be employed sometimes as a substitute for sarsaparilla.

Dose—A teaspoonful of the root, cut small or granulated, to a cup of boiling water. Drink cold, one cupful during the day, a large mouthful at a time; of the tincture, 5 to 20 min.

its leaf, and its conspicuous yellow flowers, which appear in succession from June to October. The herb is the part used. It should be collected when in flower, dried quickly and kept excluded from the air. When fresh it has a peculiar, heavy, rather disagreeable odor, which is in a great measure dissipated by drying. The taste is herbaceous, weakly saline, bitter and slightly acrid.

Properties and Uses—This plant is said to be diuretic, and cathartic, and has been used freely as such. It is most conveniently employed in infusion. The fresh plant is sometimes applied in the shape of poultice or fomentation, to external condition; and an ointment made from the flowers has been employed for irritations of the skin. The flowers are used in Germany for dyeing yellow.

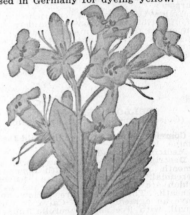

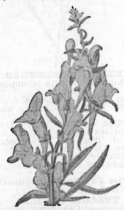

YELLOW TOAD FLAX
(Antirrhinum Linaria)

Common Names — Toad Flax, Snap Dragon, Butter and Eggs.

Part Used—The herb.

Description—Toad flax is a perennial herbaceous plant from 1 to 2 feet high, with numerous narrow linear leaves and a terminal crowded spike of large, yellow flowers. It is a native of Europe but has been introduced into this country and grows wild in great abundance along road sides and in fields and meadows throughout the middle states. It is readily distinguishable by the shape of

YERBA SANTA
(Eriodictyon Californicum)

Common Names—Mountain Balm, Consumptives' Weed, Tarweed, Bearsweed, Holy Herb.

Medicinal Part—The leaves.

Description—This evergreen shrub is a member of the Waterleaf family, 3 to 4 feet high. Stem smooth but exudes a gummy substance. The leaves are glutinous, 3 to 4 inches in length, alternately on stem, oblong, or oval, lance-shaped, narrowing gradually to a short, stalk; margins toothed except at base; upper surface smooth with depressed veins; the under side contains a network of prominent veins and is covered with a resinous substance making them appear as if varnished. Flowers whitish or pale blue in clusters at top of plant. The seed capsule is oval, greyish brown and contains small reddish brown shriveled seeds.

Properties and Uses—Yerba Santa is an excellent expectorant and valuable in spasms of asthma and throat and bronchial irritations. It is also used as a tonic. It has an aromatic odor and sweetish balsamic taste.

Dose—Steep a teaspoonful of the leaves into a cup of boiling water for half an hour. Drink a half cupful at night upon retiring hot or cold—or take a mouthful 3 times a day. One or two cupfuls may be taken. Tincture, 10 to 30 min.

ZEA MAYS

Common Name—Corn Silk, Indian Corn.

Parts Used—The fresh styles and stigmas.

Descriptoin—Indian Corn or Zea Mays needs no description as it is familiar to every American family.

The stalk or styles and stigmas must be picked before it becomes dry; then carefully dried and kept in a closed vessel to prevent evaporation of the oils upon which depend much of its medicinal virtue.

Properties—Corn silk is diuretic and demulcent. It may be employed as a mucilaginous drink or as an enema, whenever its demulcent properties suggest its use.

ZEDOARY

(Curcuma Zedoaria—Ginger Family)

Part Used—Root.

Description—Plant is related to and resembles Tumeric. It is a robust perennial, native of tropical Asia. Leaves appear with or after flowers. Flowers bracteate, in large dense spikes consisting of concave to saccate persistent bracts of which the flowerless ones are sometimes elongated, and form colored terminal tuft. Flowers are pale yellow, 3 to 5 together, surrounded by showy crimson or purple bracts. the rhizomes are deep orange or reddish brown, having a camphoraceous gingery aroma.

Uses—Zedoary was formerly an important article in spice trade, but replaced by Ginger and Tumeric. It is used now, mainly for flavoring liqueurs and curries. It is also used in perfumery, cosmetics, and still in common use in the Orient as a medicinal, for its carminative, stomachic and stimulating properties.

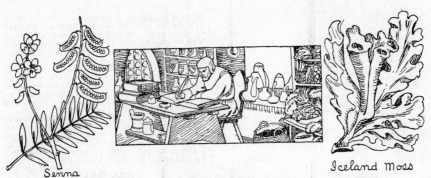

Senna

Iceland Moss

BOTANICALS LISTED UNDER CERTAIN TERMS
ALTERATIVES

ALTERATIVES: Agents which tend gradually to alter a condition.

Old-time herbalists often combined several Alteratives with botanicals listed under Aromatics, Bitter Tonics and Demulcents.

Among botanicals that may be classed as Alteratives, in this broad and general sense of the term, are:

American Spikenard rt. or berries
Bittersweet twigs
Black Cohosh rt.
Blue Flag rt.
Bull Nettle rt.
Burdock rt.
Condurango rt.
Echinacea rt.
Guaiac raspings
Red Clover flrs.

Sarsaparilla rt.
Sassafras rt.
Stillingia rt.
Oregon Grape rt.
Pipsissewa lvs.
Poke rt.
Prickly Ash bk.
Wild Sarsaparilla rt.
Yellow Dock rt.
Yellow Parilla rt.

ANTHELMINTICS

ANTHELMINTICS or VERMIFUGES: Medicines capable of destroying or expelling worms which inhabit the intestinal canal. Anthelmintics should only be administered by physicians:

Areca Nuts
Balmony hb.
Kousso flrs.
Male Fern
Melia Azedarach bk.

Pomegranate rind or bk of rt.
Pumpkin seed
Spigelia rt.
Wormseed hb.
Wormwood hb.

ASTRINGENTS

ASTRINGENTS temporarily tighten, contract, or increase the firmness of the skin or mucous membrane. They are often of value to check excessive secretions. They are

Astringents—Continued

used as external washes, lotions, gargles, mouthwashes, etc.

Astringents may be made very strongly using more botanical and longer boiling. They may be "watered down" to the strength desired. The following are considered STRONG ASTRINGENTS:

Agrimony hb.
Alum Root
Barberry bk.
Bayberry bk.
Beech Drops hb.
Bearberry lvs.
Beth rt.
Black Alder bk.
Black Cherries
Black Oak bk.
Black Willow bk.
Butternut bk.
Buttonsnake rt.
Catechu gum
Chocolate rt.
Cinquefoil
Congo rt.
Cranesbill rt.
Fleabane hb.
Golden-rod hb.
Hardhack hb.
Hawthorne berries
Heal-all hb.
Hemlock bk.
Hickory bk.
Jambul seed
Kola nuts

Logwood
Lycopus virginicus
Maiden Hair Fern
Mountain Ash bk.
Pilewort hb.
Potentilla hb.
Purple Loosestrife hb.
Queen of the Meadow hb.
Rattlesnake rt.
Red rt.
Rhatany rt.
Sage hb.
Sanicle rt.
Sampson Snake rt.
Shepherd's Purse hb.
Sumbul rt.
Sumach bk. of rt.
Tormentil rt.
Uva Ursi lvs.
Wafer Ash bk.
Water Avens rt.
Water Lily rt.
White Ash bk.
White Oak bk.
Wild Indigo bk.
Witch Hazel Twigs

Mild Astringents

Blackberry rt.
Black Birch lvs.
Celandine
German Rue

Rosa gallica petals
St. John's Wort
Sweet Fern hb.

* * * *

"Alum Root or Cranesbill root is powerfully astringent, without bitterness or unpleasant taste. Boiled in water and mixed with sugar and milk, it is easily administered to children."

"American Weeds and Useful Plants"
Wm. Darlington, M.D., 1859

"The root of Tormentil is a powerful astringent and contains (except galls and catechu) more Tannin than any other vegetable. A decoction is used in the form of gargle. Boil 1 teaspoonful of root in a pint and a half of water until reduced to one pint."—English Health Magazine

BITTER TONICS

BITTER TONICS are used for temporary loss of appetite. They stimulate the flow of saliva and gastric juices—therefore assist the process of digestion:

Angostura bk.
Balmony hb.
Barberry rt. and bk.
Bayberry lvs.
Black Berry lvs.
Black Haw bk.
Blessed Thistle
Bogbean hb.
Boldo lvs.
Cascarilla bk.
Chamomile flrs.
Chiretta hb.
Columbo rt.
Condurango rt.

Dandelion rt.
Fringe Tree bk.
Gentian rt.
Goldenseal rt.
Goldthread rt.
Hops flrs.
Mugwort hb.
Quassia chips
Sabattia—Amer. Century rt.
Serpentaria rt.
Turkey Corn rt.
Wild Cherry bk.
Wormwood hb.
Yellow Root rt. (Xanthorrhiza)

* * * *

COLUMBO ROOT: "Of all bitters the least objectionable is the Columbo root, for, whilst it acts as a bitter tonic, it does not stimulate like other bitters. It should be prepared: 2 teaspoonful of the root—pour upon it a pint of boiling water. Take a wine glass full of this infusion every morning, half an hour at least, before breakfast." —John Reitch, M.D., 1842

YELLOW ROOT: "A strong pleasant bitter; sits easy on the stomach."—Hand 1820

QUASSIA: A bitter wood which is a good, simple, stomachic tonic. It is best taken in the form of a tea. ½ oz. of it may be boiled for an hour or two, in a pint of water. Dose—half a wineglassful, 2 or 3 times daily.

CHAMOMILE: This is a plant with bitter and aromatic flowers. Of these a tea is made with boiling water. It may be taken, ½ pint daily, as a simple appetizer.

BLAND DIETETIC BOTANICALS

BLAND DIETETIC BOTANICALS: Generally non-stimulating, non-irritating, easily digestive nutritive botanicals, that are friendly to the stomach and intestines. They are especially useful for the young, aged, and during convalescence.

ARROW ROOT: A superior carbohydrate and a good source of digestible calcium, used as a light nutritious diet for children after weaning, and for delicate persons during convalescence. May be prepared as a jell, gruel, blanc-mange, beverage, in baking etc.

CAROB or ST. JOHN'S BREAD: This was said to be the food of John the Baptist and the Prodigal Son.
Carob pods have a maple-like flavor, and contain up to 50 per cent natural sugar, and for this reason, the whole pods are often eaten as candy.
Carob powder is a flavorful addition in breads, cakes, cookies and confections. It is

Dietetic Botanicals—*Continued*

becoming increasingly popular as a flavor in cold or hot milk, milk shakes and malted milk. Carob syrup, for flavoring milk beverages, is simple to prepare: Mix ⅛ cup brown sugar with ¼ cup Carob powder. Add ⅔ cup of water or milk, salt slightly. Boil 5 minutes. Add ½ teaspoon vanilla, if desired. Store in jar, in refrigerator. Add 2 tablespoonful for each cup of milk to be flavored.

Carob beverage: For each cup of beverage, use 1 or 1½ teaspoonful of Carob flour; ½ teaspoon (or less) Licorice extract, in boiling hot water or milk. Serve like hot chocolate.

CARRAGEEN or IRISH MOSS: An excellent substitute for animal gelatin. It has a remarkable property to thicken or stabilize beverages and foods. It is used to stiffen or jell blanc-mange, puddings, custards, fruit or salad moulds, etc. Carrageen is not a by-product. It contains all the natural elements characteristic of most sea plants. It is easily digested and may be given to invalids, children and the aged. Plain Carrageen, made with water or milk (either as liquid or jell) is soothing to digestive linings.

GUM ARABIC: Soluble in cold or warm water. The gum is nutritive and especially useful as a protective coating over mucous surfaces, in cases of hoarseness, minor sore throat, coughs of colds. Also recommended as a soothing demulcent for the stomach.

Recipe for beverage: 1 oz. Gum Arabic, powdered; mix well with 2 tablespoonsful honey; have a little rind of lemon; clean off the white pith, and cut the lemon in slices into a jug; then stir on it, by degrees, a pint and a half of boiling water.

ICELAND MOSS: An important article of diet in Iceland, where it is used as a bread. Iceland Moss contains about 70% lichenin starch. Boiled in sweet milk, it is a nutriment. Much of the bitter principle may be extracted by boiling the Iceland Moss in water, then discarding the first water. Boil the Moss again in fresh water for 10 minutes, in a covered vessel, and with gentle pressure, while still hot. The result is a mucilaginous demulcent liquid. It may be flavored with sugar, lemon peel, or aromatics; or milk flavored with chocolate or cocoa may be used instead of the water, by which a nourishing liquid is obtained.

OKRA PODS: Okra is valued because of its mucilaginous and non-irritating characteristics. Okra is highly recommended AS A DEMULCENT FOOD without roughage or irritation to the stomach lining. U.S. Government Bulletin #232 states: "Okra is valued in the diet, chiefly because of the nutritionally important minerals it contains. It is a good natural source of calcium and phosphorus, and a fair source of iron. Fresh green Okra is also a good source of Vitamin A. Drying Okra reduces the Vitamin A content by about half. Another value of Okra in the diet is due to its indigestible residue, some of which is considered desirable to provide bulk in the digestive tract of persons in normal health."

Dehydrated powdered Okra may be taken with water, milk, broth or other bland foods. Okra is much used in Gumbo soup, and Creole dishes.

SAGO ROOT: A nutritious starch obtained from certain palms and cycads.

Sago flour is one of the most nourishing and easily digested foods. Its demulcent properties are particulary useful in some types of digestive complaints and in fevers.

Sago jelly: Wash 1 tablespoonful of Sago, and soak it in cold water for an hour or two. Pour off this water, add more, and boil it gently until it becomes clear.

Dietetic Botanicals—Continued

Sweeten with sugar, and flavor, if desired. The addition of a sliced apple to the Sago, while the latter is cooking gives it a pleasant flavor, much preferable, it is thought, to that of any extract of wine.

SWEET ELM or SLIPPERY ELM: An important medicine, as well as food, of the American Indians and pioneers. It is still listed among recognized official drugs, and still considered one of our best emollient and demulcent medicines. It is a valuable article of diet because of its soothing influence upon the stomach and intestines. It is superior to whole milk, in its ability to neutralize stomach acids. Sweet Elm is considered one of the finest demulcents in the vegetable kingdom.

Slippery elm bark is recognized in modern times for its soothing properties. The powder, mixed with milk is wholesome and nutritious. It is easily digested. The slippery nature insures an easy passage during the processes of assimilation and elimination.

CALMATIVES

CALMATIVES: Agents used for their mild calming effect. Generally taken as a warm tea upon retiring.

Catnip hb.
Chamomile flrs.

Fennel seed
Hops
Linden flrs.

* * * *

HOPS: A Hop pillow is sometimes used for its pleasant aroma. To prepare it, fill a small pillow case with Hops, which have been sprinkled with alcohol, to bring out the active principle.

CARMINATIVES and AROMATICS

CARMINATIVES and AROMATICS: Substances of a fragrant smell, which produce upon the organs of taste, a peculiar sensation of warmth and pungency, and occasion, when swallowed, a corresponding impulse upon the stomach, which is communicated to other parts of the body.

Aromatics are useful to expel gas from the stomach and intestines. They are chiefly used to make other medicinals and formulas more palatable.

Allspice—unripe fruit
Anise seed
Angelica seed
Capsicum fruit
Caraway seed
Cardamon seed
Catnip hb.
Celery seed
Cinnamon bk.
Cloves buds
Coriander seed
Cumin seed

Eucalyptus lvs.
Fennel seed
Ginger rt.
Lovage rt.
Mace
Melilot flrs.
Mustard seed
Nutmeg
Peppermint hb.
Spearmint hb.
Valerian rt.
Wild Ginger rt.

152

Carminatives and Aromatics—Continued

ANGELICA SEED—"One of the most pleasant aromatics grown in Europe."—Whitlaw, 1829

FENNEL SEED: A very mild aromatic; sometimes made into a tea for babies' colic; more often added to Senna tea, or fluid extract of Senna, to keep the purgative medicine from griping the bowels.

GINGER: Ginger tea is an old favorite stomach warmer. A tablespoonful or two of the bruised root may have a pint of boiling water poured on it, then leaving it to stand covered for an hour or so. We don't boil aromatic teas or other preparations, because that would drive off their volatile oils, which are their active principles. Of Ginger tea, the dose is one or two tablespoonsful at a time.

CATHARTICS

CATHARTICS: Agents which promote evacuation from the bowels by their action on the alimentary canal. Cathartics may be divided into two types or groups.

1. Laxatives or Aperients are agents which are mild or feeble in their action upon the intestinal canal.

2. Purgatives are agents which induce copious evacuations of the bowels. They are generally used for more stubborn conditions in adults, or used with other ingredients to modify or increase their action. Neither laxatives or purgatives should be taken when symptoms of appendicitis are suspected, nor during pregnancy, or for other conditions that require the services of a physician.

Cathartics should only be used for occasional constipation, as continual use may develop a dependence on them.

ALOES: The drug is obtained from the liquid exuded from the leaves of Aloe vera (Curacao or Barbadoes), Aloe Perryi (Socotrine or Zanzibar), and Aloe ferox (Cape). Aloes is used for persons of sedentary habits and phlegmatic constitutions. Aloes are rarely prescribed alone—they require the addition of carminatives to moderate the tendency to griping.

AGAR-AGAR: In powdered form is often recommended for mild cases of constipation, when bulk or mechanical action is desired. It may be taken in porridge, soup, jellies, cakes or any other food. Take ½ oz. daily when needed. It takes 3 or 4 days to act, and should be continued for a week or longer until it begins to produce results. Cascara bark is added to Agar-Agar for stubborn cases of constipation.

BARBERRY bark and bark of root: Botanical contains Bitter Tonic and purgative properties.

BLUE FLAG root: A mild decoction used as a cathartic—strong decoction as emetic.

BUCKTHORN bark: This bark must be aged from 1 to 2 years. Generally taken in small doses, repeated 3 or 4 times daily.

BUTTERNUT inner bark: A gentle purgative, which does not bind. "It is one of the mildest and most certain cathartics we possess, operating without producing nausea, irritation, or pain; neither weakening the alimentary canal, nor impairing digestion." —Botanic Guide to Health, 1845

Cathartics—Continued

CASCARA bark increases secretions of the gastrointestinal canal. Like Buckthorn, this bark must be aged to modify or eliminate griping tendencies. Cascara is found very effective taken in small dosages before retiring, and taken before meals. The amount of dosage, of course, depends upon the requirement of an individual. A mouthful of a mild decoction should be enough for the average adult.

CASSIA FISTULA: The long beans of this tree contain a very interesting partitioning arrangement of seeds. The soft licorice-like flavored "partitions" have gentle laxative properties. It was an important article of trade among the ancient Egyptians. The leaves and flowers of Cassia Fistula also have cathartic properties, but they were never marketed.

CASTOR OIL: Well known for its cathartic action. Also well known and unpopular among children, and child-bearing women. The nauseous taste may be covered by Lemon, Sassafras or other essential oils.

CULVER'S ROOT, CULVER'S PHYSIC or PHYSIC ROOT: Cathartic without griping tendencies. May be taken in small doses in wine. Culver's Root was held in very high repute in Botanical Materia Medica.

JALAP root: Purgative, generally combined with other laxatives, and with carminatives such as Ginger, Cloves, etc., to modify action.

KARAYA gum: Bulk induces mechanical action. Stronger action may be had by adding Cascara, Senna or other cathartics.

MANNA: A sweet substance obtained from the trunk of the flowering ash tree, in the countries bordering on the Mediterranean. Its only important use is to open the bowels of children and delicate people, including women during pregnancy. It may may be eaten like sugar. The dose is not very definite; a little experience will show how much is required for the desired effect.

MAYAPPLE or MANDRAKE root a powerful cathartic. Generally used with mild and modifying ingredients.

PSYLLIUM seed: Tasteless, mucilaginous seeds used to increase the bulk of the feces. Seeds may be mixed with orange or prune juice and eaten without mastication. May also be mixed with a little hot water, and the resulting gelatinous mass spread on bread, or eaten with other food. Dry seeds may be placed in the mouth and followed by a swallow of water.

RHUBARB root: Cathartic principle limited to lower bowel.

SENNA, EGYPTIAN (Tinnevelly or Alexandrina) leaves: Laxative or purgative. Generally combined with aromatics and stimulants to allay its griping tendency.

SENNA, AMERICAN: Milder action than Egyptian. Preferred by many early American herbalists.

Cathartics—Continued

SENNA PODS: Mild action, almost tasteless. Used mainly for children over 7 years of age.

TAMARIND PULP: Makes a pleasant beverage that is gently laxative, quenches thirst and allays immoderate heat.

* * * *

CORIANDER seed: "Take a half or full teaspoonful of the seeds, infused along with Senna, will correct both the odor and taste of it, and the seeds are equally powerful in obviating the griping that Senna is very ready to produce."—Whitlaw, 1829

FENNEL seed is also used in the same way as Coriander seed.

DEMULCENTS

DEMULCENTS: Substances usually of a mucilaginous and bland nature, taken IN-TERNALLY for their soothing or protective coating-like properties. (For external uses see EMOLLIENTS). Demulcents may be used to allay irritation of membranes.
Demulcents have been much used for coughs due to common colds, and to relieve minor irritation of the throat.
The mildest and most soothing demulcents are marked with an asterisk (*).

Agar Agar
Arrow rt.
Cheese Plant hb.
Coltsfoot hb.
*Comfrey rt.
Couch Grass rt.
*Flaxseed
*Gum Arabic
Iceland Moss
Irish Moss
Karaya Gum
Licorice rt.
*Marshmallow rt. & lvs.
*Okra pods
*Oatmeal
Psyllium seed
Quince seed
Sago rt.
Salep rt.
Sassafras pith
Sesame lvs.
*Slippery Elm bk.
Solomon's Seal rt.
Tragacanth gum

* * * *

LICORICE: Licorice has some soothing influence over the lining membrane of the throat. By "Sympathy of contiguity" this influence extends from the gullet into the windpipe, and thus Licorice helps to soften and loosen coughs due to common colds.

FLAXSEED: This makes a good soothing drink—Flaxseed tea—for minor sore throat. Pour ½ pint of boiling water over a tablespoonful of whole Flaxseed, and stir it for a few minutes. Then let it stand covered for a few minutes more; but do not put it on the fire to boil, as that would bring out the oil (linseed oil), which is not good to drink. What is wanted in the tea is only the mucilage of the seeds. Lemon juice and sugar added will make Flaxseed tea more agreeable.

DIAPHORETICS

DIAPHORETICS are agents which tend to increase perspiration. They were commonly used in Grandmother's day as an aid in the relief of common colds.

Diaphoretics act most favorably when administered hot, before bedtime. Botanicals marked with an asterisk (*) are often referred to as "sudorifics"—agents which cause copious perspiration.

*Ague Weed hb.
Angelica rt.
Balm hb.
Blessed Thistle hb.
Canada Snake rt.
Catnip hb.
Chamomile flrs.
Elder flrs.
*Ginger rt.
Guaiac raspings
*Hyssop hb.
Linden flrs.
Lobelia

Mountain Mint (Koellia) hb.
*Pennyroyal
Pleurisy rt.
Prickly Ash bk.
Ragwort hb.
Sassafras bk. of rt.
Senega rt.
*Serpentaria rt.
Spice Bush or Fever Bush twigs
Thyme hb.
Water Eryngo rt.
Wood Sage hb.
Yarrow hb.

DIURETICS

DIURETICS. A term used for medicines or beverages which tend to increase the secretion of urine. The fastest action generally is obtained by liquid diuretics taken on an empty stomach, and taken during the day. Physical exertion retards the effects of diuretics.

Diuretics are often used with demulcents, such as Marshmallow root, Couch Grass, etc., for their soothing qualities, when irritation is present.

Diuretics should not be self administered. Their use requires the services of a physician.

Bearberry or Uva Ursi lvs.
Bilberry lvs.
Broom tops
Buchu lvs.
Burdock seeds
Button Snake rt.
Canada Fleabane hb.
Cleavers hb.
Copaiba Balsam
Corn Silk
Cubeb berries
Dog Grass rt.
Dwarf Elder bk.
Elecampane rt.

Gravel Plant lvs.
Hair Cap Moss
Horse Tail Grass
Juniper berries
Kava-Kava rt.
Matico lvs.
Pareira Brava rt.
Parsley rt.
Princess Pine lvs.
Seven Barks
Stone rt.
Water Eryngo rt.
White Birch lvs.
Wild Carrot hb.

EMOLLIENTS

EMOLLIENTS: Agents generally of oily or mucilaginous nature, used EXTERNALLY for their softening, supple or soothing qualities:

Comfrey rt.
Flaxseed meal

Marshmallow lvs. or rt.
Oatmeal

Quince seed
Slippery Elm bk.

Emollients—Continued

"The jelly or Muccilage of Quince seedes, is often used to be laid upon women's breasts."—Paradisi in Sole—1629

Flaxseed meal makes a good warm and soft poultice. Mix a sufficient portion of the meal with hot water, into a mushy mass. Spread this with a tablespoon on a piece of thin flannel or old muslin; then double in half an inch of the edge all around, to keep the poultice from oozing out. The best way to have a poultice warm when put on, is to spread it on a hot plate, close by the person to whom it is to be applied. When it is on, cover it at once with a piece of oiled silk, oiled paper, or thin rubber cloth, to keep the moisture in. Without this, it will dry up very soon.

A very little sweet oil or fresh lard put over the surface of a poultice before applying it will make it more soothing and more easily removed.

EXPECTORANTS

EXPECTORANTS: Agents used to induce expulsion or loosen phlegm of the mucuous membranes of the bronchial and nasal passages. Expectorants often are combined with demulcents as ingredients in Cough (due to cold) medicines. Strong acting expectorants are marked with an asterisk (*).

Asafetida gum
Balm Gilead buds
Balsam of Tolu
Beth rt.
Benzoin, tincture or gum
*Blood Root
Cocillana bk.
Coltsfoot hb.
Comfrey rt.
Elecampane rt.
Grindelia hb.
Gum Galbanum

Horehound—white or black hb.
*Ipecac rt.
Licorice rt.
Maidenhair Fern hb.
Marshmallow rt.
Mullein hb.
Myrrh gum
Pleurisy rt.
*Senega rt.
Skunk Cabbage rt.
Slippery Elm bk.
Wild Cherry bk.

Yerba Santa hb.

* * * *

Elecampane was mentioned by Pliny some 2,000 years ago.

Licorice was found in the 3,000 year old tomb of King Tut-Ankh-Amen of Egypt, together with fabulous jewelry and magnificent art works.

NERVINES

NERVINES or RELAXANTS: Agents which tend to abate or relax temporarily, non-serious nervous irritation, due to excitement, strain or fatigue.

Asafetida gum
Betony hb.
Catnip hb.
Chamomile flrs.
Hops flrs.

Nerve Root
Passion flr.
Scullcap hb.
Skunk Cabbage rt.
Valerian rt.

Yarrow hb.

NERVE STIMULANTS

NERVE STIMULANTS: Besides the following, stimulating alkaloids are also found in lesser known botanicals.

COCOA BEANS contain very small quantities of theobromine, a chemical similar to caffeine.

COFFEE BEANS contain approximately 0.5 to 2 per cent caffeine.

GUARANA has the highest caffeine content, approximately 2.5 to 5 per cent caffeine, and a trace of theobromine.

YERBA MATE contains the least amount of caffeine—0.2 to 2 per cent.

TEA LEAVES contain theine, in large portions—this chemical is identical to caffeine, and similar to Guarana.

Nerve stimulants are useful for a temporary "lift" when health conditions do not prohibit caffeine.

Coffee and Guarana are useful for simple headaches caused by aggravation, and other temporary conditions.

Tea is a very useful beverage when permissible.

Cocoa is one of the most nutritive of all beverages.

Yerba Mate is a very refreshing beverage.

REFRIGERANTS

REFRIGERANTS: Generally a cooling beverage.

Borage hb.	Pimpernel hb.
Burnet hb.	Raspberry fruit
Licorice rt.	Tamarind pulp
Melissa hb.	Wood Sorrel rt.

SEDATIVES

SEDATIVES often used by women for the usual minor discomforts incidental to impending menstruation (not intended for delayed menstruation.)

Black Cohosh rt.	Cramp Bark
Black Haw bk.	Motherwort hb.
Catnip hb.	Squaw Weed
Chamomile flrs.	Yarrow hb.

STIMULANTS

STIMULANTS serve to quicken or increase various functional actions of the system.

Persons of a phlegmatic temperament bear stimulants better than those of a sanguine temperament, therefore the latter require smaller doses.

Stimulants refuse to act in the presence of an excess of animal foods.

Stimulants and narcotics never act as quickly upon persons accustomed to using spirits freely, as upon those who live abstemiously.

Angostura bk.	Mayweed hb.
Bayberry lvs.	Motherwort hb.
Black Pepper	Muirapuama
Blood Root	Mustard

Stimulants—Continued

Boneset hb.
Camphor gum
Canada Snake Root
Capsicum fruit
Cascarilla bk.
Cassena lvs.
Cayenne Pepper
Cinnamon bk.
Cloves—fruit
Cocash rt.
Damiana hb.
Fever Few hb.
Fleabane hb.
Ginger rt.
Golden Rod hb.
Horseradish rt.
Hyssop hb.
Jaborandi rt.
Matico lvs.

Nutmeg
Paraguay tea
Pleurisy rt.
Pennyroyal hb.
Peppermint hb.
Prickly Ash bk.
Quaking Aspen bk.
Sarsaparilla rt.
Serpentaria rt.
Spearmint hb.
Summer Savory hb.
Sweet Gum
Sweet Shrub bk.
Vervain hb.
White Pepper
Wintergreen
Yarrow hb.
Yerba Mate lvs.
Yellow Root

* * * *

"An infusion of Savory is the warmest and most stimulating of the kitchen garden herbs."—Hands—The House Surgeon & Physician, 1820

Cayenne Pepper: "The most certain of all herbal stimulants. Produces a natural warmth."—British Herbal

VULNERARY

VULNERARY: An application for minor external wounds. Almost any green plant that does not have irritating constituents is useful for minor wounds, because of its chlorophyll content.

Applications generally are most effective when fresh herb is applied. The following have been most popularly used for many centuries in Europe and the United States:

All Heal hb.
Blood Staunch or Fleabane hb.
Calendula hb.
Centauria hb.
Clown's Woundwort hb.
Healall hb. (Scrophularia
 Marilandica)

Healing Herb or Comfrey hb. and rt.
Horse Tail Grass
Live Forever lvs.
Marshmallow hb. or rt.
Plantain lvs.
Self Heal or Heal All (Prunella
 vulgaris) hb.

* * * *

AN OLD KNEIPP MEDICINE

One of the favorite herbs of this noted physician, was Horse Tail Grass. A strong decoction of this herb was used to wash minor skin irritations.

J. E. MEYER'S DIRECTIONS FOR MAKING BOTANICAL FORMULAS

Every formula should be divided into six parts as follows:
First—3 parts Active botanicals.
Second—1 part Aromatic botanicals.
Third—1 part Demulcent.
Optional Fourth—1 part Laxative (for temporary constipation)
The above general formula gives you 3 parts of active botanicals, and 3 parts of aromatic, demulcent and laxative. In other words one-half of this formula is composed of such botanicals selected from any of the titles in the following pages, as Bitter Tonics, Alterative, Astringent, etc., and the other half of Aromatics, Demulcents and Laxative.

For example—if it is desired to make a medicine called an Alterative, you choose a box of each of three different kinds of botanicals listed under Alteratives, and one box of any botanical listed under Aromatic, and one box of any botanical under the title of Demulcent, and one box of a Laxative. If the Laxative is omitted two boxes of either the Demulcent or Aromatic may be used. The Aromatic, Demulcent and Laxative are added to modify the acrid taste or action of the more powerful botanical.

It is not good policy to attempt to make your formula a cure-all by selecting, in place of three different Alteratives, one box of an Astringent, and one box of Bitter Tonic, and one box of Alterative, as you will get a combination that will not harmonize.

GETTING THE MOST OUT OF BOTANICALS

Many medicinal preparations, flavoring herbs, or beverage herbs have been wasted or spoiled simply because the user did not prepare them, or use them, to best advantage. This naturally discourages many people from trying botanicals again.

As most botanicals are mild in action IT IS IMPORTANT THAT THEY BE GIVEN SUFFICIENT TRIAL FOR RESULTS.

See your doctor for conditions which logically require his attention.

Certain botanicals MUST be prepared right and administered correctly in order to derive benefits. For instance:

Boneset herb is an old pioneer and Indian medicine. A HOT infusion was generally taken upon retiring to induce perspiration. In the morning the COLD infusion of Boneset was taken as a mild laxative.

Powdered Slippery Elm bark is soothing to the bowels when taken as an enema. Slippery Elm is useless however, if bowels are not flushed clean before injection of botanical solution.

Chamomile or Sage are prepared like Chinese teas, when used as a beverage. As a medicine they are made into a stronger infusion. As a hair application they must be used as a strong decoction. Sage boiled in an iron kettle will make a much darker hair dye.

A weak infusion of Hops removes the aromatic properties. A stronger infusion of Hops removes the bitter tonic principle—a decoction removes the astringent properties.

Each operation gives a different result. A plant does not yield the same principles by decoction as by infusion. By decoction, the extractive, resinous, and bitter principles are obtained, while by infusion a large quantity of aromatic and volatile principles, essences, etc., are extracted.

INFUSIONS

Usually about ½ oz. of leaves or flowers to a pint of water is used for an infusion. Pour boiling water over the herb and let stand for a short time, just as you would make common tea for the table. Sometimes a little sugar or honey makes the tea more palatable. An infusion or tea should be used while fresh.

DECOCTIONS

The virtues of hard materials, such as barks, roots, wood chips, seeds, etc., must be boiled for some time, just as you would make coffee.

Porcelain or glass vessels should be used in preparing infusions and decoctions. Keep saucer over cup in which infusion is steeping: Keep cover over vessel in which decoction is boiling.

To Make ESSENCE: Take about an ounce of the essential oil of the herb and dissolve in a pint of alcohol.

To Make FOMENTATIONS: Dip cloths or heavy towels in the infusion or decoction, wring out and apply locally to part that you wish to cover.

To Make OINTMENTS or SALVE: An easy method to make a salve or ointment is to take about eight parts of vaseline or lard or any like substance and add two parts of the remedy you wish to use. Thus, if you were to make a sulphur salve you would use 8 oz. of vaseline and 2 oz. of sulphur; stir and mix well while hot and when cool you would have a regular sulphur salve ointment.

Very old method of making ointments: Boil ingredients in water until all properties are extracted. If a very strong ointment is desired, strain off the ingredients and add fresh ingredients to strained liquid and boil again. Add this watery decoction to sufficient olive oil and simmer until all the water has evaporated. Strain off the botanical (if it was boiled with olive oil). Add beeswax and enough rosin to solidify. Melt them together over a low flame and keep stirring until thoroughly mixed.

To Make PLASTERS: Bruise the leaves, root, or other part of the plant and place between two pieces of cloth, just as you would a mustard plaster, and apply to the surface you wish to cover.

To Make POULTICES: Poultices are used to apply heat (moist heat), to soothe or to draw. Usually a soft substance is used, such as soap and sugar, bread and milk, mustard, etc. Some cause a counter-irritation, some draw the blood from a congested part and thus relieve pain.

To Make SYRUPS: After preparing the substance for a tea, boil for some time, then add 1 oz. of glycerin, and seal up in bottles or cans as you would fruit.

To Make TINCTURE: Take 1 oz. of the powdered herb and add 4 oz. of water and 12 oz. of alchohol. Let stand for 2 weeks. A teaspoonful of glycerin may be added. After standing for 2 weeks, pour off liquid and bottle for use. Should the herb used have a very weak medicinal power, 1 to 4 oz. of the herb may be used for the above amount of water and alcohol.

Botanical Sources of Vitamins, Minerals and Trace Elements

All green plants contain vitamins, minerals and trace elements from infinitesimal to plentiful proportions. Seaweeds are a far richer source of iodine than any land grown plant. The root of a common wayside weed (Yellow Dock) offers one of the plant world's richest source of plant-iron. Farmers in the United States grow more than 16 million acres of Alfalfa because of the variety and abundance of natural vitamins, mineral and trace elements found in this plant.

MINERALS

All life on earth depends upon the transformation by plants, of the inorganic earth minerals to organic plant minerals. Inorganic substances may disturb the proper functioning of the organs of assimilation and elimination. Organic substances, however, such as are found only in plants are easily and quickly assimilated and do not as a rule disturb the system .

The following plants are richer in such organic salts, than many other known botanicals. Botanicals marked with an asterisk (*) are reputed to be exceptionally rich in the element under which the botanical is listed.

CALCIUM: Needed for the formation of good teeth and strong bones. Children need calcium if bones and teeth are to grow strong and well formed. Both men and women need adequate amount of calcium every day. During periods of pregnancy and lactation, women require much more calcium than normally, as they must furnish calcium for the baby.

Botanical sources: *Arrow root; *Carrageen; Chamomile; Chives; Cleavers; Coltsfoot; Dandelion root; Flaxseed; Horsetail grass; Meadow Sweet; Mistletoe; Nettle; *Okra pods; Pimpernel; Plantain; Rest Harrow; Shepherd's Purse; Silverweed; Sorrel; Toad Flax.

CHLORINE: Present in salt as sodium chloride.

Botanical sources: All plants contain more or less Chlorine in the form of Sodium Chloride.

FLUORINE: Botanical sources—Garlic; Watercress.

IODINE: Essential mineral for thyroid gland. Lack may cause simple goitre.

Botanical sources: *Bladderwrack; *Dulse; Iceland Moss; Irish Moss; *Kelp.

IRON: Most important of the blood salts; the vehicle of oxygen in the blood. Gives vitality, builds red blood cells. Lack may cause blood-iron deficiency, paleness, rundown weakened condition.

Botanical sources: Burdock root; Devils Bit; Hydrocotyle Asiatica; Meadow Sweet; Mullein leaves; Parsley; Rest Harrow; Salep; Silverweed; Stinging Nettle; Strawberry leaves; Toad Flax; *Watercress; *Yellow dock.

MAGNESIUM: Naturally present in body.

162

Magnesium—Continued

Botanical sources: *Bladderwrack; Black Willow bark; Broom tops; Carrot leaves; Devils Bit; Dulse; Dandelion herb; Hydrocotyle Asiatica; Kale; *Kelp; Meadow Sweet; Mistletoe; Mullein leaves; Okra; Parsley; Peppermint; Primrose; Rest Harrow; Silverweed; Skunk Cabbage; Toad Flax; Walnut leaves; Watercress; Wintergreen.

PHOSPHORUS: Essential mineral needed for bones and teeth.
All seeds and many fruits have a small percentage of phosphorus.

Botanical sources: *Calamus; Caraway seeds; Chickweed; *Garlic; Licorice root; Marigold flowers; *Meadow Sweet flowers; *Okra pods; Sesame; Sorrel; Watercress.

POTASSIUM: Naturally present in body.
Nearly all vegetables and legumes are well supplied with Potassium.

Botanical sources: American Centaury; Birch bark; Borage; Calamus; Carrageen; Carrot leaves; Chamomile flowers (German); Coltsfoot; Comfrey; Dandelion; Eyebright; Fennel; Mistletoe; Mullein; Nettle leaves; Oak bark; Parsley; Peppermint; Plantain leaves; Primrose flowers; Sanicle; Summer Savory; Walnut leaves; Watercress; Waywort; Yarrow.

SILICON: Naturally present in body. Is found in all plants and plant foods. However, Horsetail Grass is probably the richest source in the entire kingdom. This plant is one of the few surviving plants that grew on earth some 280 million years ago.

SODIUM: The largest source is sodium chloride or table salt.

Botanical sources: Black Willow; *Carrageen; Chives; Cleavers; Devils Bit; Fennel seed; Meadow Sweet; Mistletoe; Nettle; Okra Pods; Rest Harrow; Shepherd's Purse; Sorrel; Stinging Nettle; Watercress; *Waywort.

SULPHUR: Naturally present in body.

Botanical sources: *Asafoetida; Broom Tops; Calamus; *Carrageen, or Irish Moss; Coltsfoot; Eyebright; Fennel seed; *Garlic; Meadow Sweet; Mullein; Okra; Pimpernel; Plantain leaves; Rest Harrow; Scouring Rush; Shepherd's Purse; Silverweed; Stinging Nettle; Watercress; Waywort.

Suggestion for Using Mineral-rich Botanicals

The roots and herbs listed here may be used in any combination. For example, let us assume you desired a general formula containing, Iron, Iodine and Calcium. You could take one or two botanicals listed under Iron, one or two listed under Iodine, and one or two listed under Calcium. Take equal parts of these botanicals, and mix them; then put a heaping teaspoonful of the mixture into a cup of boiling water—let it stand until cool, and drink one to two cupsful of the tea a day. A very good combination of this kind would be equal parts of Yellow Dock root, Irish Moss and Horsetail Grass.

VITAMINS

Vitamins are manufactured within plants, and depend to some extent on the health and vigor of the plant. The controlling factors are the varieties and the conditions under which plants are grown. Cultivated plants depend almost entirely on chemical fertilizers. Seaweeds are supplied with almost unlimited elements to feed upon. Botanicals growing in the wild state, generally thrive only in virgin soils, or in soils that can supply their necessities. When a soil becomes depleted, these botanicals move on (via suckers, creepers, seeds) or are eventually crowded out by their hungry neighboring plants.

Plant vitamins and minerals are far easier to digest than vitamins and minerals of fish or animal origin.

VITAMIN A: Needed for night vision and functioning of cells of skin and mucous membranes. Vitamin A is stored in the body, but under stress and strain, a surplus is rapidly dissipated.

Botanical sources: *Alfalfa herb; *Annato seed; Dandelion; *Lambsquarters; *Okra Pods; *Paprika; Parsley herb; Watercress.

VITAMIN B^1 (Thiamine): Needed for growth and maintaining normal appetite.

Botanical sources: Bladderwrack; Dulse; Fenugreek; Kelp; Okra; Wheat Germ.

VITAMIN B^2 or Riboflavin: Needed for normal growth of children; good nutrition of adults.

Botanical sources: Bladderwrack; Dulse; Fenugreek; Kelp; *Saffron.

VITAMIN B12: Is essential for normal development of red blood cells.

Vitamin B-12 also acts as a growth factor for children. It helps put weight on underweight children.

Botanical sources: Alfalfa; Bladderwrack; Dulse; Kelp.

VITAMIN C: Needed for healthy teeth and gums; prevents scurvy.

Vitamin C is destroyed by heat, cooking, low temperatures and oxidation. This vitamin is not stored in the body. A fresh supply must be provided daily.

Botanical sources: Buffalo Berry; *Burdock seed; Capsicum; Coltsfoot; *Elder berries; Marigold; *Oregano; *Paprika; Parsley herb; *Rose Hips; Watercress.

VITAMIN D: Needed for building and keeping good bones and teeth: Prevents rickets. A limited amount is stored in the body.

Botanical sources: Annato seed; Watercress; Wheat Germ.

VITAMIN E: Abundant in many plants seeds. The need for Vitamin E in human nutrition has not been established.

Botanical sources: Alfalfa; *Avena Sativa; Bladderwrack; Dandelion leaves; Dulse; Kelp; Linseed; *Sesame; Watercress; *Wheat Germ.

Vitamins—Continued

VITAMIN G (B²): Essential in preventing a deficiency disease.
Botanical sources: Hydrocotyle Asiatica.

VITAMIN K: Necessary in the physiological process of blood clotting.
Botanical sources: *Alfalfa herb; *Chestnut leaves; *Shepherd's Purse.

NIACIN (Another B-Complex vitamin): Prevents pellagra.
Botanical sources: Alfalfa leaves; Blueberry leaves; Burdock seed; *Fenugreek; Parsley herb; Watercress; *Wheat Germ.

VITAMIN P (Rutin): Believed to be of benefit in strengthening tiny blood vessels.
Botanical sources: *Buckwheat; German Rue; Paprika.

Botanical Sources of Hormones

Aletris root, Alfalfa herb, Clover, False Unicorn root, Licorice, Pleurisy root, Sarsaparilla, Tropical Yam root and Wheat Germ.

Physiologically related compounds have been found in Alder leaves, Elder flowers, Garlic, Linden flowers, Nettles, Pussy Willows and other botanicals.

* * * *

"Whatever elements nature does not introduce into vegetables, the natural food of all animal life,—directly of herbivorous, indirectly of carnivorous animals—are to be regarded with suspicion". . . . ."The disgrace of medicine has been that colossal system of self-deception, in obedience to which mines have been emptied of their cankering minerals, the vegetable kingdom robbed of all its noxious growths, the entrails of animals taxed for their impurities, the poison-bags of reptiles drained of their venom, and all the inconceivable abominations thus obtained, thrust down the throats of human beings suffering from some fault of organization, nourishment, or vital stimulation."

—from a lecture by Oliver Wendell Holmes, M.D., delivered in 1862 before the medical class of a noted University.

* * * *

"It is the Earth, like a kind mother, receives us at our birth, and sustains us when born. It is this alone, of all the elements around us, that is never found an enemy to man. The body of waters deluge him with rains; oppress him with hail, and drown him with inundations; the air rushes in storms, prepares the tempest, or lights up the volcano; but the Earth, gentle and indulgent, ever subservient to the wants of man, spreads his walks with flowers, and his table with plenty; returns with interest every good committed to her care; and though she produces the poison, she still supplies the antidote; though constantly teased the more to furnish the luxuries of man than his necessities, yet, even to the last, she continues her kind indulgence, and when life is over, she piously hides his remains in her bosom."—Pliny, 23-79 A.D.

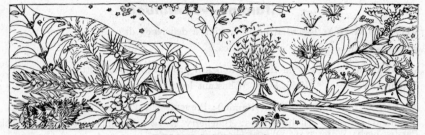

BEVERAGE TEAS

Herb teas have a place at the family table, just as Oriental teas, coffee, and other beverages—and many have qualities, flavor, aroma and goodness that are equal and oft'times better healthwise, than Oriental teas.

All herbal teas are not intended for daily use. Sassafras and Sarsaparilla are typical "spring teas"—bland flavored teas such as Bahe-Bahe, Lemon Grass, Lemon Verbena, etc., make perfect "afternoon teas" for the summer. Herby, full-flavored teas such as Sage, Dictamnus, Bee Balm, etc., taste best when there is a chill in the air, as in fall and winter.

Folks immediately become fond of some herb teas—the taste for others must be acquired.

Yarrow, Pennyroyal, Chamomile, Ginger, etc., are used to give warmth and comfort for chills, minor disturbances, or dietary abuses.

Linden, Chamomile, Calendula and Hop teas are served just before retiring, for their relaxing effect when one feels edgy or "out of sorts." Herb teas do not have the let down or depressing after-effects often characteristic of stimulants.

Some herb teas, such as Mints, Thyme, Sweet Woodruff, Wintergreen and others, leave a lingering good after-taste, after certain type meals. Warm flavored Anise or Fennel teas help relieve flatulence, after heavy meals.

Blue Mountain tea, Sweet Woodruff, Desert Tea, Damiana and other teas are wonderful when friends get together.

The essences and delicate flavors of aromatic teas gives one a refreshing change, and a certain lift after a day of close confinement and drudgery.

Some herb teas, such as Alfalfa, Betony, Clover, Linden, Nettle, etc., are served in place of Oriental teas, and coffee, when such beverages must be avoided.

Serving the right tea at the right time, and preparing them is an art in itself. Rules are simple but exact. Most tea makers agree that the tea pot should be warmed first. Put in one teaspoonful of herb per person, and one for the pot. Pour in the water as soon as it boils. Let the tea brew for 3 minutes. Then stir. After another minute pour out. Fresh drawn water is essential for good tea. Never use chlorinated, fluoridated or other chemically treated water. Never, never make teas in aluminum containers.

The flavor of many herbal teas depend mainly upon their elusive aromas, which dissipate rapidly unless a saucer is placed over the cup during steeping. Tea bags are not advisable as the bag often filters out the delicate bouquet, so essential in good herb teas.

Teas—Continued

The tea connoisseur NEVER allows tea to stand long.

To the true tea lover, any suggestion of milk or cream is unthinkable—they becloud the true tea and dull the fine aroma.

When Teas Taste Best
(Chinese Recipe)

When one's heart and hands are idle
When one's thoughts are disturbed
When shut up in one's home all day
When charming friends visit
In a quiet secluded room with old
photos, antiques, paintings, mementos,
and sweet memories.

When Teas Are Least Appreciated

At work. Watching a play. Opening
letters. During stormy weather. Going through
documents. On busy days.

AGRIMONY TEA: This humble herb has been used by the English and French country folk as tea, wherever the herb was found. The Gardeners Dictionary states: "Agrimony makes a pleasant kind of tea." It is generally infused with Licorice root and served at meals. Sweetened with honey.

ALFALFA TEA: A very good tea for daily use, but most people prefer this herb with mint, or other botanical of agreeable taste. Alfalfa is one of nature's richest sources of a variety of easily assimilated trace elements.

BAHE-BAHE TEA: A warm bland flavored tea which originated in Africa and found its way to the West Indies. The tea is much used by the native adults as well as children, and is preferred by many white European settlers. Bahe-Bahe may be used with other teas to "ease" the harsh flavors. Best served hot.

BALM or MELISSA TEA: This was an ingredient of Paracelsus' "elixir vitae" with which he wishfully (or for pelf) hoped to "renovate man and render him next to immortal." Balm has been used for ages to brew a tasty tea. In England it is flavored with a few flowers of Lavender. A little Rosemary added with Balm, "gives it character." Spearmint or a few Cloves, varies the flavor of Balm tea. Balm tea may be iced and sweetened.

BASIL TEA: A gourmet drink of exquisite odor. May also be used to add flavor and aroma to Oriental black tea.

BAY LEAF: Used as a tea in Greece and Italy. May be used to add flavor and aroma to Oriental black teas and other botanical teas.

BEE BALM or OSWEGO TEA: Used by American Indians. Still used in New England by ancestors of early colonists.

BERGAMOT TEA: Related to Bee Balm, and also used by the American Indians and early colonists, as tea. A tea with a "wild taste."

BETONY TEA: Worlidge wrote back in 1676—"The leaves of Chinese tea are a counterfeit of our English Betony, but far inferior to it."

Few, if any, herbal plants have been more praised than Betony. Antonius Musa physician to Emperor Augustus, held Betony in such high repute he wrote a long treatise devoted to this tea. Culpepper concluded that since the Emperor did not keep fools about him, Betony surely must be a worthy tea.

Betony is an excellent tea for daily use when Oriental teas must be avoided. The flavor somewhat resembles Oriental black tea. A bit of dried orange peel, or Clove, may be added.

BIRCH BARK TEA: A balsamic reminder of Indians, traders and old-time woodsmen. Add honey to sweeten.

The leaves of this tree are also used in tea, according to The Sylva Americana, 1822: "The leaves and bark, when bruised, diffuse a very sweet odor, and as they retain this property when dried and carefully preserved, they afford an agreeable infusion, with the addition of a little sugar and cream."

BLUE MOUNTAIN TEA: Martha Flint states in her book—A Garden of Simples: "On the Allegheny slopes "tea" is discriminated as "store-tea" and "yerb-tea." In Pennsylvania the population of German descent still use the leaves of the fragrant Golden Rod. This "mountain tea" has a faint perfume, pleasantly suggestive of its origin, and is sufficiently in demand to be an article of trade—gathered and cured in summer and peddled through the valleys in winter."

J. Bigelow, M.D., gives this information in his 1817 American Medical Botany: "The claims of the Blue Mountain tea to stand as an article of the Materia Medica are of a humble, but not despicable kind. Mr. Pursh informs us that this plant when dried, is used in some parts of the United States as an agreeable substitute for tea. He further states that it has for some time been an article of exportation to China, where it fetches a high price."

Blue Mountain Tea makes a golden brew, and has a delicious warm anise-like flavor and fragrance. Sweeten with brown sugar or honey. Serve hot.

BONESET TEA: A bitter brew, well known among early settlers and pioneers, who lived in cold, damp, log cabins, often with earth floors, and no windows. Sweet herbs, such as Wild Mint, Bee Balm, Sweet Fern, etc., were often added to the brew for flavor. The tea was generally taken hot as a night-cap. May be sweetened with brown sugar, or maple syrup.

BOTEKA TEA: Aromatic leaves gathered from high cool mountains of Mexico. A flavorsome tea, most popular in Sonora region. Add a little molasses, or sweeten with brown sugar or honey. A few Boteka leaves used with a good quality black tea, adds a taste and flavor "out of this world."

BUDDHIST TEA: Sold by priests to pilgrims toiling their way up to sacred Mount Omei in Szechwan province of China. Lemon may be added, and the tea sweetened.

BURNET TEA: Tea used by the French and Indians. Lemon and sugar may be added.

Teas—Continued

BRITISH HERB TEA: Recipe taken from a book on Domestic Economy, written in 1839: "Take of Hawthorn leaves, dried, 2 parts; Sage and Balm, 1 part. Mix these well together and they will make an excellent and pleasant tea, particularly wholesome for people who must avoid stimulating beverages."

CALENDULA: "The flowers are used in cooking and as a mild calmative tea."— "Venezuela Up-to-date." 1958

CASSINA or CASSENE: Indians in the Southeastern states traveled hundreds of miles to obtain a supply of Cassina. The plant is related to Yerba Mate, and has similar properties. A U.S. Department of Agriculture leaflet states—"Cassina is still being used to some extent in North Carolina and Virginia. During the War between the States, when tea and coffee were not available to the people of the South, the crudely cured Cassina leaves were extensively used by southern families and by the Confederate Army for preparing a beverage."

Cassina contains traces of caffeine. Attempts have been made to market Cassina, but as far as we know, they have not been successful, probably because of the cost of growing, harvesting and curing.

CATNIP TEA: Dr. Wm. M. Hand wrote in 1820 that "Catnip is an elegant warm cordial Aromatic." Catnip tea was a favorite beverage in many parts of Britain before the introduction of Oriental teas.

"The dried herb of Catnip, in infusion, is a highly popular medicine among the good ladies who deal in simples—and is probably often useful."—American Weeds and Useful Plants—1859.

CHAMOMILE FLOWER TEA: For ages, one of the most popular teas in the world. It is still found in many homes, European sanitoria, and served in fine restaurants in Paris. Leisurely sipping a herb tea or tissane, is, in the Frenchman's opinion the best way to top off an evening.

Dr. Schall, an old English doctor, declared that Chamomile tea was not only a preventative of nightmare, but also the sole certain remedy for this complaint.

Chamomile tea may be made in several ways. Some folks drink the tea several hours before dinner, with a little Ginger grated over the steeping brew. An after-dinner tea is made by adding Fennel seed in the proportion—2 parts Chamomile to 1 part Fennel seed. Cold Chamomile tea often gives a sense of relief after a heavy meal. Chamomile teas may be sweetened with honey. A thin slice of lemon or orange may be added too.

CINNAMON TEA: Williams, author of Useful and Ornamental Plants of Zanzibar and Pemba, states—"this is a very fragrant and refreshing tea used by the Arabs."

COSTMARY or SWEET MARY TEA: Reminiscent of Colonial days. Like all minty teas, it should not be steeped too long.

Clumps of Costmary are still found occasionally near very old home-sites.

DAMIANA: A fragrant tea from Old Mexico, held in very high repute by Spanish herbalists. Makes a sparkling golden brew with a delicious aroma and an agreeable bitterish taste.

Teas—Continued

DESERT or COWBOY TEA: This strange plant that grows in the highly mineralized soil of arid lake beds of the Rocky Mountain regions, probably has more names than any plant growing in the west. Besides numerous Indian and Mexican names, it is also known as Indian tea, Squaw tea, Mormon tea, Brigham Young tea, Teamster's tea, American Desert tea, Ephedra tea, etc., etc. The brew has a good aroma and a flavor quite different than other botanical teas. A noted botanist wrote—"this tea has long been used as a beverage among both Indians and Mexicans, and is really quite delicious."

DICTAMNUS or GAS PLANT TEA: An old Colonial Garden plant, related to citrus fruits. Italians call the plant limonella, because the leaves and seed pods have a strong lemony-like scent. The flavor of the brewed leaves is not liked by everyone. Both pink and white varieties of this attractive small shrub are used to make tea.

DITTANY TEA: Darlington's "Flora Cestrica" recommends this native American herb as a pleasant tea. The aroma of this herb somewhat resembles a mixture of Thyme and Bay Leaf.

ELDER FLOWERS TEA: An English favorite, the tea is often combined with Peppermint, and taken hot before retiring.

FENNEL SEED TEA: An agreeable tea for children, and the aged, when taken warm and slightly sweetened.

FENUGREEK TEA: Generally used when tea and coffee are prohibited. Used by ancient civilization bordering the Mediterranean.

FIVE FINGER TEA: Used mainly as a beverage by the pioneers and rustics living close to nature in the valleys, hills and mountains of Kentucky, Tennessee and Ozarks. It is a small sprawling wayside weed, resembling Wild Strawberry.

FLAX SEED TEA: Used mainly for its soothing demulcent properties. Recipe: Whole Flax seed 1 ounce; white sugar 1 ounce; Licorice root ½ ounce; lemon juice 4 tablespoonsful. To this add 1 quart of boiling water, let stand in a hot place for 4 hours, then strain off the liquor.

FRAGRANT HYSSOP: A sweet scented herb found in Minnesota, the Dakotas and the northwest. Commonly used where the herb is found, mainly by elderly folk, for its particular flavor.

GALANGAL: "A Practical Guide for the Perfumer" year 1868, states: "The Chinese prepare from it a very sweet essence, used to perfume the tea of the Emperor, and great officers of the Court."
According to east Indian sources, this strong flavored root is used by the Tartars to "make a kind of tea." Galangal is used mainly as a spice. This writer believes it is best used to give bouquet to Oriental tea, or added to bland herb teas such as Alfalfa, Strawberry leaf, etc., to heighten the flavor.

GINGER TEA: A favorite in grandmother's day. Used as a warming tea for chills caused by dampness or cold weather. Tea also used when stomach was upset by eating green fruit or other articles of diet.

In the British West Indies, a few cloves or a dash of nutmeg is added to Ginger Tea.

GRINDELIA or GUM PLANT: A resinous plant with a strong scent. Tea was used by the Indians, but the flavor is too medicinal for most tastes.

GROUND IVY TEA: In olden times, Ground Ivy was in great request for tea, and we were accustomed, in childhood to take it, as it is still occasionally drunk in villages."—Anne Pratt—Flowering Plants of Great Britain.

Some like Ground Ivy tea with a squeeze of lemon, or a few leaves of Melissa or Lemon Verbena. Sage, Lavender Flowers, or Rosemary are also used singly with Ground Ivy tea. Ground Ivy tea may be sweetened with honey. Licorice improves the flavor of Ground Ivy tea. As this root has sweetening properties, no other sweetener is necessary. Ground Ivy tea should not be steeped long.

GUARANA: This botanical makes a beverage more like coffee or chocolate. Guarana contains more caffeine than any other known plant in the vast vegetable kingdom. It is three times stronger than coffee. Guarana is made from the seeds of a vine growing in the jungles of South America. The Guarana seeds are ground up with water and Cassava flour and moulded into rolls or cakes, then dried over a fire of aromatic, resinous branches, kept smouldering from 30 to 60 hours in a drying shed, filling the compartment with fragrant smoke.

Guarana contains from 2.5 to 5 per cent caffeine compared to 0.5 to 2 per cent in coffee and 1 to 5 per cent in tea.

Guarana is useful in keeping awake for long drives, flying, or for work requiring safety and alertness. It is not for habitual use. The flavor is somewhat like chocolate. May be served hot, cold, or carbonated.

HAWTHORNE TEA: Leaves used in Germany in place of Oriental green teas. Leaves are also mixed with Black Currant leaves, or garden herbs, such as Balm, Sage, etc.

HOP TEA: Used mainly as a bitter, to improve appetite and digestion. Taken warm upon retiring, it helps induce sleep.

HOREHOUND TEA: Was brought westward by early pioneers and soldiers. V. K. Chestnut states in his book "Plants used by the Indians of Mendocino County, California" (U.S. Dept. of Agriculture publication)—"It (horehound) is especially abundant at the old military headquarters in Round Valley, and is there commonly known as soldier tea."

English herbalists recommended the tea for children because of its mildness and pleasant flavor.

Horehound tea, sweetened with honey and made hot with Cayenne, to which a teaspoonful of vinegar is added, is often drunk hot at bedtime.

Horehound candy was very popular in grandmother's day.

In England, black Horehound is used in the same way as common (white) horehound.

Teas—*Continued*

HYDRANGEA THUNBERGII: The Japanese use the leaves of this shrub as tea—they call it AMA-TSJA or "Tea of Heaven."—Archer's, Profitable Plants

INDIAN MINT TEA: When the white man came to America, he found the Indians drinking a mint tea in the same way as white folks had done in Europe for many centuries before. The plant has a distinctive mint fragrance similar to American Pennyroyal.

JUNIPER TEA: The berries are used in the manufacture of gin. An old English doctor advised: "avoid the gin and make a tea." This beverage is used commonly in Bohemia.

LABRADOR or SWAMP TEA: Chippewa Indians call this tea MUCK-I-GO-BA in memory of a Chief's son who saved the tribe from extinction. According to legend, at some remote age, the Chippewa suffered famine after extreme weather conditions destroyed their crops and game disappeared. To appease the Great Spirit, the Indian medicine men concluded that Muck-i-go-ba must walk in the big swamps for many suns. After the decreed time had lapsed, the medicine men followed, and wherever Muck-i-go-ba had walked they found strange bushes with evergreen leaves. They found no other sign of the Chief's son. The leaves of this bush were brought back and brewed into a warm fragrant tea for all the tribe. It soothed their stomachs and aching bones, so they thanked the Great Spirit for this wonderful gift. Labrador tea was used by many different tribes, frontiersmen, hunters, trappers and pioneers, wherever the bush was found. The tea is rose colored and has a mellow seasoned flavor. There is something about this tea that "suggests or blends" in with the old Indian legend.

LANTANA or BAHAMA TEA: Lantana camara, once known as Lantana pseudothea. Occasionally used by natives where shrub is found. However, the strong scent and flavor is not appreciated by most people.

LEMON GRASS TEA: A delightful afternoon tea, when served piping hot. Mario of the famous Pergola du Gosier, Guadeloupe, French West Indies, served Lemon Grass tea with his exquisite cuisine. The time—the place—and the tea were "out of this world." If you must sweeten, use a little honey. Aristocrats of Old Europe, once grew Lemon Grass in their hot houses, in order to keep a supply on hand for tea. In Grenada, British West Indies, natives add a clove or two, to each cup of Lemon tea. Natives in Trinidad "ruin" Lemon Grass tea with milk.

LEMON VERBENA: The following excerpt was taken from New Remedies, printed in 1878: "Lemon Verbena seems to have excellent qualities to recommend it other than that of fragrance, for which it is cultivated." The author of a recent work, entitled "Among Spanish People," describes it as being systematically gathered in Spain, where it is regarded as a fine beverage. It is used either in the form of a cold decoction, sweetened, or five or six leaves are put into a teacup, and hot tea poured over them. The author says that the flavor of tea thus prepared "is simply delicious, and no one who has drunk his Pekoe with it, will ever again drink it without a sprig of Lemon Verbena."

Teas—Continued

LICORICE: The roots of this plant yield a substance known as glycrrhizin, which is reputed to be 50 times as sweet as cane sugar. Although so much sweeter than sugar, it has the remarkable power to quench thirst, where other sweets increase thirst. Cold Licorice tea is used in place of water in many European industries, especially in iron and steel mills, where workers must endure considerable heat.

LINDEN or LIME FLOWER TEA: A Continental favorite, known as "tilleul" in French restaurants. The tea has bouquet somewhat resembling sweet jasmine. Use brown sugar, or honey, for sweetening. Serve with lemon, if iced. The hot tea is usually taken before retiring. A very soothing tea when nerves are taut from a day's aggravations.

MUGWORT: The Encyclopaedia of Arts and Science (1743) states—"An infusion of the stalks and flowers of Mugwort is recomemnded to old people for its mildness, instead of tea." A modern source mentions Mugwort being used as a common tea in Cornwall, England. Mint or Pennyroyal may be added. Mugwort tea should not be steeped long. Sweeten with brown sugar if desired.

NETTLE TEA: One of the oldest countryside beverages of England, believed to have been introduced by the Roman invaders.

Nettle tea is generally taken 4 times a day. The first cup taken upon arising, 2nd and 3rd are taken between meals, and the 4th cup taken upon retiring. The tea may be taken hot or cold. It is made like Oriental teas—sweetened and flavored with lemon to taste. The English are lovers of good tea—they often mix Nettle with Oriental type teas.

According to a British Health Magazine, "The addition of Nettle leaves to ordinary tea, in the proportion of one part Nettle to three parts tea, makes a cup of tea which will be appreciated by the connoisseur. The dried leaves should be rubbed through a coarse sieve, added to tea, and thoroughly mixed. The flavor is improved if this mixture is stored for some time before using. Friends, unaware of the mixture, have declared it to be the nicest tea they ever tasted."

NEW JERSEY or LIBERTY TEA: This was the tea used in place of Oriental tea, during the American Revolution. The "Boston Gazette," printed in 1768, states: "In 1768 tea made from a plant or shrub grown in Pearsontown, about 20 miles from Portland, Maine, was served to a circle of ladies and gentlemen in Newbury Port, who pronounce it nearly, if not quite, its equal in flavor to genuine Bohe tea. So important a discovery claims attention, especially at this crisis. If we have the plant, nothing is wanted but the process of curing it into tea of our own manufacture."

New Jersey tea is no longer used, or offered, for sale.

OLD MAN TEA, LAD'S LOVE or SOUTHERNWOOD TEA: Like other artemisias, this tea has a bitterish taste, with a slight suggestion of lemons. This herb was once used with Vervain, in ridiculous love potions.

ORANGE, LEMON or BERGAMOT MINT TEA: A dark brew, with a perfumed minty aroma. Try with a squeeze of lime or a bit of cloves. Sweeten with honey. Adds aroma to Oriental black tea.

Teas—Continued

PARSLEY TEA: A good source of vegetable iron and trace elements. May be enriched with Alfalfa, Yellow Dock root, Watercress, etc.

PARAGUAY TEA: See Yerba Mate.

PENNYROYAL TEA: In grandmother's time folks went out into the fields to gather their herb, and kept bunches of it hanging in the rafters of the attic for winter use. How often we took this hot minty tea upon retiring, when we were "out of sorts." "Common Sense in The Household" (1883) states: "Pennyroyal tea will often avert unpleasant consequences of a sudden check of perspiration, or the evils induced by ladies' thin shoes." An English variety of Pennyroyal is also used as tea, sometimes mixed with a few Lavender flowers.

PEPPERMINT TEA: A wholesome tea for young and old. Peppermint is an age-old beverage enjoyed by our grandparents, their parents, and many generations before them. Even the aboriginal people brewed teas from mints found growing in their native lands.
Peppermint tea deserves a come-back because of its real merit as a table tea. It deserves a place on the modern table. The use of Peppermint tea is so harmless that it can be given to children (one or two tablespoons of warm Peppermint tea, sweetened with sugar or honey). Peppermint tea may be used alone, or made in various ways. Lemon may be added, sweetened if desired, or added with other healthful tea herbs such as Alfalfa, Clover flowers, Linden flowers, etc.

PERSIMMON TEA: Professors C. Vinson, and F. Cross report that a good tea can be made of chopped Persimmon leaves—better than real tea—we are assured, because it contains the scurvy-preventing vitamin C.—from an old Science magazine.

PIPSISSEWA or PRINCESS PINE: Used by the Indians, early fur traders, pioneers, etc. A beautiful reddish tea with a flavor much too bitter for modern "sweet tooth" tastes.

PSORALEA physodes: Aromatic tea used in southern California by early settlers. A related species also used as tea in Chili, S.A. Found only in the native markets of Chili.

RASPBERRY LEAF TEA: This tea is an old stand-by in Europe for pregnant women. The tea is used in place of ordinary tea and coffee.
"We have known families in America to use Raspberry Leaf tea instead of Oriental tea; and we have no doubt that if the young leaves of this plant were gathered and sent to China, or some other distant part, and thence returned to England bearing some strange and unfamiliar name, it would sell as well as any other tea, and prove much more wholesome in the end."—Botanic Guide to Health, 1845.

RED CLOVER FLOWER TEA: A delicate flavored tea, that was very popular in grandmother's day and the "Eighties." Unlike most other teas, Red Clover flowers should be boiled for a short time. Sweeten with honey. Some folks like a few Chamomile flowers in this tea. Serve hot or cold. A good tea for daily use.

Teas—Continued

ROSEMARY TEA: Arabian physicians probably were the first to recommend this fragrant herb as a tea. Some folks add a few Lavender flowers, and a bit of lemon and honey.

ROSE HIP TEA: This is the fruit of a wild rose, well known for its natural Vitamin C content. Rose Hip tea has been long used in northern Europe, where the berries are found.

SAGE TEA: A heartening brew, if not made too strong. Sweeten with maple syrup, brown sugar, or honey. This tea is sometimes flavored with a squeeze of orange, lemon, or a dash of rum, pinch of mace, or cinnamon. In parts of Europe, Sage tea is mixed with equal parts of Melissa. In early Dutch trading days, the Chinese preferred Sage tea to their own native tea, and gave traders twice the quantity of their choicest tea in exchange.

SARSAPARILLA TEA: A well known Early American brew, which was eventually developed into a variety of concoctions. The following is a simple and good combination: 1 part Sarsaparilla; 1 part Sassafras; ½ part Virginia Snake root. Prepare like tea, but allow longer steeping time. Place saucer over cup to retain heat longer. Sweeten with brown sugar, maple syrup, or honey.

SASSAFRAS TEA: The old custom of drinking Sassafras tea in spring still is practiced by many folks, and finding favor with youngsters too. The aroma of this brew is as refreshing as the fragrances of new leaves, flowers, and the invigorating air of spring. The "Spring Tea" custom is of Indian origin.

Sassafras tea is made mainly from the bark of the roots, however, teas were also made from other parts of this tree. An encyclopaedia printed in 1743 states: "People gather the flowers to use them as tea." Another source claims Sassafras leaves make a wholesome sort of tea." Choctaw Indians gather the leaves in the fall (after they turn red) to make "file" to flavor foods. File is used to-day in New Orleans, mainly in Creole Gumbo dishes.

SLOE BERRY TREE: "The young tender leaves afford, in the opinion of Dr. Whithering, the best substitute for the foreign teas" (Oriental green tea).—The Domestic Encyclopaedia, 1802.

SPEARMINT TEA: Possesses properties similar to Peppermint, but milder and more fragrant. Flavor generally preferred by children.

Spearmint tea is also useful for nausea, and bad mouth taste following vomiting.

SPEEDWELL TEA: The plant was formerly very extensively used both in Sweden and Germany as a substitute for tea, and it had the old French name of "The de L'Europe"—while Danish writers of former days positively asserted that it was the identical tea of China. The Germans still prize the Speedwell tea, and Professor Martyn says "that it forms a more grateful beverage than the Chinese tea."

SPICE BUSH TEA: Many folks living off the beaten track in the mountains of Kentucky, Tennessee and the Ozarks still make a brew of Spice Bush Twigs. In order to extract the flavor, this tea must be boiled 5 to 10 minutes to extract the essence. The tea is fragrant, spicy and pleasant. Sweeten with brown sugar or maple syrup.

SUMACH BERRIES: Sumach bushes add a magnificent array of luscious orange, reds, and violets to our Fall colors. The crimson berries were then gathered by the Indians and early settlers, to make a pleasant acidulated beverage. Sweeten with honey.

SUMMER SAVORY: Dr. Hands wrote in 1820—"this tea is the warmest and most stimulating of the garden herbs."

SWEET BAY, (Laurus glauca): The Seminoles use the leaves of this for making a tea which they consider very wholesome.—"Across the Everglades" by H. Willoughby, 1900.

SWEET ELM or SLIPPERY ELM: Pour 1 cup boiling water over 1 teaspoonful of cut Slippery Elm bark. When cold, strain, and add lemon juice and sugar to taste. Slippery Elm tea can often be retained in the stomach, when other teas may not agree. A tea for the young and old.

SWEET WOODRUFF, WALDMEISTER, or MASTER-Of-The-WOODS: This is a small plant found beneath the pine forests of Germany, and other parts of Europe. The herb acquires a vanilla-like aroma upon drying. The tea is fragrant and palatable. Withering, English writer declared the tea exceeds even the choice teas of China.

This writer believes the tea is one of the most agreeable and most delightful of all herb teas. Woodruff is also used to flavor Swiss candies, German wine, liqueurs, etc. A pinch of the herb adds a delicate flavor to Oriental black teas.

TEA MIXTURE: One ounce each of the following: Agrimony, Melissa, Tormentil, Wild Marjoram, and Meadow Sweet. To this add ¼ ounce each of Red Roses, Cowslip flowers and Currant leaves. Mix thoroughly. Add milk or sugar if desired. Recipe taken from an old herbal.

TEA TREE (Leptospermum scoparium): According to history, the leaves of this tree were first used by sailors of Captain Cook, and other early navigators. Still used in Australia and New Zealand. Marketed only locally in the far East.

TEA-VINE or YERBA BUENA: A small vine with a fine indescribable fragrance. Used medicinally by California Indians. Called "good herb" by the Mission Fathers, and is still used as a tea by Spanish-Californians, who call it Yerba Buena del Camp.

THYME TEA: Make like Oriental tea. Best when iced and served with lemon. Thyme adds a pleasant variation of Oriental type teas, as well as other herb teas, such as Alfalfa, Red Clover, Strawberry, Raspberry, etc. If you must sweeten, use brown sugar or honey. Old-time herbalists recommended Thyme as a warming tea for the aged.

WILD GINGER TEA: Used by the Indians in the Great Lakes region, especially after bad tasting foods, such as fish, questionable meats, etc. Wild Ginger makes a pleasant tea, with a tiny bit of Jamaica Ginger and orange.

Teas—Continued

WILD MARJORAM TEA: "Medical Botany" states—"The leaves of Wild Marjoram, when dried, are used instead of tea, and are said to be exceedingly grateful."
The flavor of this tea resembles a blend of Thyme, Rosemary and Sage. Sweet Marjoram tea is more sagey.

WINTERGREEN TEA, PIONEER TEA, TEABERRY, CHECKERBERRY, BOXBERRY, MOUNTAIN TEA, CANADIAN TEA: "The people inhabiting the interior colonies steep both the sprigs and berries in beer, and use it (Wintergreen) as a beverage."—From Travels Through the Interior Parts of North America, in the years 1766, 1767 and 1768, by J. Carver, Esq., 1779.
"Quantities of Wintergreen leaves were exported to France and sold as a tea. Sels, one of the most distinguished botanists of the 18th Century, informs us that the leaf of this plant has a closer resemblance in flavor to that of Chinese tea than any other that is known. Halle, another Botanist who repeated the experiment of Sels, assures us also that it not only resembles Chinese tea in flavor, but it has all its agreeable qualities, without any of the injuriously stimulating properties which are attributed to the Chinese beverage."—"The Domestic Dictionary & Housekeepers Manual" —1842.
Rafinesque also extolled this tea. He wrote in 1828—"A very agreeable and refreshing beverage, much preferable to imported China teas."
Wintergreen tea is rose colored and has a natural sweet flavor without adding sugar or honey. The tea leaves a lingering pleasant after-taste. May also be used to flavor Oriental black tea.

YARROW TEA: A favorite medicinal brew of the old herbalists. Used as a beverage mainly by Swiss mountaineers.

YERBA MATE or PARAGUAY TEA: Millions of South Americans drink Yerba Mate, and its use is becoming very popular. Yerba Mate has stimulating properties resembling tea and coffee, but has a lower tannin content than Oriental type teas. Yerba Mate is a green leaf tea, and is often preferred by those who drink green type Oriental teas.
There is also, a toasted type Yerba Mate, that is preferred by most people in South America, and by lovers of black type Oriental teas.

YERBA SANTA: A popular tea of the old Spanish settlers in California. A writer of ethnobotany states: "The California Indians drink a tea of Yerba Santa, either alone or mixed with Horehound, in place of store tea." Jaeger, author of Desert Wild Flowers, concludes "It is rather peppery, but is pleasant to the taste." The dried leaves leave a remarkable sweet after-taste when chewed. Yerba Santa tea was used medicinally for common colds.

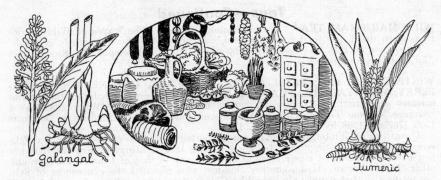

Galangal

Tumeric

SPICES AND FLAVORING HERBS

An old maxim on cookery:
"Never employ one spice
If more can be procured."

A noted physician wrote more than a century ago: "Capsicum (red pepper pods) taken into the stomach, will excite a sense of heat and pain; in like manner will a quantity of black pepper; but if an equivalent quantity of these two stimulants be given in combination with each other, no such sense of pain is produced, but, on the contrary, a pleasant warmth is experienced, and a genial glow felt over the whole body; and if a greater number of spices be joined together, the chance of pain being produced is still farther diminished."

*   *   *   *

FLAVORING HERBS: Many cooks are still unfamiliar with culinary herbs. The art of using these wonderous aromas and flavors lies almost entirely in one word—SUBTLETY. No dish should taste so strongly of herbs that the original flavor is lost. Poultry dressing, meat loaf, and hamburger should not reek of Thyme, Marjoram, Sage or other flavoring herbs. Salads should not be so filled with herbs that the concoction resembles a spring tonic.

THERE SHOULD BE ONLY A SUGGESTION OF FLAVORING HERBS—sufficient to give a simple perked-up taste to the natural food, and an appetizing aroma.

Bland foods and full flavored foods must be taken into consideration with certain type herbs. The strength of some herbs goes much further than others. In one way, Sage is similar to Garlic—its powerful aroma "takes over" completely unless used with utmost discretion The length of time it requires to cook foods must also be taken into consideration. Flavoring herbs are generally added to foods shortly before they are finished cooking, otherwise their aromatic principle and flavor may be dissipated by heat.

Herbs that are mixed in dressing and meat loaf, of course, are not cooked too long because they are incased in the food. One adds flavoring herbs to roasts, stews or soups, just before they are removed from heat. One may also use a bouquet garni in soups or stews. This is a combination of herbs, either tied together in a bouquet, or

Spices and Flavoring Herbs—*Continued*

tied loosely in a cheesecloth bag so that it may be removed when the desired flavor is obtained.

A pinch of dried herb is GENERALLY SUFFICIENT for a dish serving four. To soften dried herbs to be used in melted butter, mayonnaise and cold dishes: Place dried herb in strainer. Pour only enough hot water over to soften. DO NOT STEEP.

It is difficult to give exact directions for the use of flavoring herbs. It is rather like the directions in an old cook book—"a little ingenuity added to almost anything at hand, will make a good dish." So with herbs. One can constantly try new flavors in almost infinite combinations. Cooks who have tried flavoring herbs rarely are ever without them. Flavoring herbs add new interest and new flavor (and aromas) to almost all types of cooking. In addition to perking up the flavor of foods, they might be considered valuable healthwise for folks who must abstain from salt.

ALLSPICE: Cakes, cookies, pumpkin and fruit pies, plum pudding, gelatin desserts, mince meat, baked apples, peaches, apricots, cherries, bananas, fruit salads, tomatoes, red cabbage, beets, spinach, pumpkin, sweet potatoes, spaghetti sauce, pot roasts, spiced beef, corned beef, etc.

ASAFETIDA or ASAFOETIDA: Called "devil's dung" by Europeans but used widely in India for seasoning foods. Indians call it "food of the gods." If used with utmost discretion it may prove useful in some dishes, such as sauces, gravies, stews, etc.

BASIL: A 1783 record states: "The French are so infatuated with the flavour and qualities of this herb, that its leaves come into the composition of almost all their soups and sauces." French chefs call this Herbe Royale. It has a scent and flavor of blended spices with none of the irritating effects of spices. Parkinson wrote that "the smell of Basil is so excellent that it is fit for a king's house." Basil is particularly good with all tomato dishes, tomato soups, tomato juice, tomato sauce, and all salads containing tomatoes. Basil gives bouquet and flavor to stews, chopped meats, sausage and meat sauce for spaghetti. Basil is excellent in mixtures, such as Parsley, Tarragon, Thyme, Marjoram, Savory, etc.
Basil Vinegar: Steep 1 ounce of the herb in 1 quart of hot (not boiling) good cider vinegar, and allow to stand (covered) for 10 days to 2 weeks. Shake occasionally. Strain and bottle for usage. To increase the strength of Basil vinegar, reheat vinegar after straining off old herb, and add new herb, and allow to stand a few more days.

The French have developed several varieties of Basil, small leaf, large leaf, curly leaf, purple, bush type, etc. All may be used the same way.

BAY LEAF: Soups, stews, beef roasts, corned beef, stuffings, salad dressings, pickles, spiced vinegar, etc.

BORAGE: Beautiful star-like fresh blue flowers enhance cold drinks, fresh salads, mold salads, etc.

BOTEKA: Used like Bay Leaf in Mexico. Aromatic and more peppery—also used as a tea, and to flavor Oriental black tea.

CALAMUS: Used like Ginger, in foods in India. Also mixed with Ginger. Calamus is more perfumy and not as snappy as Ginger.

Spices and Flavoring Herbs—Continued

CANELLA or WHITE CINNAMON: Used like Cinnamon—the flavor is bitterish. Natives of the West Indies mix White Cinnamon with Capsicum, to make a sauce for meats. This recipe is said to be of very ancient Carib Indian origin.

CAPERS: Flavor buds pickled. Use as a condiment in chicken salad, milk sauces and veal stews.

CARAWAY SEED: Used in rye bread, salt rolls and sticks, cottage and cream cheese, cole slaw, tomato salad, soups, Hungarian goulash, veal, lamb, mutton and chicken stew, fish chowder, pork hocks and kraut. Seeds are used with French fried potatoes and boiled potatoes covered with sour cream.
Caraway is a basic ingredient of Kümmel cordials. It is used medicinally as a carminative and pleasant stomachic.

CARDAMON SEED: Used to flavor and give appetizing aroma to Christmas cookies, Danish pastries, coffee cake, candies, sliced oranges, fruit salads, grape jelly, spiced wines, liqueurs and non-alcoholic beverages. Syrians, Turks and Arabians use one or two of these seeds to each cup of coffee. The French use Cardamon with their demitasse.

CASSIA BUDS: Pickling, preserving, spiced fruits, mincemeat, and spiced wines.

CAYENNE PEPPER: A mixture of Red Pepper and spices. Adds "pep" to barbecues, sauces, fish, cheese, salad dressings, egg dishes, etc.

CELERY SEED: Used to flavor mayonnaise, French dressing, catsup, cream cheese, salads, cabbage and beet dishes, potato and tomato dishes, soups, pickles, meat loaf, hamburgers, sauces and gravies.

CHERVIL: Delicate flavored fresh leaves used like Parsley, in salads, soups, meat, garnish, herb butter, etc.

CHILLIES, RED PEPPER, CAPSICUM: Indispensable flavoring ingredient in the food of people in tropical countries. Used in pickles, sauces, chili con carne, tamales, ginger ale, and medicine, and with other spices to form Cayenne Pepper.
Chillies are an excellent source of Vitamins A and C.

CHIVES: The chopped fresh blades have a mild onion flavor. They are sprinkled upon (to enhance and flavor) cottage cheese, cream cheese, new potatoes, salads, soups, stews, omelets, etc.

CINNAMON: Breads, cakes, cookies, pies, waffles, french toast, pancakes, doughnuts, fruit breads, rolls, custard, bread, puddings, rice or tapioca puddings, plum pudding, and with many fruits. It is also used with beans, beets, squash, pumpkin, sweet potatoes, rice, ham glaze or sauce, pork roast, pot roast, Hungarian chicken, etc. Cinnamon is used in mulled wine, cider, grape juice, spiced punch, milk drinks, tea, etc.

CLARY SAGE: Not as strong as Sage. The minced fresh leaves used in soups in

Spices and Flavoring Herbs——Continued

France. Flowers are used to flavor wine. The fresh leaves of Clary were formerly dipped in milk, then fried in butter and served as a delicate salad.

CLOVES: Bread, cakes, fruit cakes, gingerbread, cookies, plum pudding, mincemeat, cake frostings, fruits of all kinds, tomatoes, beets, beans, sweet potatoes, winter squash, ham, pork, sausage, beef stew, gravies, and sauces. Also used as a tea; to flavor Oriental black tea, hot mulled wine, fruit juices, etc. Like Cinnamon, Nutmeg and Ginger, it has countless uses.

Natives of the British West Indies mix Cloves with pepper to flavor small native fish.

CORIANDER SEED: Used to flavor bread, pastries, confections, green salads, cream soup, curries, pickling, gravies, sauces, stews, poultry dressing, roast pork, hot dogs, etc. It is much used to flavor cordials, gin and liqueurs. In parts of South America, people are so fond of the flavor of Coriander, that they put it into almost all their dishes.

In the Far East and West Indies, a curious scented weed known as Erygium foetidum is used in place of Coriander to flavor rice and other dishes. Burkill wrote "an exceedingly little of it is not unpleasant in curry." The herb is most popular with the Chinese and East Indians.

Coriander seeds are a source of calcium, iron and vitamin A.

COSTMARY: A species of "mum," with minty fragrance. The French use fresh minced leaves in soups, salads and meat broth.

History of Esculent Plants (1783) states: "The whole plant (Costmary) has an agreeable smell which to many is far preferable to any of the mints. It is formerly cultivated in gardens for the purpose of mixing with sallads, and it is a pity it is not continued, as from its sensible qualities, it seems superior to many aromatic plants now in credit."

CUMIN SEED: Much used in Mexican cookery, and as an ingredient in chili powders. Used in cookies, pastries, bread, deviled eggs, rice dishes, cottage cheese, and cream cheese for an appetizer or spread. Cumin is also an important ingredient in curries.

Cumin seeds are much used in India to flavor foods and curries. The flavor of the seeds are improved by parching just before using. Cumin seeds contain a fair amount of calcium, iron and vitamin A.

CURRY: A mixture of savory seeds and spices. There are many types of Curries—northern tastes generally prefer the mild types. Few flavors combine so tastefully with so many different foods. A dash on roast chicken, lamb chops, in french dressing, cream of mushroom, chicken or tomato soup, adds a delightful smack. Curry adds variation to mayonnaise, dressings and sauces. It may be added to melted butter, used with vegetables, in salads etc. Curry may be used to flavor biscuits, muffins, corn bread, eggs, seafoods, soups, baked beans, rice, meats, stews, hash, chowders, gravies, etc. Dust a little Curry on bananas, fruit salads, chicken salads, tomato juice, cream cheese spreads, etc.

Suggestion: When following curry recipes, use only one-fourth as much as recipe calls for—you can add more later, if desired.

Spices and Flavoring Herbs—Continued

CURRY-LEAF or KARAPINCHA: This is a small tree that grows at the foot of the great Himalayan mountains. The pungent leaves are offered in all markets in Ceylon. The dry leaves are used in curries and mulligatawny—the fresh leaves in soups and salads—also may be used in meat sauces, gravies, etc. The aroma of Curry-leaf is exotic and indescribable.

DILL SEED: Used in cream cheese, appetizers, salads, root vegetables, sauerkraut, cream soup, potato soup, vinegar, pickles, gravies, sauces, sausages, boiled fish, etc. The herb is used in pickling.

FENNEL SEED: Used in black bread, rolls, pastries, sauerkraut, sweet pickles, soups, roast pork, sauces, fish, etc.
Fennel seeds are also much used in purgatives to allay griping tendency.

FENUGREEK SEED: Used in India in curries, and in Egypt as a condiment. The whole seeds, soaked in water, yield an emollient mucilage used for minor digestive troubles. The ground seeds are used in live stock condition powders, to fatten animals for live stock shows.
Fenugreek extract is used with other aromatic materials to make artificial maple flavoring.

FILE: Made of leaves of Sassafras, gathered in the fall, after they have turned red, when they acquire a sweetish taste and gelatinous characteristic. Thyme, Marjoram, one or the other, or both, are often added to File. Used in Creole and gumbo dishes, especially in soup, and dishes containing chicken, lobster, or shrimp.

GALANGAL: Aromatic, spicy and pungent, resembling mixture of pepper and ginger. Used as a spice, flavoring vinegar, sauce, and Russian liqueur, known as "Nastoika." Tartars flavor their tea with a pinch of this root.

GARLIC: Vegetables, salads, meats, garlic butter, garlic toast, rolls, soups, meat sauces, meat stock, poultry, etc.

GINGER: Gingerbread and cookies, cakes, apple and pumpkin pies. Baked fruits, applesauce, fresh or canned pineapple, papaya, grapefruit, sliced bananas. Basting butter or margarine, sweet potatoes, winter squash, pumpkin, beets, carrots. Steak, pot roast, barbecue marinades, corned beef, lamb, pork, veal, chicken, turkey, stews, pickles, relishes, sauces, etc.
Besides being used in many other foods, it is used in many beverages, such as ginger ale, spiced punch, spiced tea, etc.
It is important that Ginger is seasonal fresh, as the root literally "evaporates" (dioxidizes) and loses much of its good qualities with age.

GRAINS OF PARADISE SEED: Pungent and aromatic seeds, rivaling pepper in popularity during the Middle Ages. The seeds are used as a substitute or adulterant for black pepper, and to give false strength to wines, beer, spirits and vinegar.

HORSERADISH: Roast beef, oysters, oily fish, salad dressings, prepared mustard, sauces for shrimp, meats, etc.
In the tropics there is a fast growing tree, called Horseradish tree. Its soft spongy

Spices and Flavoring Herbs—*Continued*

roots have a remarkably sharp flavor similar to the plant. The bark of roots are used like horseradish.

JUNIPER BERRIES: Ripe flavor, with a tang of pine. A few berries used with all types of wild meats, as well as beef, pork, mutton and sauerkraut.

LEMON GRASS: Delicate sweet lemony flavor, used in spice mixtures, sauces, pickles, and to flavor tea and wine. The white center of the succulent fresh stems is used to impart a flavor to curries.

LEMON VERBENA: Adds a delicate aroma to fruit salads, punch, wine cups, jellies, puddings and Oriental tea.

MACE is the outer covering of Nutmeg kernel. It has a very mild flavor. Used like Nutmeg. According to an Indian source Mace is a powerful metabolic stimulant.

MARIGOLD: Fresh or dried flowers used in soups, broths, salads, yellow cake.

MARJORAM: Adds "character" to many foods. Often used with or in place of Thyme and combinations of Sweet Basil, Savory, Sage, etc. Marjoram is used to add flavor to sausages, chopped meat, lamb stew, lamb roast, pork roast, poultry stuffing, fish, butter and eggs. A common saying among beginners, "when in doubt, try Marjoram."

MINT leaves: Peppermint or Spearmint (hybrid species too) used in cold drinks and juleps. Spearmint is used to impart a delicate aroma to fruit salads, new potatoes, peas, jelly, vinegar and sauces.

MUGWORT: Used by Germans sparingly, on fatty meats, pork, goose and duck.

MUSTARD SEED: Black or White. Black Mustard seed is STRONGER than white. Some folks mix the two types together. A wide assortment of mustard sauces are made from these seeds. It is also employed in making pickles and curries. One of my favorite recipes: Mix equal parts of ground Mustard with Sage, and rub on a pork roast before it is put into oven.

NASTURTIUM FLOWERS: "The flowers of this kind (double) are much better to garnish dishes than those of the single; but for use, the single is preferable to this in salads, being of warmer taste; as is observed of all single flowers, that they are preferable to the double of the same kinds, for medicinal or other uses, as being much stronger in smell and taste; for the multiplicity of petals deprive the flowers of the organs of generation, in which are contained the essence of the flower."—from Gardener's Dictionary—1737.
  Young foliage and flower petals add flavor and aroma to soups, salads and canapes. Seeds are used to season mixed pickles.

NIGELLA: Seeds have a warm, aromatic taste, and are employed in French cookery under the name of quatre épices or "four spices." Seeds sprinkled over bread like Poppy or Sesame seeds. Called Black Cumin in the Far East.

Spices and Flavoring Herbs—*Continued*

NUTMEG: Cakes, cookies, bread, doughnuts, apple pie, fruit and custard pies, fruits, spinach, string beans, carrots, summer squash, cauliflower, sweet potatoes, succotash, chutney, catsup, desert sauces, meat, meat balls, meat loaf, beef stew, sausages, etc.
  In Africa and the West Indies the aromatic seeds of Calabash Nutmeg are used by natives to flavor foods.

ORANGE MINT: A highly fragrant mint, used to flavor teas, preserves and sweet dishes.

OREGANO: Warm aromatic flavor. An integral part of most Mexican and Spanish dishes, meats, stews, soups, etc. Oregano is also much used by Italians in spaghetti sauce.

PAPRIKA: This gives that sweet flavor to so many Hungarian dishes. Used both for color and flavor in cheese mixtures, butters, egg dishes, fruit salads, dressings, meats of all kinds, soups and vegetables. A very rich source of Vitamin C—four or five times as much as lemons.

PARSLEY: May be used generously with all meats, fish, fowl, and eggs. Also with peas, tomatoes, beans, cabbage, soups and salads.

PEPPERCORNS: One or two berries used with beef, pot roast, corned beef, gravies, in pickling, etc.

PERILLA: French use this herb to flavor and aromatize soup. Chinese use it like mint to flavor foods. Perilla has a warm flavor, somewhat like Anise.

PINEAPPLE SAGE: Fresh leaves add a delicate aroma to jellies, fruit salads and puddings.

POPPY SEED: Used mainly as a topping on cookies, breads, rolls, and as a filling in Hungarian coffee cakes. Also used in meat or poultry stuffing—sprinkled over soups, with peas, turnips, deviled eggs, etc.

ROSEHIPS: Adds color, flavor and Vitamin C to foods and beverages. Rosehips have a delicate fruity flavor. Sprinkle on foods and beverages.

ROSE GERANIUM: One or two leaves in bottom of baking dish, freezing tray, fruit cup, fruit punch, jellies, ice cream, etc., adds a delicate suggestion of roses.

ROSELLA: Pods of Hibiscus sabdariffa. Gathered immediately after flowers have fallen, before seeds form. Cherry-red pods have a sharp acidulated flavor, used for jelly, flavoring puddings and sauces. Grown in the tropics.

ROSEMARY: Used to flavor hams, salt meats, roast beef, veal, lamb, gravies, sauces, poultry and rice. When using dried herb, allow leaves to steep several hours to soften before cooking. When using on meats that require long cooking, sprinkle the herb upon food about an hour before it is finished cooking, to capture full bouquet of this herb. Long cooking destroys the fine flavor of culinary herbs.

Spices and Flavoring Herbs—*Continued*

Rosemary vinegar: Place ½ ounce of the dried herb in 1 quart white wine vinegar and allow to steep about 2 weeks (longer if stronger flavor is desired). Use vinegar with meats, stews and fish dishes.

RUE: A favorite flavor of Balkan races. Used with discretion on cottage cheese, and in salads, soups, sauces, etc.

SAFFLOWER or FALSE SAFFRON: Used like genuine Saffron. Spanish color soups, olives and other dishes with Safflower. Polish Jews use it in almost all their dishes, according to an old record.

SAFFRON: Most expensive spice in the world. Said to be the richest known source of riboflavin, or Vitamin B-2. Used in breads, cakes, fancy rolls or buns, rice dishes, meats, poultry, shellfish, soups, eggs, sauces, etc. Aids digestion of fatty meats, such as pork, duck, goose, etc., adds flavor too. Also used in sausage, poultry stuffing, cheese spreads, etc.

SALAD BURNET: Fresh herb has "cool" cucumber-like flavor. Use fresh leaves in summer salads. Garnish meat like Parsley. Try a single leaf on canapes.

SALAD MINT: Unlike other sweet scented mints, Salad mint has a flavor resembling a mixture of Celery seed and Garlic. A few fresh minced leaves go well with fresh salads, sauces, vegetables, cheese spreads, etc.

SAVORY: An aromatic and slightly peppery flavored herb. It is also known as bohnen kraut or bean herb, because it is used to flavor so many bean dishes, either dried or fresh beans, peas and lentils. Used also with vegetable dishes, such as cauliflower, eggplant, squash, cabbage, turnips, etc. Summer Savory (annual), and Winter Savory (perennial) are used in the same way.

SESAME SEED: Used to impart a delicate nut-like flavor to a variety of foods. Sprinkled on cookies, breads, rolls, confections, sweet sauces for deserts, fruit salads, salad dressings, cream cheese, garnish on soups, etc. Try Sesame seeds in casseroles instead of bread crumbs. Sesame is the main ingredient in Oriental candy known as halvah.

SMARTWEED: Fresh young leaves used for flavoring foods by the Malays. Leaves have a biting taste. Smartweed is common in Europe, as well as the U.S.A. It is generally found growing in moist soils.

SPANISH THYME: A relative of our fancy and colorful Coleus. Juicy leaves have a Sage-Thyme like flavor. Only the fresh leaves are used in all types of cookery where either Sage or Thyme are used. This writer enjoyed many excellent seafood dishes in the French and British West Indies, where the herb was minced and mixed with onions and Parsley, then inserted in a slip cut into filets of kingfish, dolphin, flying fish, etc. Herb also used in mayonnaise sauce for fish. Spanish Thyme is also known as Oregano de Espana, Sage, and other names in the West Indies.

STAR ANISE: Sweet anise flavor. Used like spice in China and Japan. Also used

Spices and Flavoring Herbs—*Continued*

to flavor liqueurs and spirits. Esteemed by Orientals as a digestive and breath sweetener.

TARRAGON: Appetizingly piquant! A MUST in French cookery. Herb used to flavor fish, meats, meat sauces, tartar sauce, mustards, cream sauce, soups, pickles, salads, etc. Tarragon vinegar is "out of this world." Recipe: Add an ounce of dried or fresh herb to 1 quart of good cider vinegar. Allow to stand from 10 to 14 days.

THYME: Favorite flavoring herb of French chefs. Thyme is the main ingredient of bouquet garni, a combination of herbs tied loosely in a cheesecloth bag, so that the bouquet can be removed from the soups or stews, when the desired flavor is obtained. Thyme or Thyme mixtures may be used to flavor poultry stuffing, meats, stews, sausages, strong cheeses, tomato juice, mixed vegetable juice, etc. A pinch of Thyme adds a pleasant variation to Oriental tea. Thyme blends well with Marjoram. The Persians nibble this herb as an appetizer. There are numerous species of Thyme— Thyme vulgaris is most popular for culinary uses.

TONKA BEANS: Closely resemble Vanilla in aroma, and are often used as a substitute. Tonka extract is used mainly to flavor cocoa, ice cream and candies. It is used in considerable quantities, to flavor snuff and tobaccos, and in the manufacture of perfumes. Ladies and gentlemen in grandmother's day often carried the beans for their subtle fragrance. The beans were a "must" in old fashioned sachets, potpourri and fragrant mixtures. Tonka extract is made like Vanilla extract.

TURMERIC: Used to flavor and color mustard, mayonnaise, pickles, sauces, curries and many other foods. Also used to color ointments and other pharmaceutical preparations. An Indian source states Tumeric is a good intestinal sedative, and has disinfectant properties.

VANILLA: One of the most popular flavors in the world—its use is almost unlimited. The extract is easily made by steeping pods in plain (not flavored) brandy, or rectified spirits. Extract improves with age. The Vanilla pods are still good after steeping. Put minced pods in ice cream.

WINTERS BARK: Little used except to add certain flavor to meat sauces.

ZEDOARY: Resembles Tumeric. Used as a spice in curries and to flavor liqueurs. Also used in medicine, perfumery and cosmetics.

Spices are Powerful Germicides

In summer the greater part of India (and, of course, Pakistan) has a shade temperature in the region of 100 degrees F. Freshly killed meat bought in the early morning will start to putrefy soon after mid-day if steps are not taken to preserve it, and even cooked meats are barely edible after 12 hours.

The ancients discovered by a process of trial and error that if meats were cooked in certain spices, they would not putrefy for days, and if cooked in special ways in Mustard oil, as in the case of vindaloo, not for weeks or months. They learned to bring together these spices in a multitude of combinations, and it is some of these that form the basis of the Curries.

Spices are Powerful Germicides—*Continued*

Cinnamon is an extremely powerful germicide. Some years ago, the scientist Cavel infected beef tea with water taken from the collecting tank of a sewage system. To one sample was added Cinnamon oil diluted to 4 parts in 1000; to another, oil of Cloves diluted to 2 parts in 1000. The germs in each sample were destroyed. But when carbolic acid was used the strength of the solution had to be increased to 5-6 parts in 1000 to be equally effective.

Yet how many people realize that Clove and Cinnamon oils are more powerfully antiseptic than carbolic acid?—Curries of India by Harvey Day.

SPICES FOR SEASONING ALSO PREVENT FOOD RANCIDITY

Certain spices prevent food's edible fats from turning rancid according to scientists of India. Previously it has commonly been assumed that spices were added to foods, particularly in tropical countries, to cover up rancidity or decay. They report that Cumin, Caraway or Fennel seeds, Cinnamon, Nutmeg, Cloves, Pepper, Turmeric and red Chillies are among the spices that will preserve fats even under very severe oxidation tests.

HERBS CONSIDERED NECESSARY WITH FOODS IN OLDEN TIMES

The following is taken from Phillips "Kitchen Garden" printed in 1831:

"French epicures keep their fish in Fennel herb to make them firm. In France the herb is used in all fish soups. It was formerly the practice to boil Fennel with all fish, and it never would have been discontinued, had its virtues been more generally known.

The American Indians also believed herbs were necessary with certain foods. The best known botanical was the root of Wild Ginger. It was eaten with foods of poor flavor. Wild Ginger root is mentioned in several early American accounts. One record, written in 1782, tells after being captured by Indians, the author made an escape —then found his way back to civilization, feeding upon weeds, roots, berries and raw meats. He wrote: "When food sat heavy on my stomach, I used to eat a little Wild Ginger root, which put all to rights."

In 1902 the following excerpts appeared in a cookery magazine, under the title "Medicine In Food."

There is a great deal of truth in the old saying that "the best doctor is the cook." The value of herbs and spices as medicine has never been disputed, special virtue being accredited to some.

Why is mint served with pea soup? The reply is, to give it flavor—which the pea soup often lacks, in spite of the vegetables boiled in it; but this mint at the same time helps correct the natural tendency that peas have to produce flatulence. Mint, whether green mint as used in cooking, or its twin brother Peppermint, are well known and universally acknowledged remedies for flatulence. Thyme, Sage, Marjoram, and other herbs possess a similar virtue.

Summer Savory is a MUST in bean dishes in Germany. It is known in that country as bohnen kraut—the bean herb. An Herbal printed almost 400 years ago, tells why it is recommended with this particular food: "Summer Savory is very good and necessary to be used in foods. It makes thin, marvelously prevails against wynde (gas)— therefore it is with much good successe Boyled and Eaten with Beanes, Pease, and other wynde pulses." In modern American cooking, beans are generally cooked with pork, making both more difficult in digestion.

Sweet Marjoram "does something" for foods besides adding flavor. Another old book tells us "Sweet Marjoram is chiefly used as a condiment in cooking, to diminish, by its excitant qualities, the heaviness of pork, goose and other fat foods." Sage is also used for fat meats.

BOTANICALS USED TO COLOR FOODS, COSMETICS, AND PHARMACEUTICAL PREPARATIONS

ALKANET: Roots yield a beautiful red or crimson, when soaked in fats, oils, alcohol, ether, etc. Steeped in water, they yield a brownish hue. Alkalies render the color blue. Used to color wines, medicines, oils, pomades, lipstick, etc.

ANNATTO, ACHIOTE, or LIPSTICK PLANT: An orange-red dye is obtained from a film covering the seeds of this West Indian bush. The dye matter may be removed by soaking seeds in fats and straining off the seeds when all available color is removed. Dye may also be obtained by placing the seeds in warm water. The dissolved coloring matter settles to the bottom. Seeds and water are removed, and the dye sediment is formed into cakes. The dye is tasteless.

Annatto is used mainly to color butter, margarine, cheese, soups, rice, etc. In the South Pacific. Annatto is mixed with Turmeric. A Puerto Rican Recipe: Fry 1 part Annatto seeds, with 2 or 3 parts lard, Crisco or Spry. Strain into jar. Use to color stews, gravy and soups.

Amazon Indians use the dye to decorate their faces and bodies.

The bark of the root of Annatto also appears to have some value as a dye, but I find no record of its use.

COCHINEAL: Actually a parasite that lives upon certain species of Opuntia cacti. It produces beautiful scarlet shades, used to color fatty foods, cosmetics, pomades, etc.

CHLOROPHYLL: A green substance found in all plants. The coloring matter of leaves is easily extracted by bruising leaves with alcohol. Powders which are to be given a green color, may be mixed directly with powdered dried leaves of spinach, celery, parsley, etc. The green substance is used to color candies, cookies, cakes, sherbet, fruit molds, salad molds, and many other foods and pharmaceutical preparations.

HENNA: One of the oldest and most reliable botanical dyes. Used the world over to dye hair, and by the Egyptians and Asiatics, for dyeing finger-nails an orange hue. Used to color cosmetics, shampoos, brilliantines, etc.

LOGWOOD: An infusion in hot water, yields a purplish-red color. Used to color wines, and combined with burnt sugar, to color brandies.

MADDER: Roots are the source of a variety of colors, including scarlet red, alizarin red, turkey red, madder red, madder purple, madder yellow and madder brown. Roots are soluble in water, ether or alcohol. Madder has the singular property of imparting its color to the animal fluids when given along with food. In this way it tinges the milk, urine, and even the bones, thus affording proof that the digestive process does

Botanical Colors—*Continued*

not in all cases, destroy the natural properties of the substances taken into the stomach.

Madder is used in food coloring, in cosmetics, lotions and pharmaceutical preparations.

An interesting note from a 1821 book of "Useful Knowledge": "Cows are remarkably fond of the Madder plant, and when they freely eat of it, their milk becomes red, yet the cream which it affords, makes a yellow butter."

MARIGOLD FLOWERS: Used to make a reddish violet hue. Put ½ ounce of flowers in a jar, and pour on a small quantity of boiling water. Allow to steep until desired shade is acquired.

Fresh or dried petals also used in soups, broths and salads. In France, the flowers are put on bottom of pan in which yellow cake is baked.

RED HIBISCUS: Flowers afford a red dye, used in the Far East in cookery, etc. A related species known as Black Malva flowers, yields a lovely lavender shade.

RED SANDERS, RED SAUNDERS or RED SANDALWOOD: Wood yields a bright red dye for coloring tinctures and other preparations.

RHATANY: Root yields a reddish-brown when steeped in alcohol.

SAFFLOWER or FALSE SAFFRON: The flowers contain two kinds of coloring matter—the one yellow, which is soluble in water—the other carthamin red, which being of a resinous nature, is insoluble in water, but soluble in alkalines carbonates. The yellow color is never converted to any use, as it dyes only dull shades. The other is a beautiful rose-red, capable of dyeing every shade, from the palest rose to cherry red.

Safflower is used like Saffron to color foods.

According to a century-old record—"Japanese ladies kept Safflower in little round porcelain cups to paint their lips. If the paint is applied very thin, the lips appear red; but if it be laid on thick, they become of violet hue, which is here considered as the greatest beauty."

SAFFRON: Makes beautiful shades of yellow. Put a pinch of Saffron in a jar, and add a small quantity of boiling water. Allow to stand in a warm place for 5 or 6 hours—then strain off. Saffron also yields its fabulous color in melted lard, olive oil, alcohol, etc. Saffron is very expensive, it takes the 3 stigma of some 75,000 flowers to make 1 pound of Saffron.

Saffron is used in breads, cakes, fancy rolls and buns, rice dishes, meats, poultry, fish, shellfish, eggs, sauces, etc., also used in cosmetics and medicines.

TURMERIC: Makes golden yellows, used in curries, mustard, sauces, bakery goods, confections, etc. Steep a small amount of powdered Turmeric in a little gin, alcohol or hot water.

Also used to color ointments and other pharmaceutical preparations. Women in Sudan use Turmeric as a cosmetic. Turmeric color cannot be used for articles containing alkali, which changes it to brown, for this reason it is used as a test for alkali.

ZEDOARY: Related and similar to Turmeric, however, color is darker and less brilliant. Used to color liqueurs, medicine and cosmetics.

Food colors may also be obtained from the juice of spinach, beet roots, mulberries, blueberries, elderberries, pokeberries, flowers, etc.

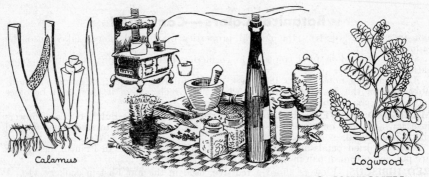

Calamus

Logwood

BOTANICALS USED IN WINES, CORDIALS, WHISKEY, BITTERS, ETC.

In former times, flavored liqueurs were made in the home kitchen, just as one once made their own butter, sauces, pickles, colors, medicinals, cosmetics, and other household needs. The recipes for many famous products originated in the humble kitchen.

The botanical kingdom offers unlimited possibilities. The easiest method of preparing flavored brandies and liqueurs in the kitchen, is by simple steeping. Aromatic principles are generally extracted by short steepings. Long steeping extracts bitter virtues. If this is not desirable, use more botanical for aromatic extract, and repeat steepings with fresh botanical. Leaves, flowers and strong flavors generally require less steeping time than hard materials, such as dried berries, seeds, barks, roots, gums and resins. When a recipe calls for a variety of ingredients, such as leaves, barks and fruits, better flavor may be obtained from each by separate steepings—either one after another, or in individual batches. Botanicals or fruits may be steeped either in Brandy or spirits, according to ingredients or taste.

Theophrastus wrote (Inquiry Into Plants) more than 2200 years ago, the following: "Wine does not linger on the palate for any length of time, but merely touches it, so that, while it makes one conscious of its own pleasant taste, it does not make the palate feel the bitter unpalatable taste of the perfume (fragrance): in fact the odor of this acts as a sort of relish (bouquet) to the draught. This effect indeed it has on wine which is sweet and especially needs the addition of perfume, because it has no relish of its own; while with other wines the reason is that, as the effect of the mixture, the two odors combine, as it were, to form one. Wine indeed, as was said before, has a special property of assimilating odors."

. The following list is by no means complete. Almost any botanical with a peculiar flavor, fragrance or action, such as spices, savory seeds, culinary herbs, etc., were used in the manufacture of many secret formulae.

ALKANET root: Makes beautiful deep red color. It does not impart its color to water, but to alcohol and fats. Used for coloring port wine and bitters. Acid renders deeper red; alkali changes color to blue.

ANGELICA root or seed: Used in the manufacture of gin, cordials, and other liquors. Root or seed have mellow aged-like flavor and fragrance.

Wines, Cordials, etc.——*Continued*

ANGOSTURA: "NEW REMEDIES" published in 1878 lists the following recipe for Angostura Bitters: Angostura bark, 4 oz; Chamomile flowers, 1 oz; Cardamon seeds, ¼ oz; Cinnamon bark, ¼ oz; Orange peel, 1 oz; raisins, 1 pound; proof spirit, 2½ gallons. Steep for a month—press and filter.

BALM herb: Used in wine and cordials, for its delicate aroma and flavor.

BASIL leaves are used to give mulled wine a delicate, spicy flavor.

BURNET herb: Gerard wrote "this herb being put into wine, yeeldeth a certaine grace in the drinking." Coles wrote "two or three stalks of this herb put into a glass of French wine, gives a wonderful fine relish to it."

CALAMUS root: Used for its fragrance and flavor, mainly in cordials and bitters. Yields its virtues in boiling water or spirits. The root is used like Ginger in India.

"Calamus imparts at once an aromatic taste and an agreeable bouquet or odor to the liquid in which it is infused. It is used by the rectifiers to improve the flavor of gin, and is largely employed to give a peculiar taste and fragrance to certain varieties of beer."—The Chemistry of Common Life, A. H. Church, 1879.

CANELLA bark: Steeped in red wine in Guadalupe, to be taken for colds. Canella is also known as White Cinnamon.

CARAWAY oil or seeds: Used to flavor cordials. Century old recipe: "A warm and pleasant cordial may be made with these seeds by steeping about an ounce of them in a pint of brandy for a fortnight, and then adding a pint of sugar syrup."

CARDAMON seed: A highly aromatic seed with warm and slightly pungent taste. Properties extracted by water and alcohol—more readily by the latter. Seeds are also chewed to conceal "tell-tale" breath, and as a breath sweetener.

"Cardamons are used in England to give strength to spirits and beer, and are extensively mixed with gin, in conjunction with Capsicum and Juniper berries, which, however is an illegal practice."—Mrs. R. Lee's—Trees, Plants and Flowers, 1824.

CATECHU: Is used in all kinds of liquors where a rough astringent taste would be desirable. The mode of using is to reduce it to a powder, and work it into a paste with some of the liquid, and then add it to the mass. One ounce or less, is sufficient for 1 gallon of liquor.

CHAMOMILE flowers: Used in South America "to aromatize wine, making a rather exotic tonic, and good tasting beverage" according to the publican "Venezuela Up-to-date," 1958.

CLARY: Raisin wine, made with fresh flowers of this herb, give it a distinctive flavor. Old recipe to sweeten wine: "In 30 Gal. of wine, infuse a handful of the flowers of Clary. Then add a pound of mustard seed, dry ground, put it into a bag and sink it to the bottom of the cask."

"In England, Clary (Salvia sclarea) is said to give an intoxicating quality to beer. Saffron also—the dried stigmas of the Crocus sativus, has a similar effect."—The Chemistry of Common Life, by J. Johnston, 1879.

Wines, Cordials, etc.—Continued

CLOVES: Cloves steeped in wine, was a very old recipe given to stop vomiting, and improve the appetite.

CORIANDER seed: A cordial may be made by steeping ¼ oz. of crushed Coriander seeds, and a small piece of Cinnamon in a pint of brandy. After 2 or 3 weeks strain off botanicals and add 1 pint of sugar syrup.

CORSICAN MINT: Used to flavor Creme de Menthe.

CUBEBS: The odor of this berry is agreeably aromatic; the taste warm, bitterish, and camphorous, leaving in the mouth a peculiar sensation of coolness, like that produced by the oil of Peppermint. Used as an ingredient in gin bitters.

DAMIANA: Aromatic leaves employed to flavor liqueurs.

FLAXSEED: The mucilage of this seed is obtained by boiling, and is used for giving a body to wines.

FLOWERING DOGWOOD: The ripe fruit is steeped in brandy and used as a stomachic in domestic practice.

GARDEN SAGE: "The leaves, flowers and seed, put into a vat with ale, while fermenting, greatly increase inebriating quality."—Universal Herbal, 1820.

GENTIAN: Is intensely bitter, without being nauseous, and the bitter principle is extracted by water and alcohol. Gentian enters largely into different formulas for bitters. Better known in Europe as Enzien.

GINSENG root: Used in Pioneer days as a cordial, made by steeping in wine and spirits.

GRAINS of PARADISE: "This plant is used to give a heating quality to beer, being a wicked adulteration, rendering it to some constitutions highly imflammatory, especially to children at the breast, by receiving the poisonous contents through the milk of their nurses*."—Whitlaw's New Medical Discoveries, 1829.

* In olden times, some women were available for weaning purposes.

Another authoritative source states: The pungent seeds are used chiefly for flavoring cordials, and for imparting an artificial strength to spirits, wine and beer.

HOPS: Used in great quantities in the manufacture of beer. Also used for furnishing the bitter principle of fine brandies, rum, etc.

HYSSOP: Peculiar flavor of leaves and flowers used to flavor wines and liqueurs.

JAMAICA GINGER: Used with other spices in a great number of liquor formulae. A Polish recipe: Steep ½ oz. of cut Ginger in whiskey, and allow to stand for a week or more (according to taste). Strain. Take a nip when having chills, or in colds.

JUNIPER: The berries impart their substance to water and alcohol and are used mainly in the preparation of gin.

Wines, Cordials, etc.—*Continued*

KAVA-KAVA: Roots have a delicate sassafras-like flavor. Used in the Pacific South Sea islands to make a ceremonial drink.

LEMON GRASS: Used to give delicate fragrance to cordials and white wine.

LOGWOOD CHIPS: Makes a deep red color, bordering on purple. Imparts its color to water and alcohol. Used in coloring wines—and combined with burnt sugar to color brandy.

MASTIC gum: Used by the Turks in making liqueur known as Raki.

MEADOW SWEET: The leaves of this lovely old fashioned herb gives a pleasant odor to wine and other liquors. Flowers and leaves have an almond-like aroma.

OAK bark: Red or Black oak are best suited for the manufacture of liquors, both for coloring. The bark is best suited for brandies, as it yields a fine brown color, and its bitter principle adds a pleasant taste to the liquor. The color can be obtained either by infusing in water or spirits.

ORANGE peel: A simple recipe: Place peels in a bag and suspend in those liquors where this odor would be desirable. Orange peel also enters into the composition of various formulas for bitters. (NOTE: Do not use peel of dyed oranges.)

ORANGEMINT: Used to give cordials a fine bouquet.

PERSIMMON: A century-old record states "The fruit is sometimes pounded with bran and formed into cakes which are dried in an oven, and kept to make beer, for which purpose they are dissolved in warm water with the addition of hops and leven. It was long since found that brandy might be made from this fruit, by distilling the water, previously fermented, in which they have been bruised. This liquor is said to become good as it acquires age."

ORRIS root: Has a pleasant odor, resembling that of violet, and a bitterish, acrid taste. Used in fine brandies and cordials, either alone or in combination with other botanicals.

QUASSIA chips: The wood is inodorous, and has a pure bitter taste, which is surpassed by that of few other substances in intensity. It imparts its bitterness, with a yellow color, to water or alcohol.
Quassia is sometimes used in the place of Catechu to impart a bitterness without astringency to liquors, but is used more extensively in the manufacture of bitters.

ROSEMARY: A noted English physician wrote at the turn of the century "Rosemary wine, taken in small quantities, acts as a quieting cordial." The wine is simply flavored by steeping the leaves in white wine and removing the herb when the desired flavor is obtained.

SAFFRON: The following appeared in a cook book printed in 1842: "Saffron is frequently added to liqueurs in France, in the belief that it has a tranquillizing effect on the nerves of the stomach." It is also used to color liquors.

Wines, Cordials, etc.—Continued

SLOE berries: Used to flavor cordials and in the manufacture of sloe gin. Berries infused in currant or raisin wine, imparts a beautiful red color and pleasant rough, subacid taste, resembling that of Port wine.

SPIKENARD berries: Carver wrote in 1779—"These are of such a balsamic nature, that when infused in spirits, they make a most palatable and reviving cordial."

WILD CHERRY: "The fruit is employed to make a cordial, by infusion in rum or brandy, with the addition of a certain quantity of sugar."—Sylva Americana, 1832.

WILD GINGER: Early Americans steeped the roots in either whiskey or brandy. Wild Ginger root contains only a suggestion of the hot Jamaican type ginger, so it may be used more freely.

WINE, AROMATIC: 1 teaspoonful of Wormwood; 2 teaspoonsful each of—Peppermint, Thyme, Hyssop, Sage, Lavender and Sweet Marjoram, 2 pints Port Wine. Steep until desired flavor is obtained, then strain.

WINES in COOKERY: Steep according to strength desired, with sherry wine any one of the following: Curry, Cayenne, Basil, or ragout spice mix which is made by combining 1 oz. each of dry mustard, black pepper and grated lemon peel, and a pinch each of Allspice, Ginger, Nutmeg and Cayenne pepper.

WINE, SPICED: To 3 quarts of white wine add: 1 oz. Cinnamon; ¼ oz. Canella; 1 level teaspoon of each of the following: Nutmeg, Ginger, and Galangal. Allow to steep 2 to 4 days, according to strength desired. Shake occasionally. Strain and add 1 pound lump sugar.

WOODRUFF or MASTER of the WOODS herb: Germans made a May wine (Maitrinke) by steeping Woodruff herb, with slices of orange or lemon peel, in dry white wine. The herb may be strained off when the desired strength is obtained.

WORMWOOD: Used with Cardamon, Angelica, Fennel and other aromatic botanicals, in the making of Vermouth. It is also much used in wines and bitters. The ancients mingled Wormwood in wine and drank it before or after a binge, to counteract the effect.

VIRGINIA SNAKEROOT: Used to flavor bitters. The bitter principle is yielded to either water or alcohol.

YARROW: "The leaves of Yarrow or Milfoil (Achillea Millefolium) have the property of producing intoxication. These are also used in the north of Sweden by the Dalecarlians to give headiness to their beer."—The Chemistry of Common Life, by J. Johnston, 1879.

ZEDOARY: A spicy root, resembling Turmeric. Used to flavor liqueurs and bitters.

NEW FLAVOR TO COFFEE

Old French aristocrats steeped a piece of vanilla bean in their coffee, to add a delicate flavor. This custom originated in Martinique, French West Indies.

Poorer people made a vanilla-like flavored coffee by infusing a handful of oats in a quart of boiling water, for a quarter of an hour. This water was strained off and discarded. The oats were then boiled in another quart of water for half an hour, and strained clear. The coffee is then made with this liquid.

In the New Orleans area and many parts of Europe. roasted chicory is added to coffee, to give it a rich smooth flavor. Roasted chicory may be used in varied amounts, to suit one's taste. The more chicory used, the less caffeine is contained in coffee.

In Arabia, the original home of coffee, a few cardamon seeds are added to each cup of coffee.

NEW FLAVOR TO CHINESE TEA

In parts of the East Indies, natives and the Dutch add a small piece of Star Anise to their tea. Star Anise has a sweet agreeable anise flavor. It is chewed by the Chinese after dinner, as a stomachic, and breath-sweetener.

To impart a fine flavor to ordinary tea, place rose petals in the tea canister, or add one drop of the attar of roses on a piece of soft paper, to every pound of tea, and keep the canister closely covered—taken from 1875 recipe book.

In Germany teas are often made weak and flavored with a little rum, cinnamon, canella, or vanilla.

In Spain, a few leaves of lemon-verbena are placed in the cup, and the hot tea is poured over them.

Bahe-Bahe is related and similar to lemon verbena, and may be used in the same way, to flavor Oriental teas.

The English sometimes use a few mint leaves with their green tea.

A little Ginger, or a teaspoon of brandy, is added to Chinese tea when the stomach is upset, or enfeebled.

In parts of China, a pinch of Ginger and salt are always added to each cup of tea.

A report from a tea connoisseur: "I add a few Boteka Leaves to a good quality black tea. The taste and flavor of this mixture is something that 'John Public' should hear about."

From an 1877 Cook Book: The flavor of Sage is so agreeable to some persons, that they put a leaf in the tea pot to flavor the tea, and they say that tea so flavored, is a fine refresher for a weak stomach.

ZEST TO MILK

Add a dash of any one of the following powders: Allspice; carob; cinnamon; cloves; mace; nutmeg; Raja curry.

Rose hips are an excellent natural source of Vitamin C, which is often lost in our daily diet, through heat and other methods of preparing foods. Stir powdered Rose hips in cold milk, for a new flavor and Vitamin C.

HERBS WITH LEMON OR LIMEADE

Top your lemon or limeade with any one of the following FRESH sprigs: lemon balm; lemon verbena; rose geranium. These herbs give a delightful "whiff" to ade (like mint julep) when you put your mouth to the glass.

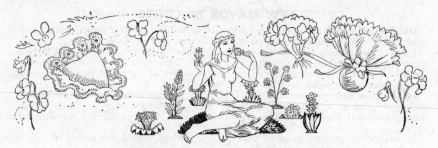

BOTANICAL PRODUCTS USED IN
POTPOURRI, SACHETS, POMANDERS, ETC.

The oldest civilized people known in history—Egyptians, Assyrians, Persians, Babylonians, and the Jews, as numerous passages of the Bible prove, used dried portions of plants and resins as perfumes and incense. The ancient Greeks and Romans kept urns filled with scented botanicals to keep the air of their homes permanently perfumed. Dry perfumes still have numerous uses around the modern household. Potpourri mixtures add a pleasant factor to stuffy rooms, especially during gloomy winter days, when their delicate natural fragrances awaken sweet memories of summer days in the flower or herb garden—of piny woods—or fields of flowers. Our forefathers, ages ago, stressed on such seeming trifles, to spread silent radiance around the household.

Grandmother made up dainty bags or pads, and filled them with scented botanicals, to be stored with clothes and linens, in boxes, chests, drawers, trunks, etc., to keep them sweet, and also keep them free from the depredations of insects. Certain scents also powerfully resist moulds that ruin leathers, books and clothing.

The delicate natural fragrances of botanicals "build up" in little used rooms, closets or closed containers. Certain botanicals, such as Calamus root, Khus Khus, Vetiver, Orris, Gum Benzoin, Gum Storax, etc., retain their aromatic principles for a prolonged period of time—these are called FIXATIVES. The fragrances of many botanicals are more elusive and require the addition of fixatives, to help retain their scents.

Some Potpurri and Sachet recipes include the addition of essential oils, in order to obtain a stronger scent, or a particular fragrance. Most essential oils (volatile oils) vaporize and lose their scent rapidly. Botanical fixatives, such as those mentioned above, are also used with essential oil recipes, to help retain their fragrance.

Sachet and Potpourri mixtures are best when they are allowed to stand for six weeks or more, in a closed container, so that the fragrances become mellow and completely blended. When made properly, mixtures improve with age, and compare with the finest natural perfumes. Fresh ingredients may be added to old mixtures to heighten their fragrance. The "life" of old Potpourri mixtures (dry types only) may also be prolonged by storing with clothes, linens, etc., in CLOSED containers.

AMBROSIA or CHENOPODIUM: Leaves and seed have a peculiar herby scent—used mainly as a blender.

ASAFETIDA: A resinous gum. In the crude state it has a most objectionable odor, but when the impurities are removed by maceration with alcohol and filtration, the

Potpourri, Sachets, etc.—*Continued*

resulting liquid, which contains the gum-resin and essential oil, is valued (in traces) as a component of certain types of oriental perfumes. Its odor is very tenacious.

BACHELOR BUTTONS: Flowers used only to add color to mixtures.

BALSAM of PERU: Useful in perfumery as a FIXATIVE for heliotrope, lotus and tilleul. Use also like Gum Benzoin and Gum Storax for dry perfumes.

BALSAM of TOLU: Excellent perfume FIXATIVE for amber, acacia, honeysuckle, champac, wallflower, etc. Use also like Gum Benzoin and Gum Storax for dry perfumes.

BASIL: Spicy scented leaves used in mixtures. Purple Basil is most colorful.

BAY LEAF: The same kind used in cookery. Subdued fragrance useful to obtain a carnation-like aroma, when mixed with other spicy ingredients.

BENZOIN: Gum used as a FIXATIVE—it should be finely ground. Use about 1 oz. of gum for 2 quarts of flowers, leaves, or mixture. Gum Benzoin is often used with Gum Storax.

BLACK MALVA: Dark purple flowers, used only for color effect.

CARDAMON: Whole seeds are very fragrant. Creamy white seeds may be stained for color effect.

CALAMUS: A perfumy root that is used in fragrant and repellent mixtures. The root is also used as a FIXATIVE to retain and prolong the aromatic principles of other botanicals, or fragrant oils.

CALENDULA or MARIGOLD: Yellow flowers, used only to add color.

CARAWAY: Ingredient in old-fashioned recipes.

CEDARWOOD CHIPS: Repellent—used also as a base for scented mixtures. Cedarwood retains its aroma for some time, so it may also be used as a FIXATIVE, if its strong aroma does not overcome all other aromatic botanicals.

CINNAMON: Both ground, or sticks, are used in fragrant spice and carnation-type mixtures.

CLARY SAGE: Leaves and flowers are more highly scented, than common Sage.

CLOVES: A powerful fragrance in medicine, teas, sachets, potpourri, pomanders, etc.

CORIANDER: Often used in old-fashioned recipes.

COSTMARY: Used mainly to scent linens. Also called Bible-leaf, because leaf often was used as a page marker.

DEER'S TONGUE: The dried herb has a sweet vanilla-like aroma. Often found hanging in cabins of negroes living in Southeastern states, where the herb is found. The scent of this herb is stronger than Sweet Woodruff.

GAS PLANT: Heavy lemony scent—used in mixtures. Seed pods are attractive in mixtures.

Potpourri, Sachets, etc.—*Continued*

GERMAN RUE: An important nosegay herb of Old England. Citizens held little bouquets of this herb close to their noses, during plagues, when they suspected they were in immediate danger. Nosegays of Rue and Rosemary, or Rue with other herbs, are still placed on the Justice's bench in English courts, the custom arising in 1750 during an epidemic of jail fever at Newgate.

GOBERNADORA: A heavy scent, used only with lighter fragrances.

HOLLYHOCK: Assorted colored flowers—used only to beautify mixtures.

KHUS KHUS or VETIVERT: The roots of this grass, when dried, acquire a very pleasant aroma resembling Sandalwood with a whiff of Myrrh. Bundles of the dried root are widely sold in the West Indies by the natives, as a repellent against cucarachas (roaches) and other insects. In India the roots are manufactured into awnings, blinds, sunshades, but principally used for screens, which during the hot season, are placed in doorways and windows, and are better known as tatties, which when wetted, diffuse a refreshing perfume, and the evaporation of the water at the same time, cools the air. Khus Khus may be used in mixtures. It is one of the best FIXATIVES for dry or liquid perfumes. Khus Khus blends well with rose combinations.

LAVENDER: Flowers. Probably the most popular of all scented herbs in Elizabethan days. The flowers were used alone, or in mixtures for color and aroma.

LEMON SCENTED GERANIUM: "A friend once told me that when she was a small child, she remembers her grandmother carefully picking the old leaves from this plant and putting them in a cloth bag in the linen closet. To this day, the wood retains the pleasant fragrance."

LEMON VERBENA: The leaves have a delicate and delectable sweet lemony scent. Use only with the most delicate fragrances.

LIFE EVERLASTING: Bundles of this herb were hung in the old-time log cabins, for their fine scent, and medicinal uses. The herb was also used by pioneers as stuffing for pillows.

MARJORAM: Herb and flowers have a piny aroma—blends well with pine, woodsy, and herb garden blends.

MINTS: Use sparingly in mixtures. Orange mint is most perfumy and colorful, and by far the best for Sachets and Potpourri.

MULLEIN: Golden flowers, used only to add color to mixtures.

ORANGE: Peel, leaves and flowers are used in Sachets and Potpourri. Peels may be used as a FIXATIVE.

Parkinson wrote in 1629, "The dryed rinde of Orenges, by reason of the sweete and strong sent, serveth to bee put among other things to make sweet powders."

ORRIS: Root. This is one of the best of all dried botanicals used. The odor resembles violets. Improves with age. May be used alone, or in mixtures for Sachets, Potpourri and Pomanders. A wonderful FIXATIVE.

Potpourri, Sachets, etc.—*Continued*

PATCHOULI: Leaves. Famous Indian shawls were scented with these leaves when shawl was not in use. Saris too, were kept in a box with Patchouli leaves.

PERILLA: Leaves have a subdued anise-like scent. Blends well with spicy mixtures.

ROSE: Doubtless the most popular of all flowers. Leaves, buds and petals are used in Sachets and Potpourri. The most fragrant petals are those from pink or darker colored flowers. Rosa damascena (Damask rose), Rose gallica and Rose centifolia (cabbage rose) are excellent sources for petals. Damask rose is the best source of rose leaves. Gruss an Terplitz rose is an excellent source for rose buds, as the bush is ever-blooming.

ROSE GERANIUM: The old leaves of this plant have an aroma resembling roses. Women of Malay and other parts of the far East hide the leaves in their hair, for their delicate aroma. Excellent in mixtures with other delicate scented leaves and flowers, such as Lemon Verbena, Lavender, etc.

ROSEMARY: One of the oldest and most popular of all fragrant herbs. The incense-like aroma suggests ancient rituals and ceremonies. Used with Rue during plagues, in Old England.

SAFFLOWER: Golden red flowers, used only to color mixtures.

SAGE: Leaves used to enhance herby, and special type mixtures.

SANDALWOOD: Chips or raspings are used in Oriental type mixtures, and as a base and FIXATIVE for Rose Sachet and Rose Potpourri mixtures.

SASSAFRAS: Used as a repellent in Colonial times.

SOUTHERNWOOD: The French call this herb Garde-robe, and use it as a moth repellent. It is also used to give linens a fresh clean aroma.

STORAX: Gum, used as a FIXATIVE. It should be finely ground. Use 1 oz. of gum for each 2 quarts of flowers, leaves, or mixture. Gum Storax may be combined with Gum Benzoin.

SUMBUL: Root. Has penetrating odor of musk. Used only in mixtures for Sachets and Potpourri.

SWEET FERN: The aroma suggests pine forests. Used by Indians to line their baskets when they went berry picking.

SWEET MELILOT: The tiny white or yellow flowering varieties acquire a sweet vanilla-like fragrance upon drying. Flowers may be used alone or blended into mixtures.

SWEET VERNAL GRASS: Used by Indians to make scented baskets.

SWEET WOODRUFF: Suggests a field of new-mown hay.

TANGERINE: Peels used like orange peel.

Potpourri, Sachets, etc.—*Continued*

TONKA or TONQUIN BEANS: Long lasting fragrance resembling vanilla. Blends well with spicy, fruity and flowery fragrances. A recipe book printed in 1878 states: "When snuff-taking was much more general than at present, a Tonka bean was generally kept in the snuff-box for the sake of the agreeable fragrance which it imparted to the snuff. Now, however, the uses of Tonka beans are mostly confined to the preparation of elixirs, of perfumes either for fluid extracts, for handkerchiefs, or for sachet powders. They are often, however, to be seen in hosiers' shops, where they are sold for placing in drawers with linen. The Creoles fully appreciate the fragrance of these seeds, and make use of them not only for their perfume, but also for putting in chests or drawers for the purpose, they say, of driving away insects."

WINTER SAVORY: Used as a flea repellent. Fido may appreciate a pillow made of this herb.

WORMWOOD: Used in great quantities during the Middle Ages by wool cloth manufacturers, to protect their goods from moths. Used occasionally in mixtures.

English Potpourri Recipe

1. Make a mixture of dry Rose petals, Lavender flowers, and any other fragrant flowers available.

2. Make another mixture of the following: 2 oz. Cinnamon; 4 oz. Orris; 2 oz. Cloves; 4 oz. Benzoin Gum; 1 oz. Cardamon seeds; 1 drachm (1 teaspoonful) otto of Rose. Mix these ingredients thoroughly in 6 pounds of coarse salt. Place a layer of mixture No. 1, in a wide-mouth earthern jar. Over this place a layer of mixture No. 2. Repeat this process until the jar is filled. Press down tightly and allow this to stand and mellow for 3 months before using. Mix ingredients thoroughly after the time specified, then place mixture in Potpourri jars.

Another recipe: To 1 pound of dried Damask Rose petals, add ¼ pound each—common salt (not iodized), coarse salt, and brown sugar; ½ oz. each of Storax, Benzoin, ground Orris, Cinnamon and Cloves. Rose Geranium, Lemon Verbena, Orange or other aromatic leaves may be added to the mixture. Put ingredients in jar, stirring frequently with a wooden spoon. Allow aroma to "build up" in closed rooms, clothes closets, etc. Keep jar covered when doors of rooms, etc., are left open.

Spice Potpourri

Half a pound of common salt (not iodized); half a pound of coarse salt; half an ounce each of Nutmeg, Cinnamon, Cloves, Allspice, Benzoin, and borax; half an ounce of Orris root pounded separately, and mixed afterwards, together with the salt; some lemon and orange peel dried and pounded, and half a drachm (½ teaspoonful) of musk, if available.

Sweet Jar Recipe

Use the leaves of Lavender, Lemon Verbena, Sweet Marjoram, Rosemary, Bay and Orange, and the flowers of Violet, Clove Pinks, Lavender, Roses, Jessamine, Wallflowers, Heliotrope, Myrtle, Mignonette, Balm of Gilead, Carnations, or other available material.

Gather the above on a dry day; carefully pick the petals from the buds and stems; spread them open until perfectly dry, and put them in paper bags until you make

Sweet Jar Recipe—*Continued*

your jar. Then begin with a layer of the dry leaves and petals and a layer of the spice mixture, and so on until it is filled. Cover it two days, and then mix up the whole together from the bottom of the jar. It should be frequently mixed after the jar is made.

Another recipe: 2 oz. Lavender flowers; 2 oz. Orris root; 1 oz. ground Rosemary, and 5 drops Oil of Rose. Mix well.

Rose Pot Pourri

Gather Damask rose petals when rose is at the peak of bloom. Pack them in a glass jar which has a tight cover. Between every 2 inch layer of petals, sprinkle 2 teaspoons of salt. Add more layers of petals and salt to the jar each day until it is full. Keep in a dark, dry, cool place for one week. Then spread out the petals on a paper towel and loosen them carefully. Mix the following ingredients thoroughly and sift well through the petals in a large bowl:

½ oz. violet scented talcum powder
1 oz. Orris root
½ teaspoon Mace
½ teaspoon Cinnamon
½ teaspoon Cloves
4 drops oil of Rose Geranium

Add the following very slowly:

20 drops Eucalyptus oil
10 drops Bergamot
2 teaspoons alcohol

Repack the mixture in the jar, cover lightly and set aside for 2 weeks to ripen. It will then be ready to distribute in rose jars.

Another: An old recipe, warranted to be good, and which calls for great care in the gathering of the petals. It is said to remain fragrant in open bowls for 2 years if occasionally stirred, but in the closed pot pourri it will remain fragrant much longer. Pluck the rose petals early in the morning; with them have an equal quantity of lavender blossoms, and put them all in a large earthenware bowl; add ½ pound crushed Orris root, and then to every 2 pounds add 2 ounces each of bruised Cloves, Cinnamon, Allspice and salt; let the whole stand for about 2 weeks, thoroughly mixing it every day with your hands, and then it will be ready for use.

Ceylon Sachet

Two parts Khus Khus; 2 parts Damask Rose petals; 1 part Patchouli; 1 part Mace.

Clove Pink Sachet

2 oz. Orris root; 1 oz. Lavender flowers; ½ oz. Patchouli; ½ oz. Deer's Tongue; 2 teaspoonsful Cloves; 1 teaspoonful Allspice; 10 drops each of Oil of Rose; Orange flower and Lavender and 15 drops of Sandalwood. Mix.

Frangipanni Sachet

¼ pound Sage; ¼ pound Sandalwood; 3 pounds Orris root; ¼ pound Khus Khus, and 30 grains each of Oils Neroli, Sandalwood and Rhodium.

Another recipe: 2 pounds Orris root; 2 oz. Khus Khus or Vetiver; 2 oz. Sandalwood; 1 drachm (1 teaspoonful) Oil of Rose and 1 drachm Oil of Sandalwood.

Sachets—Continued
Heliotrope Sachet

1 pound Damask Rose petals; ½ pound Tonka beans; 2 oz. Vanilla pods; 2 pounds Orris root; ½ oz. Heliotrope Oil.

Rose Sachets

1 pound Damask Rose petals; ½ pound finely rasped Sandalwood; ½ oz. Rose oil.
Another recipe: 1 pound Damask Rose petals; 2 or 3 oz. Rose Geranium leaves; ½ pound rasped Sandalwood, and ¼ oz. Rose oil.
Another: 1 pound rasped Sandalwood, ¼ oz. Rose oil.
Another: 8 oz. Sandalwood, 1 pound Damask Rose petals, and 2½ drachms (2½ teaspoonsful) Oil of Rose. Mix.

Spicy Sachets

2 oz. each of dry Damask Rose petals and Lavender flowers; 1 oz. Orris root; 2 teaspoonsful each of Cloves, Allspice and Cinnamon.
Another recipe:—Used as a repellent against moths—Take 1 oz. each of Tonka beans; Caraway; Cloves; Mace; Nutmeg; Cinnamon, well ground; add 6 oz. of Orris root and mix well.

Verbena Sachet

½ pound lemon peels; ½ pound orange peels; ¼ pound Caraway seed; 1 pound Verbena leaves; 40 grains Verbena oil and 1 oz. each of Oil Bergamot and Lemon.

Violet Sachets

Wheat starch, 4 pounds; powdered Orris root, 1 pound. Mix together and add attar of Lemon, ¼ oz. Oils of Bergamot and Cloves, each 1 drachm (1 teaspoonful.)
Another: 1 pound powdered starch; 3 oz. powdered Orris root; 20 drops Oil of Lemon; 10 drops Oil of Lavender; 5 drops Oil of Cloves. Triturate well together, and sift through a fine sieve.
Another: Drop 12 drops of Oil of Rhodium on a piece of loaf sugar; powder this well in a glass mortar, and mix thoroughly with 3 pounds of Orris root. This will resemble Violet perfume. If more oil is added, a Rose perfume will be produced.

Wild Flower Sachet

½ pound Calamus root; ¼ pound Caraway seed; ½ pound Lavender flowers; ¼ pound Marjoram; 1½ oz. Cloves; ¼ pound Orange mint; ½ pound Damask Rose petals; 2 oz. Rosemary; ¼ pound Thyme.

To Extract the Delicate Odors of Flowers

The essential oils of many flowers cannot be separated by means of the still; and yet these flowers yield the most penetrating perfumes. Among these is jasmin. To impregnate oil with the odor of these flowers, the following plan is resorted to. Bits of cotton cloth are saturated with oil of Ben. The advantage of using this oil is that it does not become rancid; fresh Olive oil is, however, more generally employed except by first rate perfumers. A saturated bit of the cotton cloth is laid upon a tray* of

* Use a metal or glass tray, so the delicate perfume of the flowers is not absorbed by the other articles or substances. DO NOT use plastic trays.

Extract Odors of Flowers—Continued

flowers and covered with another layer of flowers equally thick; upon this is laid another mass of oiled cotton and another layer of flowers, and so on until a vessel is filled, or a sufficient pile raised. Sometimes cotton wadding is substituted for the cotton tissue. After a day or two the flowers must be changed, and this change repeated until the cotton has acquired a strong odor of the flowers. The oil is then pressed out and put into bottles.—From The Magazine of Domestic Economy, 1840.

Century Old Method for Collecting the Odors of Flowers

Roses, and all flowers containing perfumed oils, may be made to yield their aromatic properties by steeping the petals or flower leaves in a saucer or a flat dish of water, and setting it in the sun. The petals should be entirely covered with water, which, by the way, should be soft or rain water. A sufficient quantity should be allowed for evaporation, and the vessel should be left undisturbed for a few days. At the end of this time a film will be found floating on the top. This is the essential oil of the flower, and every particle of it is impregnated with the odor peculiar to the flower. It should be taken up carefully and put in tiny vials, which should be allowed to remain open until all watery particles are evaporated. A very small portion of this will perfume glove boxes, apparel, etc., and will last a long time.

Jennings, author of The Family Cyclopaedia (1822) highly recommends salt with roses. He states: "Roses, and other flowers whose fragrance only is wanted, and which is not injured by the flowers being bruised, are best preserved with salt. Roses, for example, if well rubbed or pounded with one-fourth of their weight of common salt, and placed in a jar, will retain their odour for years. From such roses almost all the rose water sold in the shops is made; indeed, we believe the water distilled from salted roses is even more fragrant, it will certainly keep better, than that which is distilled from the fresh-blown rose."

WONDROUS SCENT FROM AUTUMN FIELDS

"Perhaps the herb Everlasting, the fragrant immortelle of our autumn fields, has the most suggestive odor to me of all those that set me dreaming. I can hardly describe the strange thoughts and emotions that come to me as I inhale the aroma of the pale, dry, rustling flowers. A something it has of sepulchral spicery, as if it had been brought from the core of some great pyramid, where it had lain on the breast of a mummied Pharaoh. Something too, of immortality in the sad, faint sweetness lingering so long in its lifeless petals. Yet this does not tell why it fills my eyes with tears, and carries me in blissful thought to the banks of asphodel that border the River of Life."—Oliver Wendell Holmes.

* * * *

As the scent of new-ploughed ground, the odor of woodlands, the fragrance of flowers, have power to recall the vanished years of childhood, so grateful memory breathes a perfumed air which sweetens and keeps fresh the thought of those we love, even though they be dead.

* * * *

The aroma of Vanilla, Tonka, Heliotrope or Rosemary are soothing—the smell of Musk, Calamus and spices were once believed to arouse amourous tendencies. Old herbalists had great faith in scents of herbs as a means to health.

OLD FASHIONED DENTIFRICES

The book "Personal Beauty" published by doctors D. Brinton and G. Naphey, in 1870, extolls (probably with exaggeration) Areca Nut in this quaint recipe: "This nut is brought from Java, and its charcoal in powder is probably the best dentifrice in the world. It sweetens the breath, whitens the teeth, removes the tartar, and gives the gums and lips an attractive red color. About as much of the charcoal should be used as can be held on the point of a knife. It should be placed in the mouth on retiring at night, and gently rubbed into the interstices of the teeth. In the morning it is to be carefully rinsed out. The only objection to charcoal is, that it occasionally leaves a dark line at the base of the teeth. This can be prevented by attention, and by keeping the mouth closed during sleep—a very important point to observe for all who would have sound teeth and a sweet mouth."

Doctors Brinton and Naphey recommend the following when gums are tender: Precipitated chalk, 1 lb; powdered borax, ½ lb; Myrrh, 4 oz; powdered Orris root, 4 oz. Mix and sift through fine sieve.

A century-old English recipe advises—"a mixture of honey with the purest charcoal, will make the teeth as white as snow." Use once or twice a week.

Described as "one of the best, as well as the most elegant tooth-powder" in 1822 recipe book: Take of powdered Cream of Tartar, Peruvian bark, and Myrrh, of each equal parts; mix them. If scent is desired add a small quantity of Orris root.

A recipe published in 1878 describes the following as "an agreeable and delicate dentifrice": An ounce of Myrrh in fine powder, and a small quantity of powdered Sage.

Recipe from Savory's "Companion To The Medicine Chest": "Powdered Rhatany root combined with pulverized Charcoal, in proportion of one part to three of the Charcoal, forms an excellent toothpowder."

This delectable recipe was taken from a rare old book on the manufacture of cosmetics:

Powdered Arrow root	1 pound	Oil of Cloves	10 drops
Powdered Orris root	3 ounces	Oil of Bergamot	12 drops
Oil of Lemon	20 drops		

Rub the oils with the powders until thoroughly mixed.

14 oz. of prepared chalk; 4 oz. each of powdered borax; powdered Orris root; and granulated sugar; ½ oz. Cardamon seeds. Flavor with Wintergreen, Rose or Jasmine. If color is desired, use 4 oz. rose-pink, and as much less of prepared chalk. Tooth-powders should be thoroughly triturated in a stone mortar and finely bolted.

Take of prepared chalk, 1½ oz; powdered Orris root, 3 oz; tincture of Vanilla 4 teaspoonsful; Oil of Rose, 15 drops, and of honey, enough to make a paste.

ROSE TOOTH POWDER: Take of prepared chalk, 2 oz; powdered Orris root, 1 oz; Carmine (if color is desired) 30 grains; Oil of Rose Geranium, 8 drops; attar of Sandalwood, 2 drops. Rub the Carmine with a small portion of the chalk, and then triturate all together.

OLD TIME TOOTH BRUSHES

Natural tooth brushes were very popular before the use of animal bristles, or synthetic brushes. Natives of the West Indies, Africa, and other parts of the world still use these natural brushes without additional cleansers, such as powders and pastes. The following recipes were taken from a century old cosmetic manufacturing

Tooth Brushes—Continued

book. Natural tooth brushes were tied up with ribbons in neat little bundles. Scent and color were often added to these brushes.

Brushes of Marshmallow roots: Take straight and rather large roots, and cut into lengths of 5″. Unravel (or peel) the 2 ends, and boil roots with a few sticks of Cinnamon. When tender, withdraw them carefully to prevent breakage, and soak for 24 hours in brandy, and after this, dry them in a warm oven or room. When they are to be used, they are soaked in warm water, and the teeth rubbed therewith.

Antiscorbutic brushes of Horseradish roots: These are made similarly to the preceding, except that instead of brandy, use tincture of Cloves, for macerating the root, which is afterward laid over with Gum Tragacanth, and this gum, when dry, again covered with several coats of compound tincture of Benzoin.

Alfalfa root brushes: Take roots of convenient size and strip off outer skin or bark, and dry slowly. When the roots are well dried, cut them into small pieces of 3 inch length, and upon each end thereof, strike lightly with a hammer; the fibres are thus detached and form a brush.

Brushes of Licorice root: Favorable to delicate gums. Select such root as is sound and straight, and divide into lengths of 4 or 5 inches, and after perfect dessication by a mild heat, rasp off their outer skin at ends.

All types of natural tooth brushes are soaked in warm water before brushing teeth, when one does not have the fresh natural "brush."

BOTANICAL BREATH SWEETENERS

If bad breath is due to dietary abuse (upset stomach) try drinking a cup of warm Chamomile tea.

Rubbing the teeth, and washing out the mouth with fine Charcoal powder, will render the teeth beautifully white, and the breath sweet.

Recipe of the Middle Ages: "Anise seede chewed in the mouth, maketh a sweete mouth and easie breath, and amendeth the stench of the mouth."

Lozenges for bad breath: Gum Catechu, 1 oz; white sugar, 2 oz; Orris powder ½ oz. Make them into a paste with mucilage, and add a drop of Neroli. One or two may be sucked at pleasure.

In grandmother's day, ladies chewed a bit of delicate scented Orris root to sweeten the breath.

Angelica plant derives its name for its supposed angelic virtues. "Mystical Flora of St. Francis De Sales" states—"It is said that those who chew the root called Angelica always have imparted a pure sweet mouth breath."

The perfume-like Cardamon seed is much used in the Orient as a breath sweetener. In Europe the seed is sometimes seen in fancy dishes, or in glasses in cocktail lounges and bars. Imbibers nibble upon Cardamon after drinking, in order to cover up a bad taste and an offensive tell-tale breath.

In the Orient a small piece of sweet flavored Star Anise is nibbled, the same as we nibble upon mints following a meal.

Centuries ago, Nutmegs were also popular as a masticatory. Gerarde wrote—"Nutmegs causes a sweet breath, and mends those that stinke, if they be chewed and holden in the mouth." Mace may be used in the same way. It is best simply held in

Breath Sweeteners—Continued

the mouth. Mace is a powerful metabolic stimulant. (In such cases the bad breath is masked by the nutmeg.)

GUM MASTIC: "Turkish and Armenian women use this resin as a masticatory for cleansing the teeth, and giving an agreeable smell to the breath. It is also employed to fill the cavities of* carious teeth, for which purpose it is very well adepted."—Whitlaw's New Medical Discoveries, 1829.

* Your dentist will do a better job.

Calamus root is chewed to "clear the voice" and sweeten the breath, by rustics in Europe and America.

Whole Cloves have been chewed to sweeten the breath for more than 4000 years. The flavor of Cloves is long lasting. According to "Preventive Medicine and Hygiene" Cloves have "very marked antiseptic powers and are valuable preservatives. The active antiseptic constituents are the aromatic or essential oil which it contains."

OLD TIME CHEWING GUMS

Take 4 parts Balsam Tolu, and 1 part each of Gum Benzoin, White Wax, Paraffin, and powdered sugar. Melt together. Mix well and roll into sticks.

1 # Sugar	2 oz. Spruce Gum
6 ½ oz. Glucose	1 pint water

Dissolve gum in small amount of water, then add remaining water to sugar and glucose, and boil the syrup up to a strong crack degree. Remove pan from fire, and gently stir the dissolved gum into the syrup, replace the pan on fire, boil sharply for two minutes, then pour out the liquid on an oiled slab.

12 oz. Oatmeal	¼ # Confectioners sugar
½ # Balsam of Peru	¼ # Gum Arabic

Dissolve gum in sufficient warm water to make a thick solution. Mix the sugar and oatmeal, make a bay in the center, turn in the gum, add flavoring and coloring, and work the whole to a stiff pliable paste.

Spruce Gum

Before the days of sweet flavored chewing gum, country boys gathered their gum from Spruce trees. City "kids" could buy this old-fashioned gum in drug stores, at candy counters, and general stores, at a penny a stick. Spruce gum is tangy, purple-hued, and long lasting.

Early woodsmen also chewed Spruce gum, as well as the gums of European Larch and Sweet-gum trees—not so much for the flavor, but in the belief it would harden their teeth. The gums had to be carefully chewed for about 3 days, before it was just right. If too soft, it would stick to the teeth, if too hard, it would disintegrate into a powder. These gums to-day are used for medicinal salves, incense and perfume.

Chewing Balls

The following combinations were taken from a very old apothecary book:
Equal parts of Gum Mastic and Ginger
Equal parts of Cubebs and Nutmegs
Equal parts of Ginger, Rhubarb, Mastic, Pellitory and Orris
Angelica root alone.
The powdered ingredients were added to white wax, and formed into balls. As most of these botanicals are strong flavored, very little is needed for the chewing balls.

Chewing Balls—Continued

How different these recipes are from our modern sweet gums! A variety of other flavors may be obtained from botanicals listed as "Breath Sweeteners and Chewing Botanicals."

TOOTHACHE

Temporary Relief

Oil of Cloves probably is one of the most popular toothache medicines used. The oil is put on a piece of cotton, then in the cavity of the tooth.

Oil of Origanum is also much used as a toothache medicine.

In Germany shavings of Galangal are used to relieve an aching tooth.

An English source claims the chewing of a fresh leaf of Yarrow will relieve toothache.

"Old Timer's" Recipe: Chew the root of Bull Nettle on the tooth that is hurting.

Prickly Ash tree is also known by the name of Toothache Tree, because of its reputation as a relief for toothache.

Ginger root is chewed in the West Indies to alleviate the pain of toothache.

SAGE GARGLES

For Minor Sore Throat Due to Colds

Sage has been a popular ingredient in gargles for ages. The following recipes were gleaned from herbals, and old cook books, containing home medicines:

Make a very strong Sage tea, sweeten with honey; dissolve a small bit of alum in the brew.

Pour a pint of boiling water on a small handful of the leaves of common Sage; let it stand a half hour; add vinegar sufficient to render it acid, and 2 large spoonsful of honey. To be used as a gargle, swallowing occasionally.

Make ½ pint of very strong Sage tea. Add strained honey, common salt and strong vinegar, of each 2 tablespoonsful: Cayenne pepper, 1 rounded teaspoonful. Steep the cayenne pepper with the Sage tea, strain, mix, and bottle for use.

Pour ½ pint of hot malt vinegar upon 1 ounce of Sage herb, and add 1 pint of cold water.

Boil Persimmon bark, and Sage leaves together. Strain and cool.

Take Sage, Hyssop, Gold Thread root, borax and alum. Boil all together in a half pint of water. Strain. Use as a mouth wash for canker sores. Gargle is made by adding molasses to above after straining.

Take a large handful of Sage, boil in 1 quart of the best white wine vinegar, until reduced to near 1 pint, then sweeten it well with honey. You may, if you desire, add 2 small wine glasses of port wine.

Old American recipe for common minor mouth and throat irritations: Take the flowers of Life Everlasting, Sage leaves, Golden Seal or Gold Thread roots. Make a tea and sweeten.

ASTRINGENT GARGLES

Modern English herbals recommend a strong decoction of Tormentil for use as a mouth wash, as well as a gargle. A recipe advised boiling 1 teaspoonful of the root in 1½ pints of water, until reduced to 1 pint.

A decoction of Cranesbill has been used as a gargle since Colonial times, when the Indians revealed the valuable properties of this root. Cranesbill was extolled in practically all early American herbals. Doctor W. Darlington, wrote in 1859—"Cranesbill

Astringent Gargles—*Continued*

root is powerfully astringent, without bitterness or unpleasant taste. Boiled in water and mixed with sugar and milk, it is easily administered to children."

Doctor W. Beach, founder of the Eclectic School of Medicine (believers in plant medicines) advised a decoction of Black Cohosh root as a gargle.

Another recipe: Take of Sumac berries and Golden Seal, a sufficient quantity. Make a strong decoction, strain, and add 1 teaspoonful of pulverized alum to every pint of the decoction. Gargle frequently.

Rustics in Europe still make a gargle from a decoction of Agrimony herb.

A decoction of Yellow root (Xanthorrhiza apiifolia) is used as a gargle in South Carolina, and the Cumberland and Tennessee mountains, where this botanical is found.

A strong decoction of Barberry, makes an excellent astringent gargle and mouth wash.

SOOTHING GARGLES

The dried seeds of Quince, slightly boiled, make a fine mucilaginous drink, and are also used as an emollient gargle.

Hill's Family Herbal offers this recipe: Slippery Elm boiled in water makes one of the best gargles that can be supplied by the whole list of medicines. It should be sweetened with honey.

Grandmother's recipe: Make a tea of Catnip herb. Sweeten with loaf sugar.

Dry throat may be eased with Flaxseed tea. Simmer 1 teaspoonful Flaxseed in 1 pint of water. Strain. Add lemon and honey to taste. Use as a gargle, or swallow a mouthful 3 to 5 times a day.

An English recipe recommends a gargle made with Iceland moss for dry throat.

BOTANICAL MOUTH WASHES

Herbal Mouth Wash: Take ¼ oz. each of dried Mint and Thyme; ½ oz. Cloves crushed, and ½ Nutmeg, grated. Pour on to these ingredients ½ pint of any spirits, and let the mixture stand together for 2 to 3 days, then strain off the tincture formed, and add 10 drops of Oil of Peppermint. It is then ready for use.

The tincture of Rhatany has long been recommended, mixed with an equal quantity of Rose-water, as an astringent wash for the gums, and as a breath sweetener.

Another mouth wash may be made with ½ oz. tincture of Myrrh, and 2 oz. tincture of Peruvian bark.

A good mouth wash is made by adding a little tincture of Myrrh to a glass of water.

OLD RECIPES USED TO RELIEVE HICCOUGHS

To relieve hiccoughs, suck a lump of sugar on which two or three drops of oil of Peppermint have been poured. Works like magic, according to author.

Another recipe advises sipping Peppermint tea.

Dioscorides, in the 1st century A.D., maintained that "ye decoction of ye dried leaves and seeds of Dill being drank stayeth ye hickets" (hiccough).

"Some use to eate the seed of Dill to stay the hiccough."—Parkinson's Paradisi in Sole

Recipe from a modern source: Dill, the seed bruised, 2 teaspoonsful infused in ½ pint of boiling water. 2 ounces to be taken every hour or two.

Other old recipes advise chewing Fennel or Anise seed, and swallowing the juice.

Old Recipes Relieve Hiccoughs—Continued

English recipe: Infuse 2 teaspoonsful of Wild Carrot in ½ pint of boiling water; drink 2 ounces every hour until hiccoughs cease.

From an herbal printed in 1800: Take 3 drops of oil of Cinnamon, on a lump of sugar. Repeat, if necessary, every 4 hours.

From the Family Magazine, published in 1741: "An ounce of Skirret root, boiled in a pint of good red port, and a large coffee cupful taken blood-warm, when the hiccough is troublesome, has been of service."

ADVICE from a 230 YEAR OLD HEALTH BOOK
Weight Control

A load of flesh and fat can hardly be bore by youth; but when age creeps on, and we keep the same load as in our youth, nothing can be expected but perpetual confinement; get rid therefore of your corpulency in your youth, if you design to lead your life with any comfort in years; for if you have not half the spirits in years that you had in youth, you carry double the load; and, to increase your burden when you should lay it down, is growing in folly as you grow older.

The diet of lean people, and of the corpulent, should not be the same; for we can't make lean people fat with salt meats, nor the corpulent lean with milks, creams, and jellies. If the lean are to be made fat, they must feed with smooth diet, such as almonds, millet puddings, sweet milks, jellies, creams, smooth ale, sack, chocolate, rice, and such like; to use little exercise, sleep much, and avoid cares. And if you want to make a man lean, feed him with little and give him salt meats and sour wines; let him exercise stoutly, study hard, or give him troubles for his portion; let him go late to bed, and rise early, and you may make a scarecrow of him at pleasure. Here the ladies, who study shapes, may see how to preserve them; but, I fear, few will care to purchase them at this rate.

Moderation In Middle Age

Youth is not so subject to diseases as age and green (middle) old age is the most subject to them, because they have not as yet forgot their youth, and continue to act as young men in all their enterprises, which they not being able to bear, they must suffer of course. Moderation therefore, is the only method of preserving health, to those of this age; what harm do such men not avoid, by clothing warmer, by eating less, by drinking no more than will cheer them up, by using exercise proportionable to what they eat, by insisting on a diet moderately warming, by taking a gentle purge, if they are sickish at stomach, or by fasting out too full a meal.—The Family Companion For Health—1730—The Author a member of the College of Physicians

COSMETIC CREAMS WITHOUT ANIMAL FATS
Agar-Agar Cream

Agar-Agar, 1 oz; water, 8 oz; stearic acid, 1 oz; sodium carbonate, 5½ drams; Cocoa Butter*, 1 oz; alcohol, 2½ drams.

Agar-Agar, or Japanese Isinglass, is a gelatinous substance prepared from a species of seaweed. It is not as soluble as isinglass, but dissolves in boiling water, forming a transparent jelly when cold.

Dissolve the Agar-Agar in 5 ounces boiling water and strain. To 3 ounces of water

Cosmetic Creams without Animal Fats—Continued

in a water-bath add the stearic acid and the sodium carbonate; when action ceases add the Cocoa Butter and Agar-Agar. Mix thoroughly by means of an egg beater, then remove the dish from the water bath and continue agitating until a uniformly smooth lather, measuring about three times the volume of the contained liquid, results. When nearly cold add the perfumes desired.

* Cocoa Butter is useful in perfumes, ointments, confectionery, etc. It is used in vanishing creams and in skin paint remover. Medicinally it is used in moulded sticks as the base of certain suppositories and pessaries. Cocoa Butter melts at body temperature and remains free from rancidity for a long time.

Irish Moss Cream

Irish Moss, 1 oz; distilled water, 10 oz; Glycerin, 2 oz; boracic acid, 1 dram; eau de cologne, 1 oz.

Wash the Irish Moss in a little cold water, then boil gently in the 10 ounces of water, in a closed vessel, and strain. Add the Glycerin and borax, previously dissolved in 1 ounce of water, cool, and finally add the eau de cologne.

Tragacanth Cream

Tragacanth, powdered, 2 oz; Glycerin, 8 oz; boracic acid, 1 oz; powdered borax, 1 oz; alcohol, 5 oz; distilled water, 48 oz; tincture of Benzoin, 1 oz; Oil of Bergamot, 60 drops; Oil of Orange flowers, 30 drops; Oil of Rose Geranium, 60 drops.

Soak the Tragacanth in the water for 24 hours in a wide-mouthed bottle, occasionally agitating it. Add the Glycerin, cut the oils in the alcohol and then gradually add, with constant stirring, when a thick cream results. Add the tincture of Benzoin and thoroughly incorporate.

Witch Hazel Cream

Stearic acid, 4 oz; sodium carbonate, ½ oz; Glycerin, 4 fluid drams; water, 16 fluid oz; distilled extract of Witch Hazel, 20 fluid oz.

Dissolve the sodium carbonate in the water and add to the Glycerin contained in a large pan*. Then add the stearic acid and heat the mixture on the water-bath until effervescence has ceased and a clear solution results. Keep this near the boiling point for at least an hour, stirring frequently and making up for loss of water through evaporation by the addition of more water, being careful not to add too much. Now add the Witch Hazel extract, transfer the whole to a suitable dish and beat it until the proper consistency is acquired.

* Use only enamel or stainless steel pan.

Witch Hazel Toilet Cream

Toilet creams are softer than cold creams as they contain no fats or oils. The following is a good example: Ingredients—½ oz. Quince seed; 20 grains borax; 2 oz. Glycerin; 2 oz. alcohol; 1 oz. water; 28 oz. distilled extract of Witch Hazel. Macerate Quince seed, Glycerin and extract of Witch Hazel together for about 12 hours, agitating frequently, then strain and add a solution of the borax in the water, and the alcohol.

BOTANICAL VINEGARS

VINEGAR of the FOUR THIEVES: According to an old French legend, during the plague at Marseilles, four robbers plundered the dying and the dead, without injury to themselves. They were imprisoned, tried and condemned to die, but were pardoned on condition of disclosing the secret whereby they could ransack houses infected with the terrible scourge. They gave the following recipe: Take of Rosemary, Wormwood, Lavender, Rue, Sage and Mint, a large handful of each. Place in a stone jar, and turn over it one gallon of strong cider vinegar, cover closely, and keep near the fire for four days; then strain and add 1 oz. of pounded Camphor gum. Bottle and keep tightly corked. (This is merely a legend without scientific foundation.)

Vinegar of the Four Thieves was used to wash the face and hands, before exposing one's self to infection. It is very aromatic and refreshingly cool in the sick room; so, if it can accomplish nothing more, it is of value to nurses.

More modern recipes add Garlic, Calamus, Cinnamon, Cloves and Nutmegs to the above recipe. Spices are well known for their antiseptic properties.

BALSAMIC Vinegar: For minor wounds and bruises. Take ½ oz. each of Sage, Lavender flowers, Hyssop, Thyme and Savory; 2 Garlic bulbs, and ½ cup of salt. Infuse in 1 quart of white vinegar; allow to steep 3 weeks, then strain. Wormwood, steeped in vinegar, gives almost immediate pain relief to minor bruises or sprains.

AROMATIC Vinegars: For facial wash or as a hair rinse—steep 1 oz. of any one of the following, or in combinations, in white vinegar for from 2 to 3 weeks, then strain off botanical: Lavender flowers, Rosemary, Orris, or other fragrant botanicals. Aromatic vinegars are also made with tincture of Benzoin, Balsam of Tolu, and oils, such as Lavender, Bergamot, Rosemary, Neroli, etc.

"Vinegar acquires a very agreeable colour and taste by infusing in it some petals of Sweet Violet (Viola odorata)."—Robt. Thornton's Family Herbal, 1814.

ROSE VINEGAR for the Complexion (astringent wash): Steep 1 oz. of Damask rose petals in ½ pint of white wine vinegar for one week. Strain off the leaves and add ½ pint of Rose Water to the vinegar. Wipe the face with a soft linen cloth dipped in the rose vinegar.

LONGEVITY SECRET OF A FRENCH BEAUTY

Ninon De Lenclos was that famous beauty of the old French Court who retained her youthful charms to such a miraculous degree that one of her grandsons fell in love with her when she was seventy. The circumstances were peculiar. He had never seen her before and everything ended most respectably when he found out who she was.

French historians claim they have discovered the secret formula Ninon used to keep herself looking young. She took herb baths and this is how she concocted them: "Take a handful of dried Lavender flowers, a handful of Rosemary leaves, handful of dried Mint, handful of Comfrey roots, and one of Thyme. Mix all together loosely in a muslin bag. Place in your bath, pour on enough boiling water to cover and let soak ten minutes. Then fill up tub. Rest fifteen minutes in the "magic water"—and think virtuous thoughts."

Note: Of course the above recipe has no scientific foundation.

EASY METHOD OF DYEING FABRICS WITH BOTANICALS

In recent years renewed interest is being revived in natural dyes, because for technical reasons, chemical dyes cannot be used successfully on all chemically-made fabrics. Natural dyes have a beauty, warmth and richness of their own. A new dye may offer wonderful possibilities to its discoverer. Marvelous effects are sometimes obtained by unique materials and methods. The art of dyeing is no more difficult than the making of home brews, preserving foods, or other arts, once so commonly practiced in many households. Colors used for dyeing may be obtained from plants growing in your particular area, or it may be simpler (and more durable) to use long established old-time dyes such as Indigo, Madder, Cochineal, etc. The chemicals needed as mordants are inexpensive. One does need sufficient soft water (rain or river water) available, because well water or city water generally contain chemicals that may affect dyeing processes.

Natural dyes adhere best and most firmly on wool. Silk also "takes" to natural dyes. However, cotton and linen are more difficult, so the beginner should not attempt these until quite proficient.

IMPORTANT: The majority of natural dyes are not permanent, unless the cloth be previously impregnated with what has been termed a MORDANT, which possesses a very strong affinity both with cloth and the dye, and hence serves to bind the one to the other.

Before cloth is dyed or treated with mordant it MUST be free from grease or oleous matter. Wool, which is naturally of a greasy nature, requires to be scoured before it is dyed. Silk should be washed with soap and warm water: and cotton and linen require bleaching and scouring in alkaline lye. This of course does not apply to store purchased materials that have already been treated.

It is suggested that beginners experiment in a small way, and only with wool—simple colors (no mixtures) and with one mordant, until familiar with technical actions and reactions. It may be well to make notes of all experiments.

Old-time dyers had large copper kettles for light or bright colors, and large iron kettles for dark colored goods. Enamelware kettles may serve the same purpose, when proper mordants are used. To spread mordant evenly, as well as the dye, it is important that the container is large enough so goods will not be crowded.

MORDANT recipe: For each pound of wool to be dyed, dissolve 2 oz. of alum (slightly less for light colors) and ½ oz. cream of tartar in a little hot water. Then add this to 2 gallons of SOFT water. Immerse the wool, then heat slowly to simmer, and allow it to simmer ½ hour. After this has cooled off, remove wool and squeeze gently. When excess water is removed, place wool in a clean bag and hang in a dark place for 3 or 4 days or until thoroughly dry.

Preparing The Dye Bath: The amount of dye material used, of course, depends upon the shade of color desired. If fresh botanicals are used, chop them up into small pieces, and allow to stand overnight in enough soft water to cover. On the following day, strain this through 4 thicknesses of cheesecloth. Tie strained botanicals in the cheesecloth, so no particles of dye material will come out. Boil contents of bag for ½ hour in dyed water that was strained off, plus additional soft water to make sufficient dye. Remove cheesecloth bag and hang over the brew, so dye can drip back into container it was boiled in. When luke-warm, add sufficient luke-warm soft water to make 2 gallons (for each 1 pound of wool). Rinse mordanted wool in clear luke-warm water; squeeze out (do not wring) excess water, then immerse wool in dye.

Dyes—Continued

Bring dye water slowly to boiling point. Stir wool gently, continuously with a wood paddle, to keep wool loose, so dye will adhere evenly. Allow dye bath to simmer ½ hour. If too much dye water boils away, remove wool; add sufficient hot water—stir thoroughly before immersing wool again.

Professional dyers generally have additional dye solution available, but it is VERY IMPORTANT that the fabric is removed, whether adding water, or more dye solution. Stir water or new solution thoroughly in the original solution BEFORE immersing the fabric again. Neglecting this will cause the fabric to dye unevenly.

When dyeing is complete, remove wool and rinse in clear water, of the SAME temperature as dye water. Repeat operation in slightly cooler clear water until water is completely cool and quite clear. Remember, NEVER wring out goods. When sufficient moisture is removed, roll wool in a clean cloth to absorb remaining moisture. Hang in shade until dry.

While this method is very simple, it must be followed carefully. To obtain an EVEN color it is equally as important that the cloth is MORDANTED EVENLY, as it is to spread the dye evenly about the cloth. Neither the dye nor mordant can be spread evenly over a fabric that is wrinkled and folded tightly in a container that is too small.

FAST and EASY-TO-USE natural dye materials for the beginner: Indigo (blue), Madder (Turkey red), Cochineal (bright red), Fustic (yellow), Henna (Golden orange-yellow).

OLD-TIME DYEING METHODS

The art of dyeing was brought to perfection about a century ago, before the world-wide adoption of coal-tar dyes, or so-called anilines. Many famous old recipes, treasured by families from generation to generation, have disappeared with the arrival of the Chemical Age.

The information presented here was taken from Jennings Family Cyclopaedia, printed in 1822. This book is an excellent recording of the home arts of that time. Most of the dye materials mentioned by Jennings have been used for ages, and have proven their worth. The dyeing methods are more complicated, but render more permanent and lively colors. Note especially, the recipe to obtain a colorful black, (instead of dead black).

Alum and cream of tartar were most commonly used as mordants, however, a variety of other mordants were also used to obtain permanency, and various effects. These are well explained by Jennings.

Mordants not only fix coloring matter, but they most commonly, in some degree, alter the natural hue. Thus an alum mordant, changes the dull red of madder to a bright crimson; the solutions of tin, not only fix the color of cochineal in wool, but change it from a crimson to a bright scarlet; the salts of iron, which were powerful mordants, always alter the color of dyes—the yellow of weld, to olive-brown, drab or lead color, according to circumstances; the red of madder to a violet brown, and striking a blueish-black, whenever the gallic acid is present. Hence a great advantage is most ingeniously made of mixing different mordants to produce varieties of shades; thus a mixture of the iron and alum mordant, will produce with madder, all the shades of pea color, purple and violet. With weld, brown, olive-green, and the like, so that with no more than three or four coloring materials, an almost infinite variety of dyes may be produced by a dye selection and mixture of the various mordants.

Dyes—Continued

The substances principally used as mordants are earths, metallic oxydes, tannin and oil.

Acetate of alum, answers much better than common alum. It is prepared by pouring acetate of lead into a solution of alum: an insoluble compound is formed by the lead and sulphuric acid in the alum, which precipitates, and the acetate of alum remains dissolved in the liquid.

Lime is also sometimes used as a mordant, but it does not answer so well as alum. It is employed either in the state of lime-water, or of sulphate of lime, dissolved in water.

All the metallic salts or oxydes, are mordants, but the salts or oxydes of tin and iron, are those only which are extensively used.

Muriate of tin is dissolved in a large quantity of water, to which some tartar is also usually added, the cloth dipped in the solution, and allowed to remain till sufficiently saturated. It is then taken out, washed and dried.

Sulphate of iron is dissolved in water, and the cloth dipped in it: this is commonly used for wool. It may be used also for cotton, but the acetate of iron is preferable; which is prepared by dissolving iron, or its oxyde, in vinegar.

Tannin is used as a mordant thus: an infusion of nut-galls, sumach, or any other substance containing tannin, is made in water and the cloth is dipped in the infusion, and allowed to remain till it has absorbed a sufficient quantity of tannin. Silk absorbs a great quantity of tannin. Tannin is also employed with other mordants to produce a compound mordant. Oil is also used for the same purpose, in the dyeing of cotton and linen. The mordants with which tannin is most frequently combined are, alum and oxyde of iron.

Besides these mordants others are occasionally used to facilitate the combination of the mordant with the cloth, so as to alter the shade of the color; the chief of these are tartar, acetate of lead, common salt, sal ammoniac, sulphate and acetate of copper.

The same coloring matter produces very different dyes, according as the mordant is changed; thus, if we use the alum mordant and cochineal, the cloth will be crimson; but the oxyde of iron and cochineal produce black.

All colors are obtained from primary colors, BLUE, YELLOW and RED—these may be used in a multitude of variations by using different dyes as well as mordants.

BLUE

Indigo and Woad are considered the best blue dyes. Indigo is a very permanent color, resisting the sun, air, washing with soap and most chemical agents. (Indigo plants grow very well in the Carolinas and Georgia. Woad grows well in the north as well as states mentioned.)

Indigo requires no mordant; every kind of cloth may be dyed with it as follows: Let one part of indigo be dissolved in four parts of sulphuric acid; to the solution add one part of dry carbonate of potash; and then it is to be diluted with eight times its weight of water. The cloth must be previously boiled for an hour in a solution containing five parts of alum, and three of tartar, for every 32 parts of cloth. It is then to be thrown into a water bath, containing a greater or smaller proportion of the diluted sulphate of indigo, according to the shade which the cloth is intended to receive. In this bath it must be boiled till it has acquired the wished for color. The alum and tartar facilitate the decomposition of the sulphate of indigo; the alkali answers the same purpose. There are many other methods of dyeing with indigo.

YELLOW

Weld is the substance much employed for this color; fustic, and quercitron bark are also used; and indeed these three constitute our chief yellows. But Venice sumach, Sawwort, Dyers' Broom and American Golden Rod, are occasionally used.

Almost all yellow coloring matters must be dyed by the assistance of mordants. Alum is the most common; but oxyde of tin is used for very fine yellows. Tannin is also used after alum, to fix the color more copiously on cotton and linen. Tartar is also used; so also is muriate of soda, sulphate of lime, and even sulphate of iron.

The yellow dyed by fustic is more permanent, but not so beautiful as that given by weld or quercitron. The mordant for fustic is alum.

Weld and quercitron yield nearly the same color, but as the bark yields coloring matter in much greater abundance, it is much more convenient and cheaper. The methods of using each of these are nearly the same.

Wool may be dyed yellow thus: Let it be boiled an hour or more in one-sixth its weight of alum, dissolved in a sufficient quantity of water. It is then to be plunged, without being rinsed, into a bath of warm water, containing in it as much quercitron bark as equals the weight of the alum employed. The cloth is to be turned through the boiling liquid till it has acquired the intended color. Then a quantity of clean powdered chalk, equal to the hundredth part of the weight of the cloth, is to be stirred in, and the operation of dyeing continued for eight minutes longer.

For very bright orange, or golden yellow, the oxyde of tin must be used as a mordant. And for bright golden yellows some alum must be added along with the tin: for a delicate green shade tartar must be added in different proportions, according to the shade wanted. By the addition of cochineal in small quantity, a fine orange may be obtained.

Silk is dyed different shades of yellow by either weld or quercitron bark. The proportion should be from one or two parts of bark, to twelve parts of silk, according to the shade. The bark tied up in a bag and put in the dyeing vessel whilst the water is cold. When it is heated to about 100°, the silk previously cleaned must be put in and continued in the liquor until until it is of a proper color. When the shade is wanted to be deep, a little chalk or pearl-ash should be added toward the end of the operation.

Cotton and linen should be prepared for yellow by dissolving one part of acetate of lead, and three parts of alum, in a sufficient quantity of water, heating the solution to 100°. The cloth must be soaked in the dye for 2 hours, and then hung out and dried; when the soaking and drying should be repeated; after which it is to be barely wetted with lime water, and then dried once more; the number of repetitions of the entire process must depend upon the brightness of the dye required. The dyeing bath is prepared thus: take 12 or 18 parts of quercitron bark, according to the brightness required: let them be tied up in a bag and placed in a sufficient quantity of cold water. Into this the cloth must be put, and turned around in it for one hour, while the heat is gradually raised to 120°. It must then be allowed to advance to a boiling heat, and the cloth be suffered to remain in a few minutes only afterwards.

RED

The materials employed for this color are lac or kermes, cochineal, archil, madder, carthamus, and Brazil wood.

Woolen stuffs of the coarse kind are dyed red with madder; but fine cloth is almost exclusively dyed with cochineal.

Red Dyes—Continued

Scarlet may be dyed thus: For each pound of cloth, put from fifteen to twenty quarts of very clear river water into a small copper kettle. When the water is lukewarm, put in 2 ounces of cream of tartar, and one and one-half teaspoonsful of powdered cochineal; when the liquor is ready to boil, add 2 ounces of a solution of tin made thus: take 8 oz. of clear river water, and 8 oz. of strong aquafortis, mix them together; then add half an ounce of sal ammoniac by degrees; taking care that one piece dissolves before you add a second; then put in two teaspoonsful of saltpetre; lastly, add by little at a time, 1 oz. of pure grain tin. When the whole is dissolved it is fit for use. It should be kept in a cool place closely stopped.

The dyeing materials being thus mixed in the copper, the fire should be raised under it, and when the liquor boils, the cloth after being passed through warm water that it may receive the dye equally, is to be put in and well handled in the liquor for an hour and a half; it must then be taken out and slightly washed in clean water. Then prepare a fresh water, in which must be put one ounce and a half of pure starch; and when the liquor is a little more than lukewarm, six and a half teaspoonsful of cochineal, finely powdered, must be thrown in a little before the liquor boils. Two ounces of the solution of tin must then be added. Boil the liquor after this a few minutes, then cool it a little, put in the cloth to be finished, and boil it in the liquor for an hour and a half. Take it out and wash it, and the process is completed.

For crimson, the following process will answer: Your copper being ready to boil, put in for each pound of cloth, two ounces and a half of alum, and one and one-half ounces of white tartar. Let the liquor boil a minute or two, then put in the cloth, and boil it for half an hour, when it is to be taken out and cooled in all places alike. Fill the copper again with fresh water, the former liquid being thrown away. When about lukewarm, put in about an ounce of cochineal finely powdered; when it boils, cool it down by the addition of a pint of cold water; put in the cloth, and boil for an hour, or an hour and a half, as occasion may be. It must now be taken out, washed, and hung up to dry. If a lighter shade be required, use less of the ingredients. This color is called grain crimson, to distinguish it from false crimson, obtained from Brazil wood.

Silks may be colored red by madder by means of a mixed mordant of alum and the solution of tin; but the hues from madder are seldom sufficiently bright, hence cochineal and carthamus are generally used.

To obtain shades of red, the above processes must be varied.

Cotton may be dyed scarlet by means of the solution of tin, cochineal ,and quercitron bark, but the color is too fading to be of any value.

BLACK

The substances employed to give a black color to cloth, are red oxyde of iron, and tannin. Log-wood is usually employed as an auxiliary, because it communicates lustre, and adds to the fulness of the black.

Cloth before it receives a black color is usually dyed blue, which renders the color much finer than it would otherwise be. If the cloth be coarse, blue may be too expensive. A brown color is then previously given to it by walnut peels.

The following is a process of dyeing black in the small way. Fill the copper to the brim with soft water, and when it begins to boil, add 4 oz. of logwood, 3 oz. sumach and 3 oz. of Alder bark. Boil these ingredients half an hour, and put in the cloth; keep it under the water and boil it for one hour, moving it about every 10 minutes during that period. Then take the cloth out of the liquor, and hang it out to cool.

Black Dyes—Continued

Then dissolve 6 oz. of sulphate of iron in a bowl of the boiling liquor; mix two-thirds of this solution into the copper, and check the boiling by throwing in as much water as may have evaporated; the cloth is then to be put again into the liquor, stirred as before, and boiled for one hour. It is then to be taken out and cooled again in all parts alike; in the interim add the remaining of the dissolved copperas; check the boiling as before, put in the cloth again, and boil it for 2 hours; then take it out to cool again. While cooling put into the copper two or three ounces of logwood, two or three ounces of bark, an ounce of sulphate of iron, two ounces of pearl-ash and about half an ounce of pounded archil. These must boil one hour. The boiling must be again checked as before, the cloth again put in and boiled for one hour, and handled as before. Thus the process will be completed. This process is tedious, but it will produce a very good black.

Silk is dyed black by a process not very different from that of cloth. It imbibes tannin freely, which can be given to it at pleasure, by allowing the silk to remain a shorter or longer time in the decoction.

It is by no means easy to give a full black to linen or cotton, and still less so, a durable black; the color generally yielding to the action of soap.

BROWN

BROWN, or fawn color, buff and nankin: Birch, Alder bark, and Sumach, are occasionally used for these colors, but the more common is a decoction of walnut peels, or walnut root. The best of these in dyeing fawn colors, is the bark, or rind of the walnut.

A copper kettle half full of water is placed over the fire. As soon as it grows warm, walnut bark is to be added in proportion to the cloths intended to be dyed, and the lightness or depth of the shades required. It is then to be boiled for about a quarter of an hour, when the cloths previously moistened with warm water, are to be immersed in it, frequently turned, and well stirred until they have sufficiently imbibed the color. They are of course to be aired, dried, and dressed in the usual manner.

Walnut root requires a different process: A copper kettle is filled about three parts full of soft water, into which the root is immersed, tied up in a bag. When the liquor has become very hot, the article to be dyed is to be plunged into it, repeatedly turned, and occasionally aired. The lighter stuffs are next to be dipped, until the color is completely extracted. Care must be taken that the liquor does not boil.

The process of dyeing with Alder bark, is nearly the same as that with walnut roots. It is chiefly used for worsteds, imparting shades darkened with sulphate of iron.

Sumach possesses nearly the same properties as the bark of the walnut tree. Its color is not so deep, somewhat inclining to be green, but solid and permanent.

These different substances, however, are not infrequently mingled together, and as they differ only in degrees of color, it is easy by their admixture to obtain various shades.

MIXED COLORS

As most dyes and mordants tend to destroy or change each other through chemical action, to obtain mixed colors (shades of greens, orange, violet, etc.) the goods are first dyed with one primary color, then followed by another. This process may be followed by succeeding immersions in a variety of blues, yellows or reds, to obtain subtle or intense colors.

Mixed Colors—*Continued*

GREEN: A mixture of blue and yellow. The cloth, however, is generally first dyed with blue, and afterwards with yellow, to produce the desired color. When sulphate of indigo is employed, it is, however, usual to dye the cloth at once.

VIOLET, PURPLE and LILAC are all mixtures of blue and red. Wool, cotton, and linen are first dyed blue; the two last are then galled and soaked in a decoction of logwood; but a more permanent color is given by means of oxyde of iron; they are then dyed scarlet in the usual manner; or by cochineal being mixed with the sulphate of indigo, the process may be performed at once. Silk is first dyed crimson by means of cochineal, and then dipped in a sulphate of indigo.

ORANGE is a mixture of yellow and red. If blue be added to a mixture of yellow and red, the result is an olive. Wool may be dyed orange by first dyeing in scarlet, and then in yellow. If first dyed with madder, the produce will be a cinnamon color. Silk is dyed orange by means of carthamus; cinnamon color by logwood, Brazilwood, and fustic, mixed together. Cotton and linen are rendered cinnamon-hued, by means of weld and madder; and olive-hued by being passed through a blue, yellow, and finally a madder dye.

GREYS, Drabs and Dark Browns, are all mixtures of black with other colors. If cloth be previously combined with brown oxyde of iron, and afterwards dyed yellow with quercitron bark, a drab of different shades will be produced according to the proportion of the mordant employed. And the drab may be deepened by mixing a little sumach with the bark.

LIST OF NATURAL DYES

Important: See article, Old-time Dyeing Methods—how MORDANTS are required to SET or fix a color; also how mordants may affect the dye material. Tannin-rich botanicals, such as Indigo, Mangrove, Sumach, Alder, Oak barks, etc., require no mordant to set or fix colors. The reason it is so difficult to remove stains of Oriental tea from fabrics, is due to its tannin content.

RED

BRAZILWOOD and SAPPANWOOD are derived from species of Caesalpinia. Color of either species is fugitive.

COCHINEAL (a cactus parasite): Renders shades of red and crimson, with certain mordants and mixtures.

COTINUS SUMACH: "The root serveth to dye with, giving to woll and cloth a reddish colour."—Gerarde's Herbal, 1636.

HENNA leaves yield a beautiful orange-red dye on wool, hair and fabrics. It is one of our oldest and best dye botanicals.

LOGWOOD: Purplish-red. Used mainly with tannin and salts of iron to produce black.

MADDER root: Scarlet or "Turkey red"—one of the world's oldest dyes.

POINSETTIA—the flowers (actually the bracts) yield a scarlet dye. This is the Poinsettia offered by florists at Christmas time. This probably is not a fast dye, unless a proper mordant could be used with it.

RED SANDERSWOOD or RED SANDALWOOD: Blood-red.

Natural Dyes—Continued

SAFFRON—yields a beautiful red—but is too expensive to use.

TUMERIC: Used to heighten and render brighter, the red colors dyed with Cochineal and Vermilion.

YELLOW

ANNATTO: Elusive bright yellow, formerly used to dye wool and calico goods. Now used mainly to color butter, cheese and other fatty food products.

FUSTIC is still used in quantities to dye leather, wool, silk, rayon and nylon.

GAMBOGE: Used to dye silk robes of Buddhist priests.

QUERCITRON, or bark of BLACK OAK (Quercus velutina) found in eastern U.S.A. Because of its tannin content, mordant is not needed with Quercitron. Other varieties also yield a yellow color.

SAFFLOWER: Used to dye silks, crepes and woolens.

TUMERIC: Fleeting golden yellow, once used to dye cotton, wool and silk. Now used mainly to color mustard, curries, etc. Tumeric formerly was in great request by glovers, for dyeing yellow gloves.

The following botanicals were popularly used in Colonial times, and by "do-it-yourself" moderns: Apple-tree bark, Broomsedge, Cotton flowers, Goldenrod flowers, White Hickory bark, Lily of the Valley leaves, Marigold flowers, Black Oak bark, Lombardy Poplar leaves, Privet leaves, Sunflower petals, Tulip tree leaves, Zinnia flowers, Bearberry leaves, Alfalfa seeds, etc.

ORANGE and GOLD

OSAGE ORANGEWOOD yields an orange-yellow dye. It is also much used as a base for green colors.

Broomsedge and Madder
Coreopsis flowers
Dahlia flowers
Fustic and Madder
Hollygrape root and Madder
Quercitron and Madder

* * * *

"The women in Pennsylvania and other parts of North America, in dyeing worsted a fine lasting orange colour, which does not fade in the sun, use urine* instead of alum in dyeing, and boil the dye—Sassafras root—in a brass boiler, because in an iron vessel it does not yield so fine a colour."—Encyclopaedia of Arts and Sciences, 1743

* Urine was used by the American Indians to set colors, and was also much used in the Orient, for the same purpose.

BROWN and TAN

BLACK CUTCH or CATECHU: Obtained from a tree of India and Burma. An important source of brown dye.

Natural Dyes—Continued

BUTTERNUT: "The leaves, bark or unripe fruit afford a dye of a chocolate-brown color for woolen goods, which, with that of Black Walnut, was used in the South to a great extent during the rebellion, as a dye for the uniforms of the soldiers."—C. F. Millspaugh

Black tea leaves yield a delicate rose-tan dye. The natural tannin content of the leaves set the color.

MARKING NUT tree (Semecarpus Anacardium). The juice of the nut, mixed with a little quicklime and water, is used in India for marking linen, and the bark is used to make a brown dye.

Various types of brown: Birch bark, or leaves, with Fustic; Madder and Fustic; and Goldenrod flowers and Madder.

Barks of any one of the following trees: Norway Maple, Red Maple, Black Walnut, Hickory, Black Oak, White Oak, Tupela, Red Bud, Chittam and Apple tree.

Other sources for brownish colors: Pecan hulls, Coffee Beans, Juniper berries and Black Walnut hulls.

GREEN

Green color is generally obtained by dyeing fabric with blue, then with a yellow color.

Chlorophyll

Fustic and Indigo

Goldenrod flowers and Indigo

Osage Orangewood with Indigo, or Woad.

White Hickory bark and Indigo.

BLUE

BLUE BOTTLES flowers (Centaurea Cyanus) dye blue.

INDIGO: One of the oldest and most reliable dyes for wool, silk, cotton and linen.

WOAD: Young leaves yield a light blue; mature leaves yield a darker blue, and old leaves yield a bluish black.

Indigo and Woad yield dye ONLY after botanicals undergo special processing.

PURPLE

Shades of purple are generally obtained by dyeing fabric, first with blue, then follow with a red coloring.

BLACK

ALDER bark: "Is much used of poore country diers for the dyeing of coarse cloath, caps, hose and such like into a blacke colour, whereto it serveth well."—Gerarde's Herbal, 1636

The Chinese make a black dye from red Hybiscus flowers, so common in Florida, and most of the tropical world.

The bark of Mangrove roots is a source of black dye, requiring no mordant, because of its high tannin content. Mangrove offers an almost unlimited supply of both dye and tannin, as it is found growing on the ocean shores of a large part of the tropical world.

DYE PLANTS USED BY THE INDIANS

This list of dye plants, used by the Indians, is far from complete. An entire book could be devoted to the subject. Red, yellow, and brown were the most common colors used, simply because the Indians found few plants to produce durable blue, violet, and green. Various fruits yielded such colors, but faded under outdoor conditions lived by the Indians.

RED

A bright red is obtained from the fruit of Strawberry blite (Blitum capitatum) to color clothes, wood and skins. The fruits were simply crushed and applied to materials.

The roots of common Puccoon (Lithospermum canescens) yield a red dye.

The entire plant of Bristly Crowfoot (Ranunculus pennsylvanicus) is boiled to yield a reddish dye. Oak bark is added to set the color.

Blackfoot tribes used Orthocarpus lutens to dye animal skins red.

Many tribes used the rich coloring of Bloodroot to produce bronze or deep reddish shades. Mordant is needed to set the color. Bloodroot is one of the richest of all Indian dyes.

Pokeberries yield a reddish purple dye if they are gathered before they ripen completely. Fully ripened berries yield a purplish-black dye. A small crimson fruited species, Phytolacca rivinoides, growing in Florida, and the West Indies, yields a luscious golden red color. No mordant has yet been discovered to make the color of either species durable.

RED BROWN

Ojibwa tribe used the bark of Hemlock (Tsuga Canadensis) with a little rock dust to set the color.

Hopi Indians used several species of Thelesperma to produce a reddish brown color. Sumac berries were used as mordant.

The roots of Mountain Mahogany make a rich red brown on cotton, wool and leather.

BROWN

Apparently all varieties of Alders were used, wherever the shrub was found, to produce a brown and reddish dye. Alders require nothing to set the color. The inner bark is said to be better for color—however, the outer bark may also be used.

BROWNISH-BLACK

Ojibwa Indians make use of the seed hulls of the Hazelnut, in setting the black color of Butternut dye.

YELLOW

The Flambeau Ojibwa Indians add Goldthread roots to other plant dyes, to emphasize the yellow color.

Western tribes peel off the bark of the root of Oregon Hollygrape, to obtain a bright color.

Pima and Papago tribes used Yellow Dock, and other varieties of Rumex, to obtain

Indian Dyes—Continued

a yellow dye for cotton fiber. It is said the root yields a darker color when the plant is in flower. Fresh mesquite gum was boiled with the dye to make it fast.

Blackfoot tribes used Wolf Moss (Evernia vulpina), a lichen found on old trees and decaying logs, to dye porcupine quills yellow.

Hopi Indians use the golden flowers of Rabbit bush to make a dye.

In the Midwest, Indians boiled the whole plant of Jewel weed or Touch-me-not—the yellow color was deepened or made more reddish with a few rusty nails added to the solution.

The inner bark and center pith of the stem of Smooth or Staghorn Sumac, was used to produce a warm orange-like yellow. Nothing is needed to set the color.

Other sources of yellow dye: Bark of American Crab Apple tree, roots of Hackberry, roots of Smooth Sumac, twigs and leaves of Clematis, leaves of Agrimony, and the roots of Xanthorrhiza apiifolia.

GREEN

Western tribes use the twigs and leaves of Giant Arbor Vitae to make a dye.

Desert tribes used the bark of Rabbit bush to produce a green. Neither of these dyes are fast.

INDIAN FORMULAE

RED DYE: Ingredients: Inner bark of White birch, outer and inner bark of Red-osier Dogwood, Oak bark, ashes from Cedar bark, soft water. Boil the barks in hot water. Prepare the ashes by burning about an armful of scraps of cedar bark. This should make about 2 cups of ashes, which is the correct quantity for about 2 gallons of dye. Sift the ashes through a piece of cheesecloth. Put them into the dye after it has boiled a while, then let it boil up again, and then put in the material to be colored.

SCARLET RED: Ingredients: 2 parts Bloodroot (fresh or dried), one part each of Wild Plum bark, Red-osier Dogwood and Alder. Simmer all together in soft water until color is obtained. Amount of water and materials to be used depends upon depth of color desired and amount of material to be dyed. A dark red color is obtained by using equal parts of Bloodroot and Wild Plum bark.

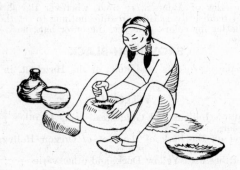

PYRETHRUM
One of Man's Oldest and Safest Insect Killers Made from Flowers

Pyrethrum is fatal to many forms of biting and sucking insects, such as flies, fleas, mosquitoes, roaches, ants, aphids, animal lice, bed bugs, lace bugs, leaf hoppers, thrips, moths, hornworms, etc.

No insect has yet developed a resistance to Pyrethrum. Resistance is a major failure of chemical insecticides. In 1946 there was one insect of "public health importance" resistant to new chemical insecticides. In 1956 there were 36 resistant insects!

Pyrethrum is non-poisonous to man and higher animals. Widespread sprayings of quick killing chemicals have damaged or killed outright, millions of fish, and has destroyed and poisoned much of the food for fish, birds and animals. Minute dosage of several new insecticides has already shown seriously to have reduced reproductive rates of game birds.

Pyrethrum is non-absorbing and non-corrosive. Some pesticides, including chlordane, dieldrin and toxephene, cannot be washed off most foods, even by using a hot detergent bath. These poisons are actually absorbed by skins of some vegetables and fruits. Vitamins and flavor are packed in the skins of most vegetables and fruits.

Pyrethrum may be used either as a dry powder, or by its burning fumes. As a dry powder it may be used pure or mixed with flour, in which form it should be puffed about the room, especially into cracks.

When ignited, Pyrethrum smolders, giving off fumes that do not harm fabrics, corrode metals, damage paintings, etc., as sulphur fumes would. Pyrethrum is used in the proportion of 1 ounce per 30 cubic feet of air space, the exposure being for not less than 4 hours.

Pyrethrum should be distributed in pots or pans, and set on fire with a little alcohol, which should first be sprinkled over it. The quantity apportioned to any one pot or pan should not exceed 1½ inches in depth, if the exposure is to be for 4 hours. Set pots or pans on brick to prevent scorching floor.

Pyrethrum is not limited to the above methods—it is often mixed with other botanicals, chemicals, and also used in liquid form.

RECIPE BY SWASHBUCKLING ARTIST OF 16TH CENTURY

The following incident occurred during the terrible sack of Rome in the year 1527.

Benvenuto Cellini, famous artist of that period, was fighting in the service of Pope Clement VII. Cellini was wounded on the battlement of the fortress of St. Angelo. His autobiography states: "A cannon shot reached me, which hit the angle of a battlement, and carried off enough of it to be the cause why I sustained no injury. The whole mass struck me in the chest and took my breath away. I lay stretched upon the ground like a dead man, and could hear what the bystanders were saying. Among them all, Messer Antonio Santacroce lamented greatly exclaiming: "Alas! alas! we have lost the best defender that we had!" Attracted by the uproar, one of my comrades ran up; he was called Gianfrancecso, and was a bandsman, but was far more naturally given to medicine thàn to music. On the spot he flew off, crying for a stoop of the very best Greek wine. Then he made a tile red hot, and cast upon it a good handful of Wormwood; after which he sprinkled the Greek wine, and when the Wormwood was well soaked, he laid it upon my breast, just where the bruise was visible to all. Such was the virtue of the Wormwood that I immediately regained my scattered faculties." (The value of Wormwood for this purpose is denied by modern medical authorities).

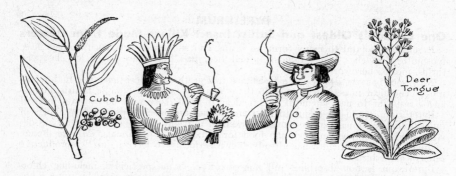

Cubeb

Deer Tongue

BOTANICALS USED IN SMOKE MIXTURES

ALLSPICE—crushed, adds fragrance to pipe tobacco.

AUGUST FLOWER: Commonly smoked in areas where it is found to help loosen nasal congestion, due to head colds.

BEARBERRY Leaves—used by Potawatomi Indians to mix with their tobacco (evidently for a milder smoke.)

BUCKBEAN—the leaves of Buckbean are smoked instead of tobacco.

CHERVIL: A very delicate scented herb used in Europe for smoking.

CISTUS CRETICUS: "Leaves grateful as a smoke."—Whitlaw, 1829

COLTSFOOT: Predominating ingredient of British Herb Tobacco—consisting of Buckbean, Eyebright, Betony, Rosemary, Thyme, Lavender and Chamomile. These are mixed, and smoked in a pipe.

CORN SILK: Used by Indians as a filler, with other smoking botanicals.

CUBEB BERRIES: Used for nasal congestion.

DEER TONGUE: Adds fragrance to pipe tobaccos.

DITTANY: Southern Indians chewed and smoked the fragrant leaves as a substitute for tobacco, according to the records of a pioneer doctor.

GINSENG ROOT: Was commonly chewed as a substitute for tobacco by early Americans. The juice was swallowed for its stomachic properties.

LICORICE: Used to flavor many types of tobacco.

LIFE EVERLASTING: Used by peasants in Europe as a pipe tobacco.

MARJORAM—the leaves were used in many old-time smoking and snuff mixtures.

MASTER-OF-THE-WOODS: Adds aroma to pipe tobacco.

Smoke Mixtures—Continued

MULLEIN—leaves are often smoked like tobacco, for temporary relief of nasal catarrh and minor throat irritation.

ROSEMARY: According to Culpepper, this aromatic herb is smoked as pipe tobacco.

SAGE—leaves have been dried and smoked in a pipe as tobacco.

SASSAFRAS bark: Used in pipe tobaccos.

SUMACH (Rhus glabra): When the leaves turn red in the fall, the Indians gather and dry them to use in tobacco mixtures.

STAGHORN SUMAC—the leaves were used like Sumach (Rhus glabra) by Indians.

STYRAX: Used to flavor pipe tobacco.

SWEET MELILOT or SWEET CLOVER—white or yellow, used to flavor tobacco and cheese.

TONKA BEANS, crushed—add sweet aroma to pipe tobacco. Also used in snuffs.

YERBA SANTA: Aromatic leaves smoked and chewed like tobacco by California Indians. The taste of Yerba Santa is peculiar, being rather disagreeable, resinous and bitter at first. This taste soon disappears and gives place to a sweet and cooling sensation, which is especially noticeable when one ceases to chew for a minute, or drinks a glass of water. As one Indian expressed it "It makes one taste kind of sweety inside."

TRY CHEWING HERBS TO DISCOURAGE CIGARETTE HABIT

A well known organization proposed the following prescription to break the fag habit: 1. Chew Gentian root or Chamomile flowers, when the desire to smoke appears. 2. Take a dose composed of ½ teaspoonful each of Rochelle salts and cream of tartar each morning before breakfast, for a week. 3. The greatest aid will be found in a change of dietetic habits. Smokers are fond of highly seasoned foods and stimulating drinks. 4. Keep away from smokers and tobacco-smoke laden atmosphere as far as possible, for three weeks. 5. Take a Turkish bath twice during the first two weeks. 6. Keep out in the open air as much as possible. Keep the mind occupied.

Note: A friend wrote he broke the tobacco habit by chewing a tiny piece of Gentian root, whenever he had the urge to smoke. Gentian root is used in many tonic preparations. An early American Herbal advises—"Those who wish to break themselves of chewing tobacco, will find Sassafras pith an agreeable substitute." However, we do not claim that everyone can overcome the tobacco habit this way.

NICOTINE-FREE HERBAL TOBACCO

The leaves of Coltsfoot, dried, form a principle ingredient in all herb tobaccos, and constitutes the chief part of their value. The best of these mixtures consists of the following plants, the proportions of which may be altered according to circumstances: Take of Coltsfoot leaves, dried, 1 pound; Eyebright and Buckbean, of each ½ pound; Wood Betony, 4 oz.; Rosemary 2 oz.; Thyme 1½ oz.; Lavender 1 oz. Some add

Herbal Tobacco—Continued

Rose leaves and Chamomile flowers. The herbs should be rubbed to a coarse powder between the hands. Those who prefer a mild tobacco, may increase the quantity of Coltsfoot, which some prefer in the proportion of one-half to the whole quantity.

TRY THIS FOR SMOKER'S COUGH

When irritation is due to excessive smoking: Mix equal parts of Hyssop; Black Horehound; Coltsfoot; and Marshmallow root. Place 3 or 4 teaspoonsful in a teapot, and infuse as ordinary tea. Drink 1 cupful as desired. Milk may be added if desired. For a persistent cough, see your doctor.

OLD RECIPE FOR MAKING PERFUMED SMOKE

Take Balm of Peru ½ ounce; 7 or 8 drops of Oil of Cinnamon; Oil of Cloves, 5 drops; Oil of Nutmegs, of Thyme, of Lavender, of Fennel, of Aniseed (all drawn by distillation) of each a like quantity, or more or less as you like the odor, and would have it strongest; incorporate with these half a dram of Ambergrease; make all these into a paste, which keep in a box. When you have filled your pipe with tobacco, put upon it about the bigness of a pin's head of this composition. It will make the smoke most pleasantly odoriferous, both to the takers and to those that come into the room, and one's breath will be sweet all day after.

Editors note: This recipe may best be used as an incense, rather than a pipe tobacco.

BOTANICALS USED AS DETERGENTS

BOUNCING BET: Fresh herb is stirred in warm soft water, until it forms a lather. Used to wash fine silks and woolens. Cleanses and imparts a beautiful lustre to materials. A common wayside weed.

LIGNUM VITAE: Fresh leaves used as soap in the West Indies.

PAPAYA: Fresh leaves used in Africa and the West Indies.

SOAP BARK: Contains more lather-forming qualities than any other plant known.

SOAP BULB or CHLOROGALUM: Fresh bulbous roots are mashed and stirred in soft water, to form a lather. Used for washing fine silks, delicate fabrics and hair. Contains neither alkali or oil. A soap made of this bulb was widely advertised as a remedy for numerous minor skin conditions. Plant found on hill slopes of California.

YUCCA BACCATA or GLAUCA: Chopped roots are tied up in a bag, then placed in warm soft water and stirred to a lather. Used for shampooing hair, and to wash woolens and cotton fabrics. Said to leave a fine sheen on hair and wool. Yucca plants are common in the southwest, New Mexico, Arizona, etc.

* * * *

HERB SCENTED CANDLES: Melt refined paraffin—add fragrant oils, powdered aromatic herbs, or incense mixtures, and stir thoroughly. Take plumbers candles or other candles and dip quickly in melted scented wax. Repeat several times until sufficient scented wax adheres to candles.

Another method: Fasten candles at their wicks with paper clips, on a stretched string or wire, then pour scented wax over hanging candles. Have a container beneath candles to catch drippings. Color may be added to scented wax, if desired.

FLAVORING TIPS

AGRIMONY herb: Flavor with Licorice root.

CONDURANGO root: Flavor with dried Orange peel.

CLOVES: A powerful flavor in almost any type tea or mixture.

CRANESBILL or ALUM root: Sweeten with honey.

FENNEL seed: Usually mixed with laxatives to counteract certain unpleasant effects.

GERMAN RUE: The flavor "takes over" when put in formulas, unless added with discretion.

GROUND IVY: Flavor with Licorice root.

HOREHOUND: Flavor with Ginger root.

LICORICE: The agreeable taste of Licorice in any form covers, to a practical extent, the taste of very many disagreeable remedies. Acrid and bitter tastes are well disguised by it. A syrup made by adding two parts of the fluid extract to 14 parts of simple syrup will disguise the bitter or otherwise unpleasant taste of a large proportion of the fluid extracts. The taste of quinine can be concealed by it.—Ellingwood's Materia Medica and Therapeutics.

PEPPERMINT: Covers the taste of some nauseous drugs and produces sensation of cool in the mouth when the breath is drawn in after taking it.

VALERIAN root: Flavor with Mace.

WORMWOOD: A powerful bitters, when the herb is fresh. Use with discretion in formulas.

KEEPING QUALITIES OF BOTANICALS

Buckthorn bk, Cascara bk, Calamus rt, Coriander seed (whole), Deer Tongue herb, Master-of-the-Woods, Sweet Grass, Orris and a few others improve after certain aging periods.

Jamaica Ginger, Tonka, Vanilla, etc., deoxidize rapidly when left exposed to air. Their properties are best retained in air-tight or glass containers.

Most botanicals (especially leaves and flowers) deteriorate, so it is important that you obtain them from a good source for best results.

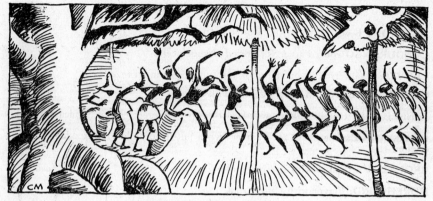

BOTANICAL CURIOS

The following are generally prized, used, or carried for their exotic shape, color, fragrance, or simply for the legends and beliefs once associated with them. The legends and beliefs of course are strictly lore and imaginary.

Many superstitions were brought with the slaves from Africa to the West Indies, then to the American mainland by way of New Orleans and other ports. Legends of Rosemary, St. John's Wort, Master of the Woods, and several others were brought from the Old World.

ADAM and EVE: A curious root, carried mainly as a love charm.

ASAFOETIDA: An old European belief held that a small piece of this powerful odorous gum, hung around a child's neck, would protect it from many diseases—especially germs sensitive to this particular odor.

BASIL, SACRED: Similar to Sweet Basil. Held in reverence, mainly by the Hindus as a divine herb, to protect body and family. On a visit to Trinidad, the author found Sacred Basil in most Hindu gardens, and as a border plant around a grave-like mound near a Hindu temple.

BASIL, SWEET: In Haiti, native merchants often sprinkle their stores with a composition made of Sweet Basil soaked in water, which according to the creed, chases bad luck and attracts buyers. The herb is often associated with Erzulie, The Haitian voodoo goddess of love.

BETH ROOT or TRILLIUM: Was used by Indian women to attract a warrior mate. Pieces of the root were cooked and secretly mixed with the food intended for the desired "victim."

BLOOD ROOT: Slave charm of Colonial times. The roots were believed to have power to avert spells wrought by villianous persons. The color of Blood roots was considered very important. Salmon shade roots were considered "queens" or "she" roots. The dark red roots, were considered "kings" or "he" roots.

BUCKEYE: Many people still carry this nut around as protection against rheumatism.

Botanical Curios—Continued

CATNIP ROOT: According to a very old European legend, chewing the root of this plant will make the most gentle person fierce and wrathful. Turneiserius tells of a hangman who was usually gentle and pusillanimous, and who never had courage to perform the duties of his wretched vocation, until he had first prepared himself by chewing this root. Catnip herb exerts powerful influence upon cats.

CURRY LEAF: According to "William's Plants of Zanzibar," Swahili people burn Curry leaf as incense, to keep devils away from their sick children.

DEVILS SHOESTRING: Long roots are formed into a collar-like necklace for teething, and also to ward off bad dreams, evil spirits, etc.

DRAGON'S BLOOD: Resin somewhat resembles dried blood. Used as a charm, as well as in voodoo mixtures.

FIVE FINGER GRASS: So-called because the leaf is divided into five segments. Plant is hung over the bed by colored folks, believing it will bring restful sleep, and ward off any evil that five fingers could bring. Used in the Old World for similar purposes.

GRAINS OF PARADISE: Generally carried in a small bag, or tiny container, and used in voodoo mixtures. The charm actually works best with foods—it is used like pepper, as a spice. Also used to flavor cordials, spirits and wines.

JEZEBEL: Named after the wicked queen of Biblical times. Generally prized by superstitious women of wicked intent. Jezebel was simply carried about by the superstitious, who dwelled upon wishful thinking. The root actually is quite harmless.

JOBS TEARS: Strung as prayer beads, teething beeds, and as an ornament. The seeds are in lovely shades of pearl gray. According to tradition, they are named after weeping Job of the Bible. The seeds are stained beautiful shades, in the West Indies, for necklaces.

JOHN THE CONQUEROR ROOT: A very popular root in our Southern states. Superstitious folk believed that if the root was carried in their pocket, the bearer would never be without money, and be blessed with luck, and even had the ridiculous belief it would make one invisible. High John, Southern John, Lesser John, etc., were resorted to when one or the other proved a failure.

JUMBIE SEEDS: Evil spirits are known as "Jumbies" in the Leeward and Windward Islands of the West Indies. Jumbie seeds are round, about 2 or 3 times larger than a pea seed, and are beautifully marked with crimson and black colors. They are strung and used as an ornament and worn also as an amulet. Natives place a few of the seeds in their kerosene lamps "to make the oil last longer."

KHUS-KHUS, or French Vetivert: Fragrant roots, used in bath of virgins in Jamaica. An interesting account is described by Zora Hurston's book "Voodoo Gods." Indians living in Trinidad believe Khus-Khus plants must be watered through August and September ONLY, on dark nights when spirits linger near the plant. The plant is widely distributed in the West Indies, where it is planted on terraces to prevent washouts. Dried roots are used in dresser drawers to keep away cucaraches (roaches)

Botanical Curios—*Continued*

and other insects, as well as to give clothing a delicate fragrance. Bundles of Khus-Khus are offered in the markets, or streets, of almost every West Indian Island.

LOVAGE ROOT: Aromatic root, used in bath water, in the belief it would make one more lovable. Cleanliness undoubtedly adds to the charm.

LUCKY-NUT: A curious shaped poisonous nut, carried about by natives in the West Indies, as a good luck charm.

MASTER OF THE WOODS: In ancient times, powerful Teuton warriors, with fierce whiskers and hairy chests, believed they needed a sprig of this dainty herb to wage a successful battle. The herb was fastened to their horned helmet, shield, or tucked in their animal skin mantle.

Master of the Woods is used in modern Germany to flavor May wine (Maitrinke). This is generally made by steeping a few branches of the herb with a slice of orange or lemon in a bottle of white wine. The herb and orange are removed when the desired flavor is obtained.

MUGWORT: An old European legend held that pillows stuffed with this aromatic herb would reveal one's entire future in dreams.

ORRIS ROOT, or QUEEN ELIZABETH WHOLE ROOT: Many whole roots vaguely resemble human forms in seated position. They are valued according to the perfection of shape. Voodoos tie thread around the "neck" of the figure and let the root hang. Wishes are fulfilled or rejected according to the way the root moves. Movement is made through unconscious or intentful action of voodoo holding thread. Powdered Queen Elizabeth root is often known as "Love Powder." It is also mixed with other "love and wooing compounds," probably for scent.

Orris root has a delightful violet-like aroma, and is used in sachets, pot-pourri, clothes closets, dresser drawers, trunks, etc., to give clothes a delicate aroma.

ROSEMARY: This delightful fragrant herb is still worn by some brides in Europe, on their wedding day. It was also a very old custom to deck the bridal bed with Rosemary.

There's Rosemary for you, that's for remembrance:
I pray you, love, remember.
Another old saying: "Where Rosemary flourishes, the lady rules."

SAMPSON SNAKE ROOT: Carried as an amulet, in the belief it would increase one's physical powers.

SAINT JOHN'S WORT: It was an ancient custom in Europe, to gather this herb on St. John's Day, the 24th of June. The herb was hung up in the windows as a preservative against evil spirits, phantoms, spectres, storms, and thunder—whence it derived its ancient name—"Devils Flight." The herb was also worn about the neck as a protective amulet.

SANDALWOOD: Used since remote ages, mainly as an incense in religious ceremonies in India and China. According to legend, King Solomon's Temple was built of Sandalwood.

Botanical Curios—*Continued*

SEA BEANS, LUCKY STONES or SACRED STONES: Names refer to both Calabar beans or species of Caesalpinia. These beans are occasionally washed ashore in the West Indies, where the ocean currents or winds carry the seed from remote islands in Africa or South America. Some of the beans do resemble stones. The fortunate native who finds these beans carries them about as some people carry a Buckeye.

SEA SPIRIT: Merely immersed in water (sometimes colored) for its ghost-like, almost transparent appearance. Sea Spirit is actually whole agar-agar.

STAR ANISE: Curious shaped aromatic seed, carried about as a luck charm. Also used to flavor foods, liquor and in incense.

SOUTHERNWOOD: For some twenty centuries, superstitious people in Continental Europe, believed that if this herb was tucked under one's mattress, it evoked sensual passions. The recipe did not state if one used a pinch or bale of this aromatic herb.

TONKA BEAN: Worn around the neck for its sweet aroma, and as a love charm or amulet.

VALERIAN ROOT: Albertus Magnus wrote in the Middle Ages, that a decoction of the roots "restored peace and harmony between husband and wife." Probably some measure of "peace" was obtained because of the reputed sedative properties of this root.

VERVAIN: A relic of ancient pagan times. Druids used the herb in a mixture to ward off the "evil eye." In the Middle Ages, the herb was very popular in witches brews.

Trefoil, Vervain, St. John's Wort, Dill
Hinder witches of their will.

Yarrow, Betony, Elecampane, Columbine, Rue, Mugwort, Celandine and Nettle were also used in witch concoctions with Vervain. It was believed the brew should contain 7 or 9 ingredients to be an effective potion. Rue was considered an antidote, or counter-charm, against witch practices. In Tyrol people carried Rue, with Agrimony, Maidenfern, Broom-straw, and Ground Ivy, in order to "sense the presence of witches." Vervain was also generally included as an ingredient of "true love powders" and philters. Marvelous cures were once attributed to this botanical.

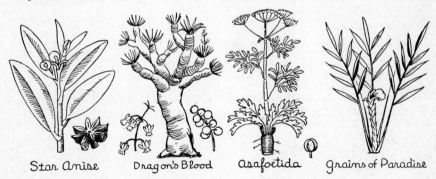

Star Anise   Dragon's Blood   Asafoetida   Grains of Paradise

Botanical Curios—Continued

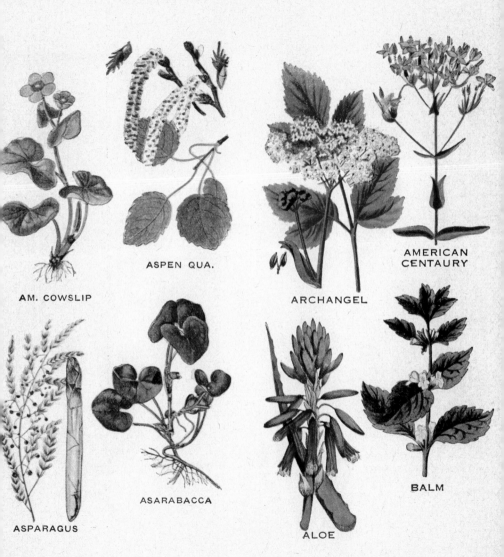

AM. COWSLIP

ASPEN QUA.

ARCHANGEL

AMERICAN
CENTAURY

ASPARAGUS

ASARABACCA

ALOE

BALM

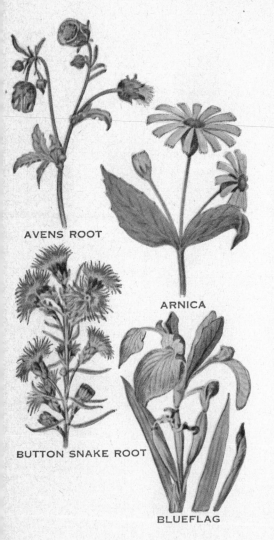

AVENS ROOT

ARNICA

BUTTON SNAKE ROOT

BLUEFLAG

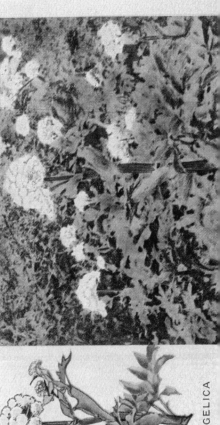

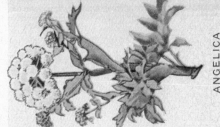

ANGELICA

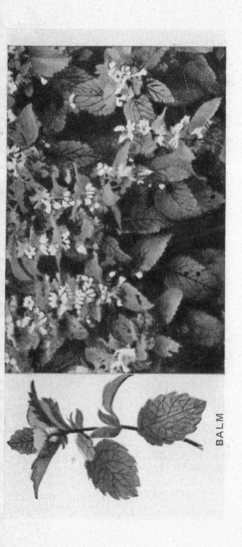

BALM

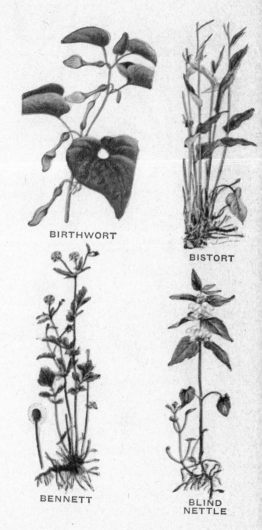

BIRTHWORT

BISTORT

BENNETT

BLIND
NETTLE

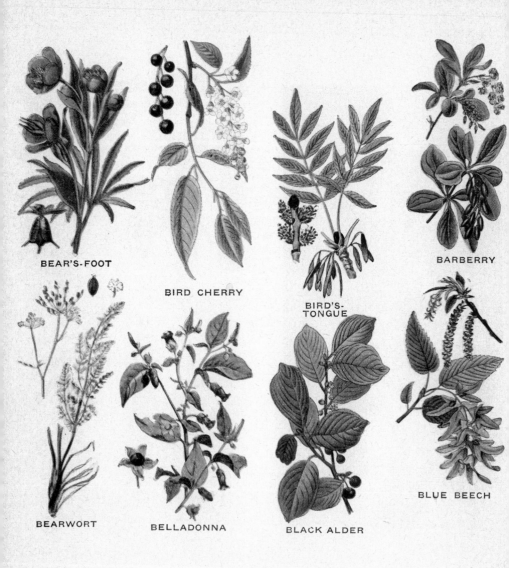

BEAR'S-FOOT

BIRD CHERRY

BIRD'S-
TONGUE

BARBERRY

BEARWORT

BELLADONNA

BLACK ALDER

BLUE BEECH

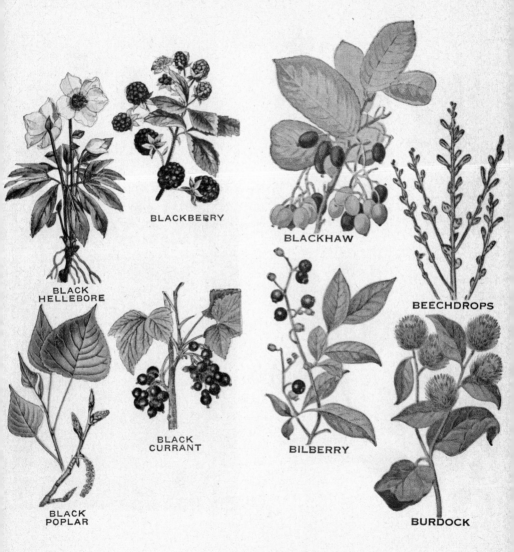

BLACKBERRY

BLACKHAW

BLACK
HELLEBORE

BEECHDROPS

BLACK
POPLAR

BLACK
CURRANT

BILBERRY

BURDOCK

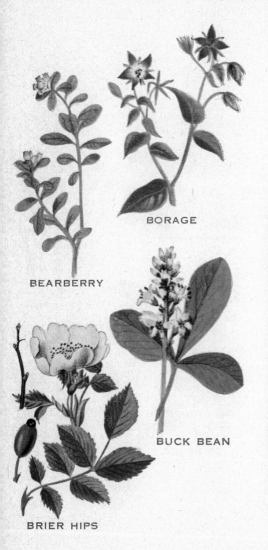

BORAGE

BEARBERRY

BRIER HIPS

BUCK BEAN

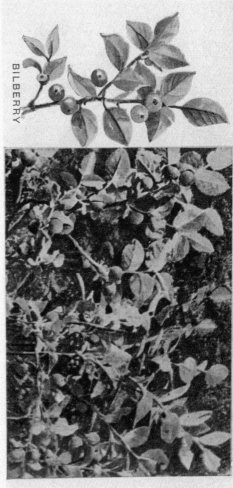

BILBERRY

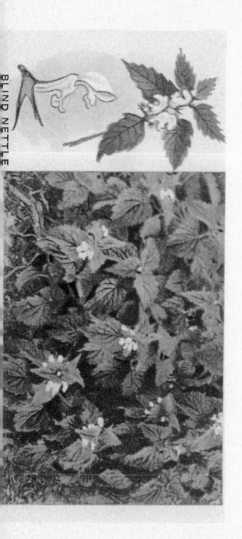

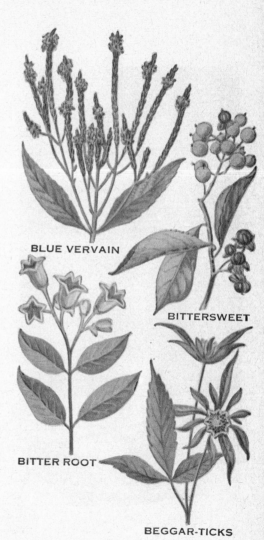

BLUE VERVAIN

BITTERSWEET

BITTER ROOT

BEGGAR-TICKS

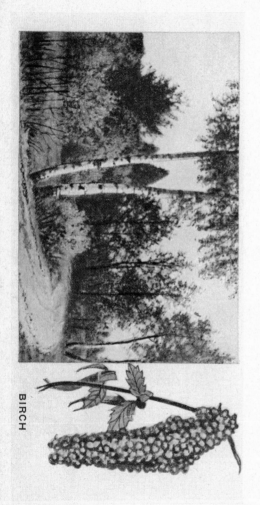

BIRCH

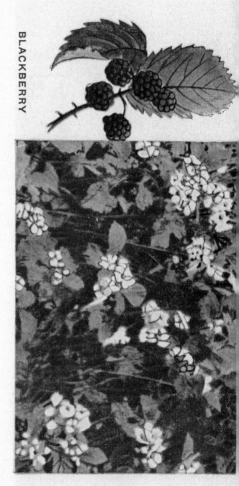

BLACKBERRY

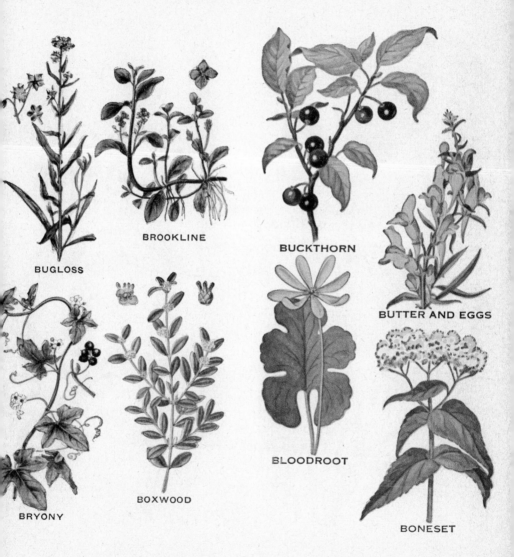

BROOKLINE

BUCKTHORN

BUGLOSS

BUTTER AND EGGS

BRYONY

BOXWOOD

BLOODROOT

BONESET

241

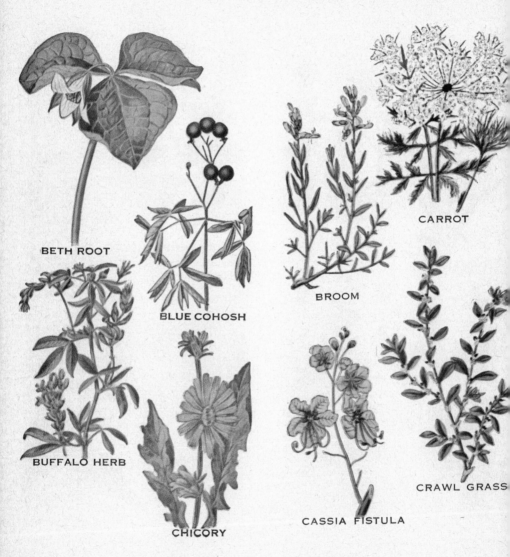

BETH ROOT

BLUE COHOSH

BROOM

CARROT

BUFFALO HERB

CHICORY

CASSIA FISTULA

CRAWL GRASS

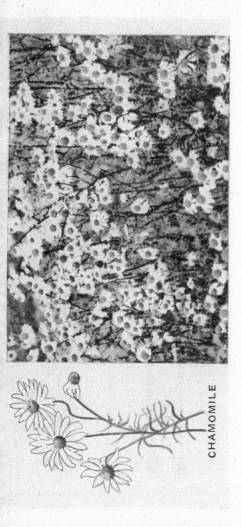

CHAMOMILE

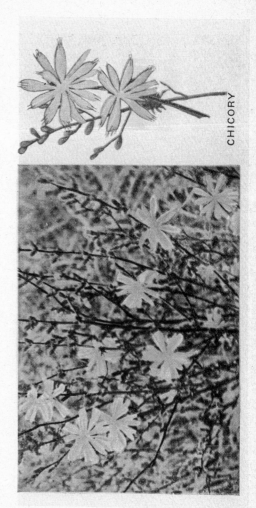

CHICORY

243

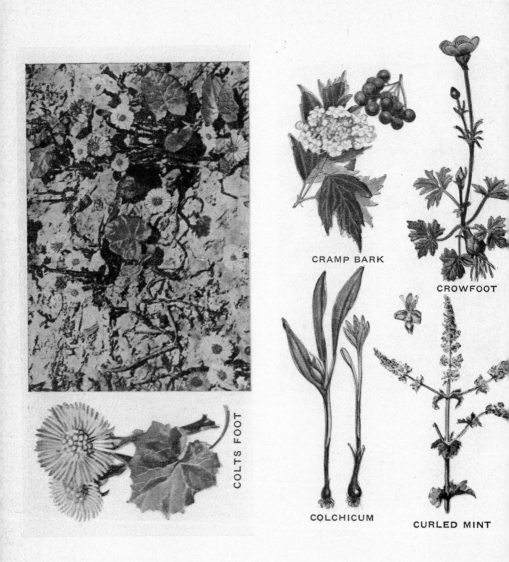

CRAMP BARK

CROWFOOT

COLTS FOOT

COLCHICUM

CURLED MINT

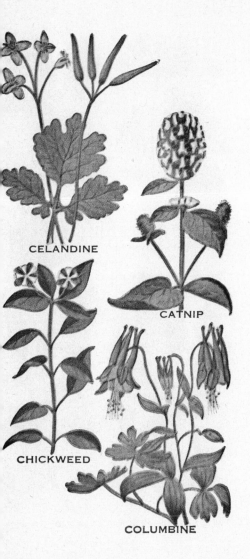

CELANDINE

CHICKWEED

CATNIP

COLUMBINE

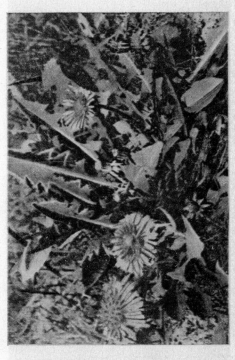

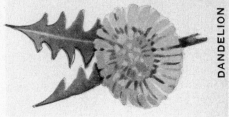

DANDELION

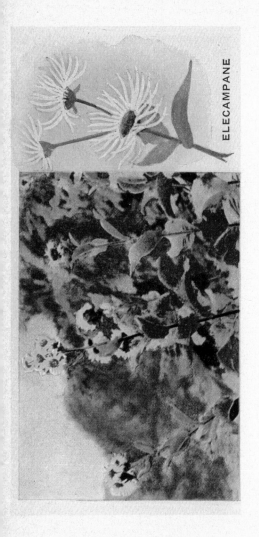

ELECAMPANE

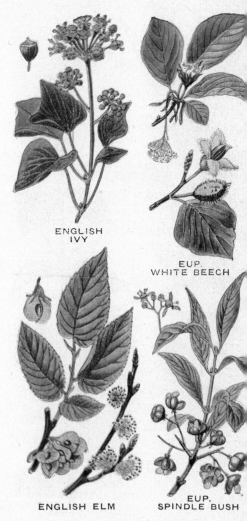

ENGLISH
IVY

EUP.
WHITE BEECH

ENGLISH ELM

EUP.
SPINDLE BUSH

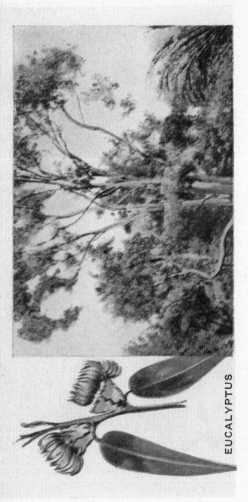

EUCALYPTUS

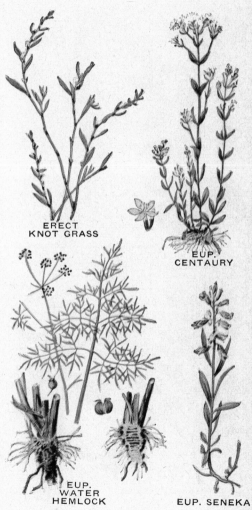

ERECT
KNOT GRASS

EUP.
CENTAURY

EUP.
WATER
HEMLOCK

EUP. SENEKA

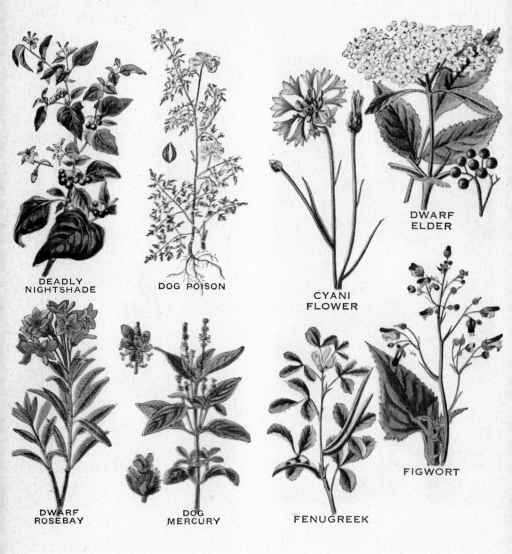

DEADLY
NIGHTSHADE

DOG POISON

CYANI
FLOWER

DWARF
ELDER

DWARF
ROSEBAY

DOG
MERCURY

FENUGREEK

FIGWORT

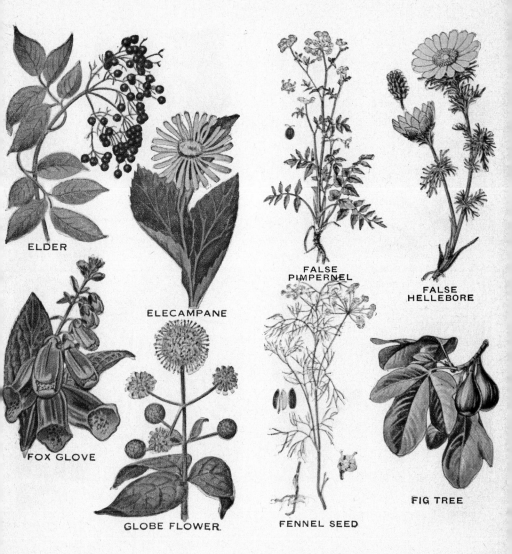

ELDER

ELECAMPANE

FALSE
PIMPERNEL

FALSE
HELLEBORE

FOX GLOVE

GLOBE FLOWER.

FENNEL SEED

FIG TREE

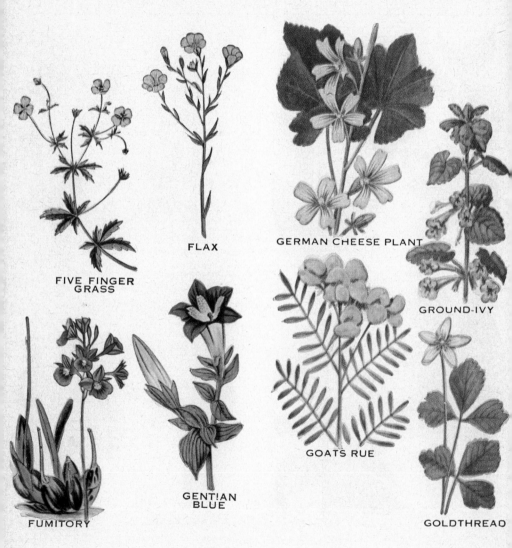

FLAX

GERMAN CHEESE PLANT

FIVE FINGER
GRASS

GROUND-IVY

FUMITORY

GENTIAN
BLUE

GOATS RUE

GOLDTHREAD

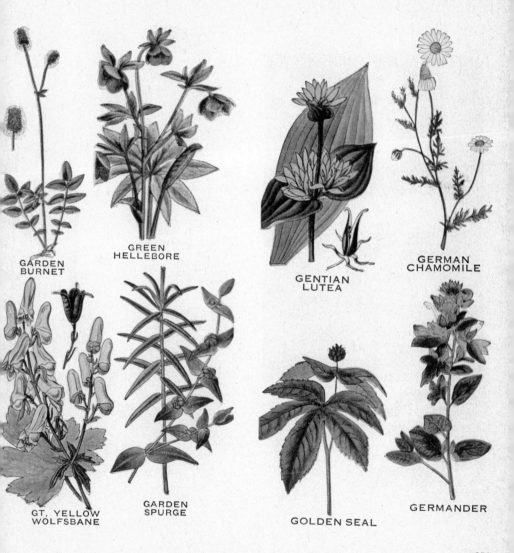

GARDEN
BURNET

GREEN
HELLEBORE

GENTIAN
LUTEA

GERMAN
CHAMOMILE

GT. YELLOW
WOLFSBANE

GARDEN
SPURGE

GOLDEN SEAL

GERMANDER

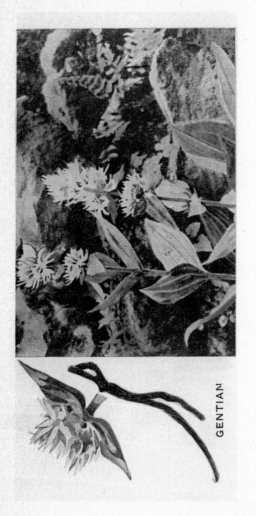

GENTIAN

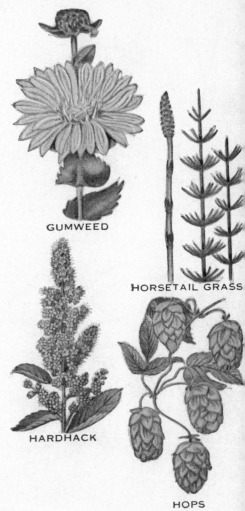

GUMWEED

HORSETAIL GRASS

HARDHACK

HOPS

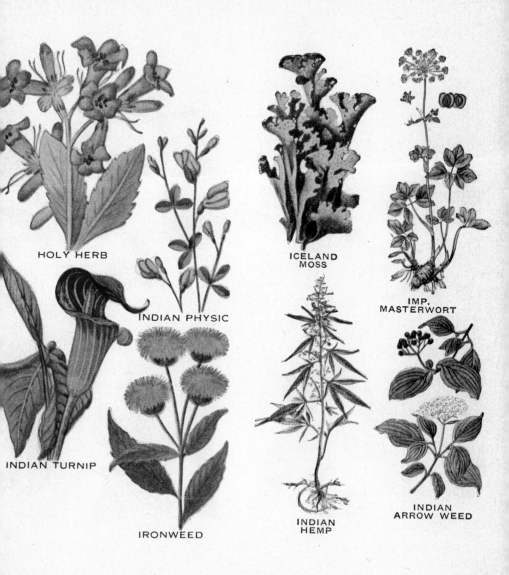

HOLY HERB

INDIAN PHYSIC

INDIAN TURNIP

IRONWEED

ICELAND
MOSS

INDIAN
HEMP

IMP.
MASTERWORT

INDIAN
ARROW WEED

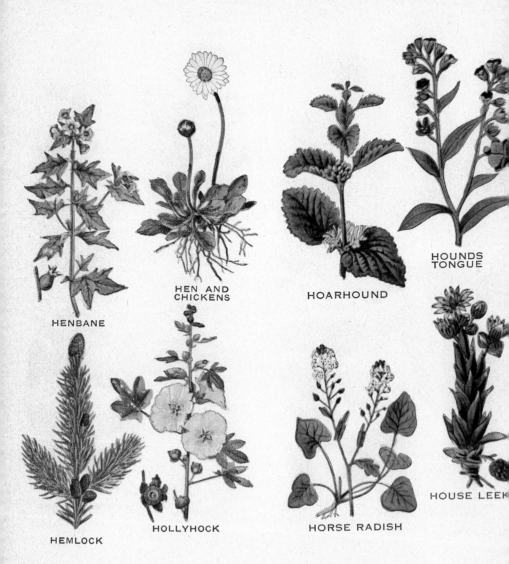

HENBANE

HEN AND
CHICKENS

HOARHOUND

HOUNDS
TONGUE

HEMLOCK

HOLLYHOCK

HORSE RADISH

HOUSE LEEK

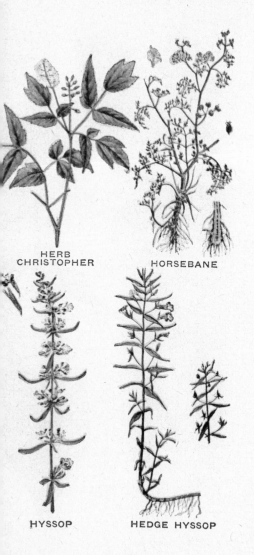

HERB
CHRISTOPHER

HORSEBANE

HYSSOP

HEDGE HYSSOP

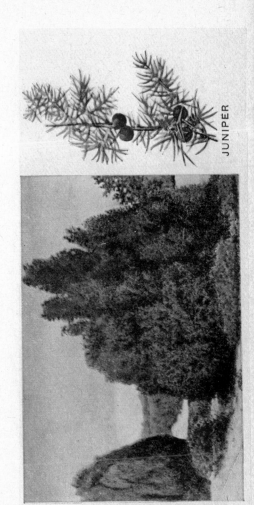

JUNIPER

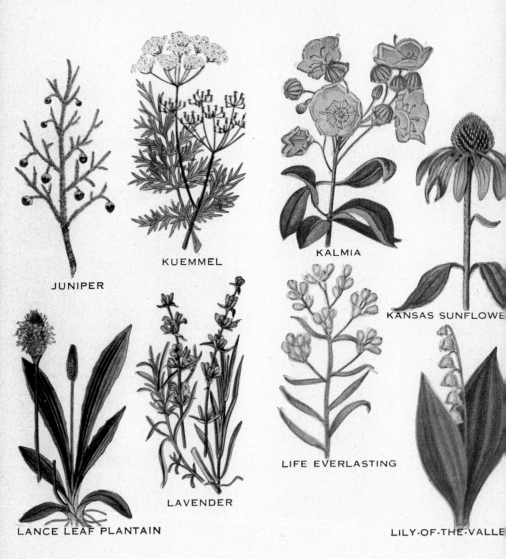

JUNIPER

KUEMMEL

KALMIA

KANSAS SUNFLOWE

LANCE LEAF PLANTAIN

LAVENDER

LIFE EVERLASTING

LILY-OF-THE-VALLE

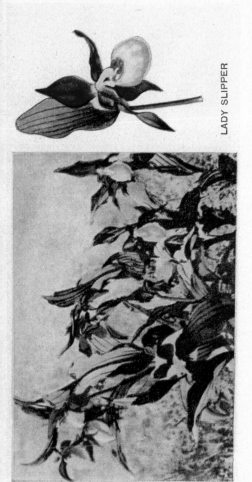

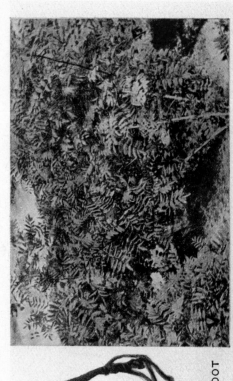

LADY SLIPPER

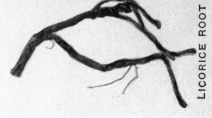

LICORICE ROOT

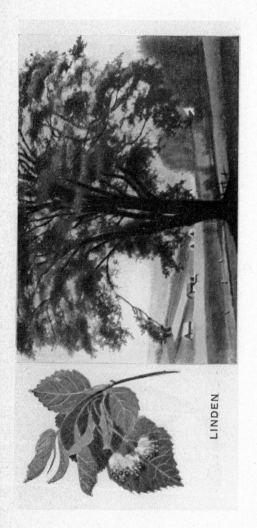

LINDEN

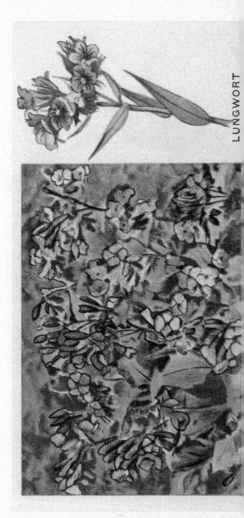

LUNGWORT

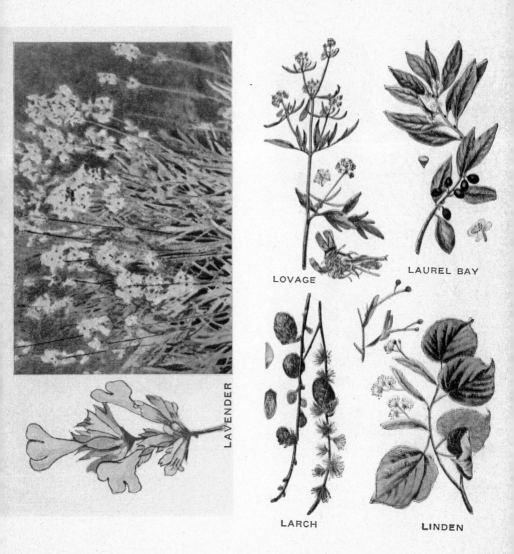

LAVENDER

LOVAGE

LAUREL BAY

LARCH

LINDEN

259

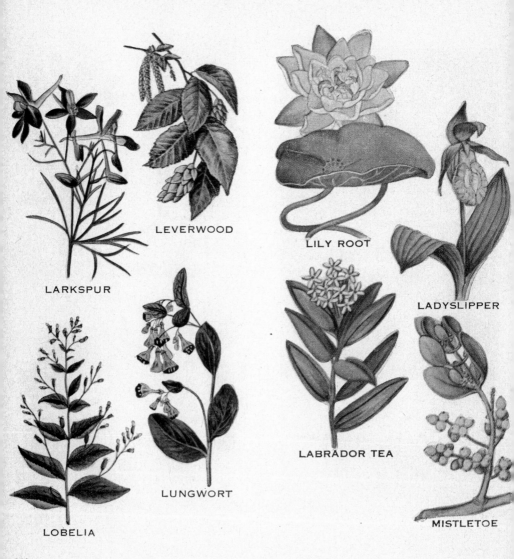

LEVERWOOD

LILY ROOT

LARKSPUR

LADYSLIPPER

LOBELIA

LUNGWORT

LABRADOR TEA

MISTLETOE

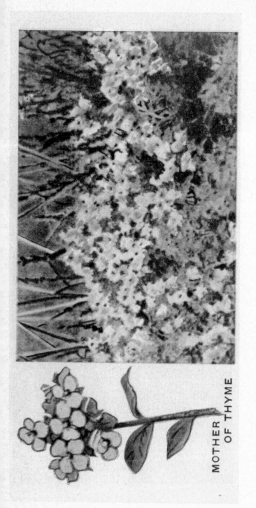

MOTHER OF THYME

MARSH MALLOW

MULLEIN

MOTHERWORT

MAY APPLE

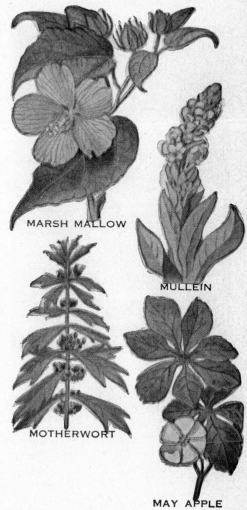

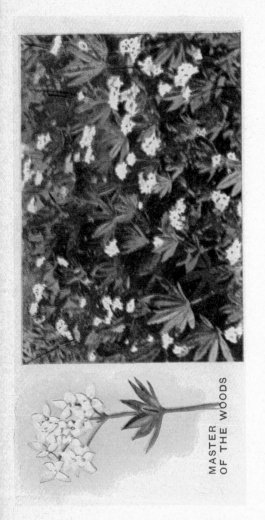

MASTER OF THE WOODS

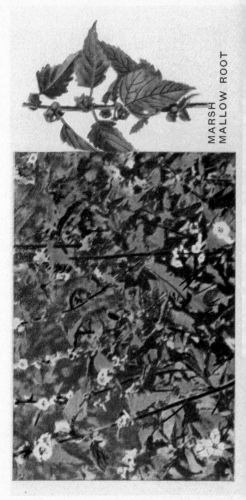

MARSH MALLOW ROOT

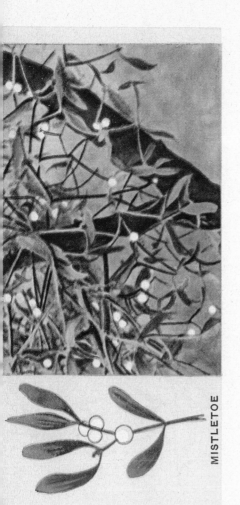

MISTLETOE

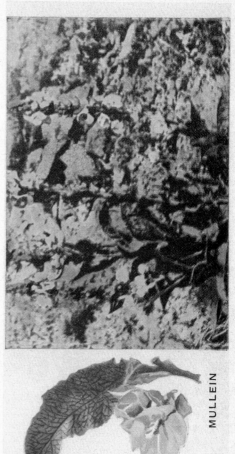

MULLEIN

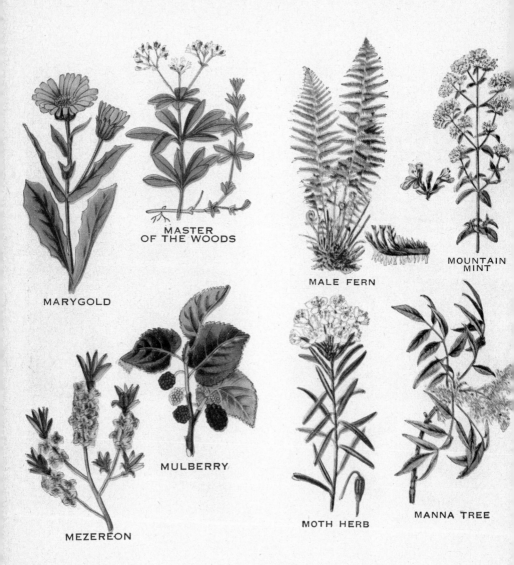

MASTER
OF THE WOODS

MALE FERN

MOUNTAIN
MINT

MARYGOLD

MULBERRY

MEZEREON

MOTH HERB

MANNA TREE

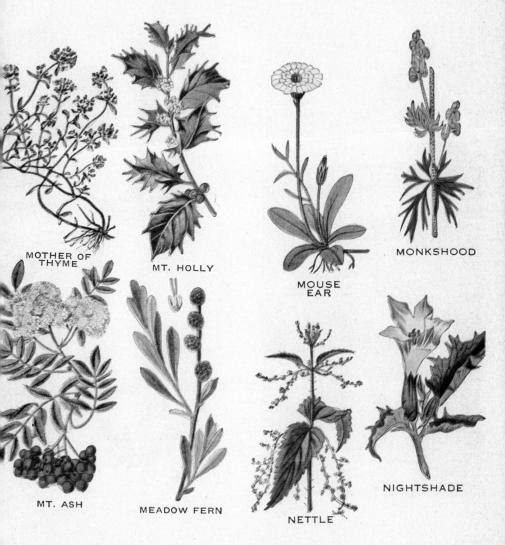

MOTHER OF
THYME

MT. HOLLY

MOUSE
EAR

MONKSHOOD

MT. ASH

MEADOW FERN

NETTLE

NIGHTSHADE

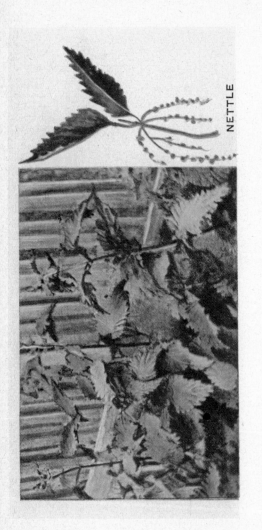

NETTLE

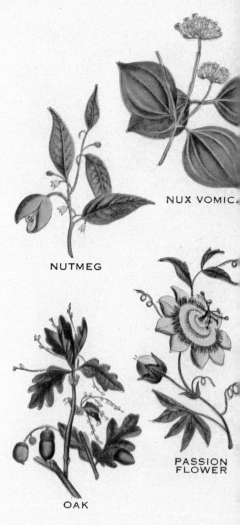

NUTMEG

NUX VOMICA

OAK

PASSION FLOWER

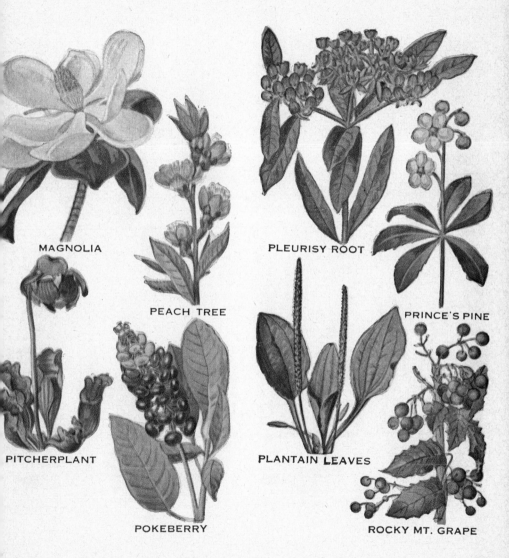

MAGNOLIA

PLEURISY ROOT

PEACH TREE

PRINCE'S PINE

PITCHERPLANT

PLANTAIN LEAVES

POKEBERRY

ROCKY MT. GRAPE

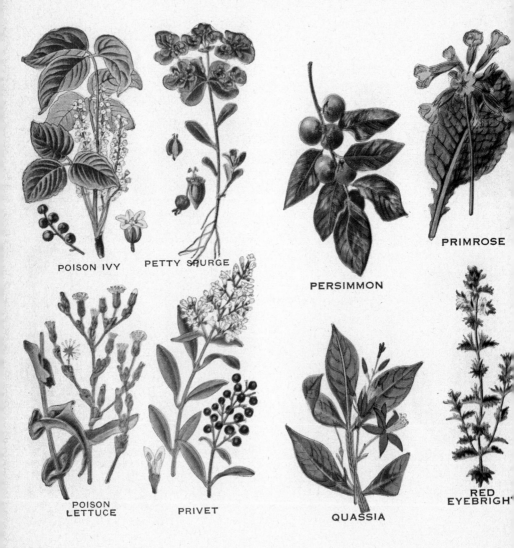

POISON IVY

PETTY SPURGE

PERSIMMON

PRIMROSE

POISON
LETTUCE

PRIVET

QUASSIA

RED
EYEBRIGH'

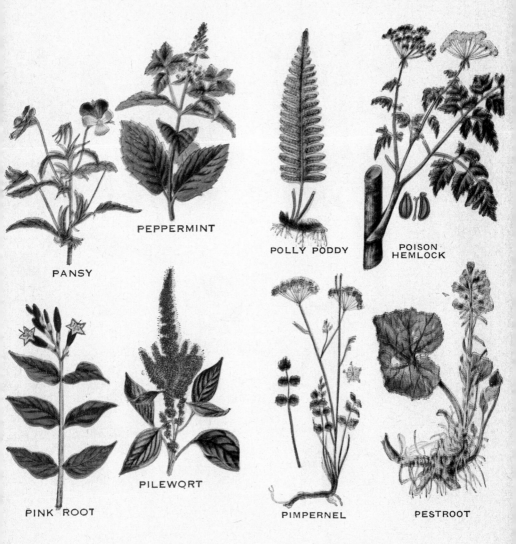

PANSY

PEPPERMINT

POLLY PODDY

POISON
HEMLOCK

PINK ROOT

PILEWORT

PIMPERNEL

PESTROOT

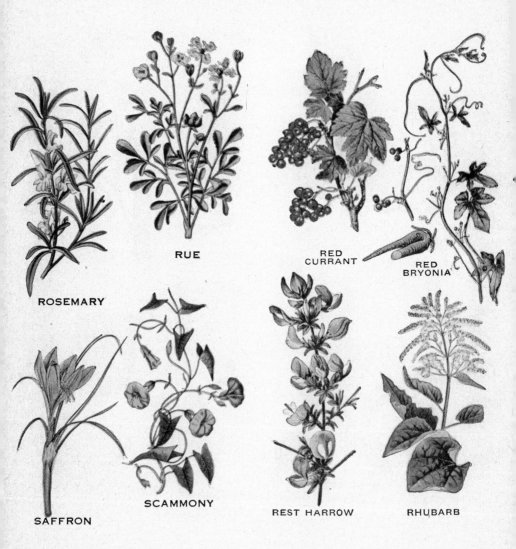

ROSEMARY

RUE

RED
CURRANT

RED
BRYONIA

SAFFRON

SCAMMONY

REST HARROW

RHUBARB

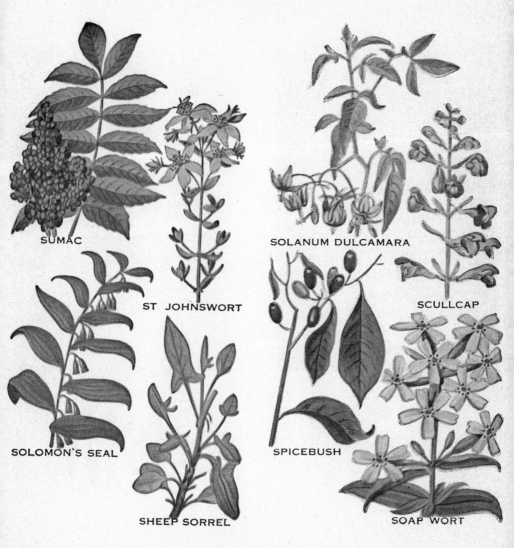

SUMAC

ST JOHNSWORT

SOLOMON'S SEAL

SHEEP SORREL

SOLANUM DULCAMARA

SCULLCAP

SPICEBUSH

SOAP WORT

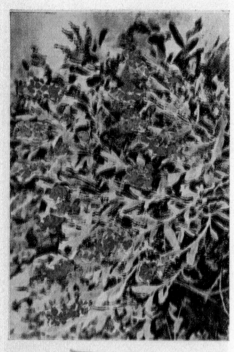

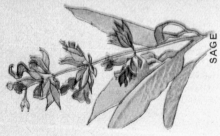

SAGE

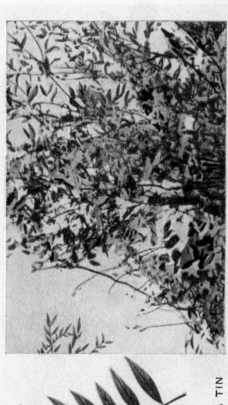

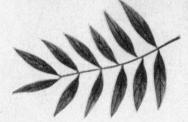

SENNA TIN

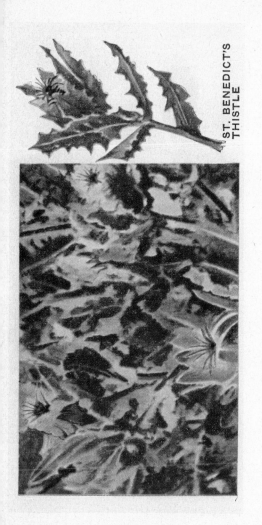

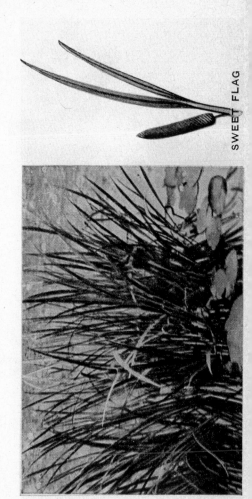

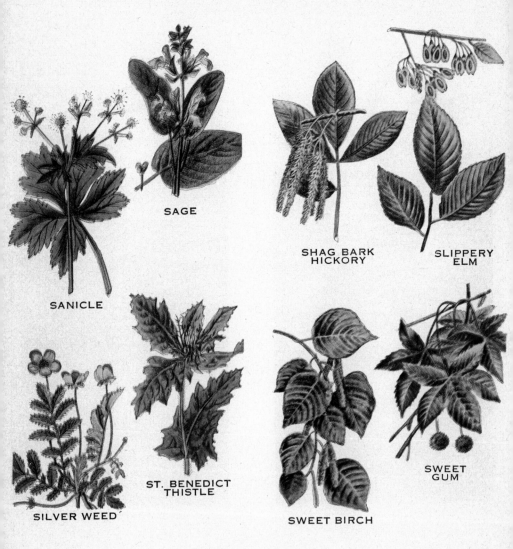

SAGE

SHAG BARK
HICKORY

SLIPPERY
ELM

SANICLE

SILVER WEED

ST. BENEDICT
THISTLE

SWEET BIRCH

SWEET
GUM

274

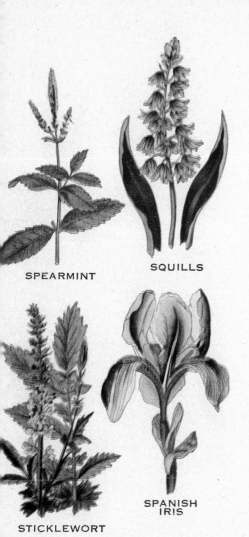

SPEARMINT

SQUILLS

STICKLEWORT

SPANISH
IRIS

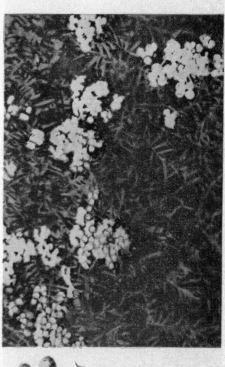

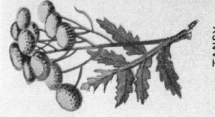

TANSY

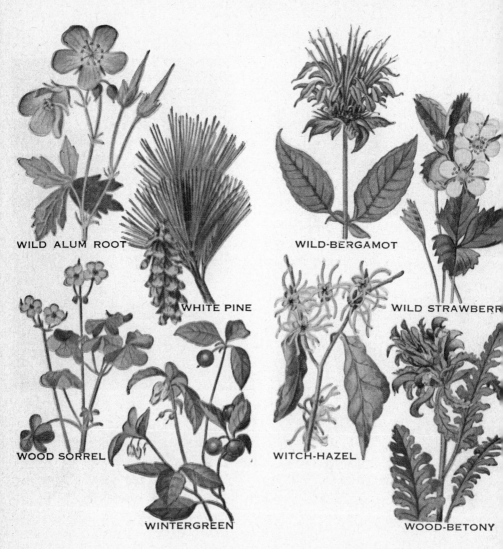

WILD ALUM ROOT

WHITE PINE

WILD-BERGAMOT

WOOD SORREL

WINTERGREEN

WITCH-HAZEL

WILD STRAWBERR

WOOD-BETONY

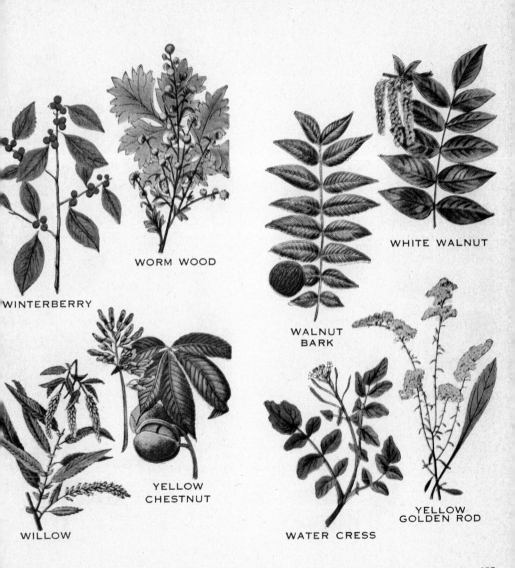

WINTERBERRY

WORM WOOD

WHITE WALNUT

WALNUT
BARK

WILLOW

YELLOW
CHESTNUT

WATER CRESS

YELLOW
GOLDEN ROD

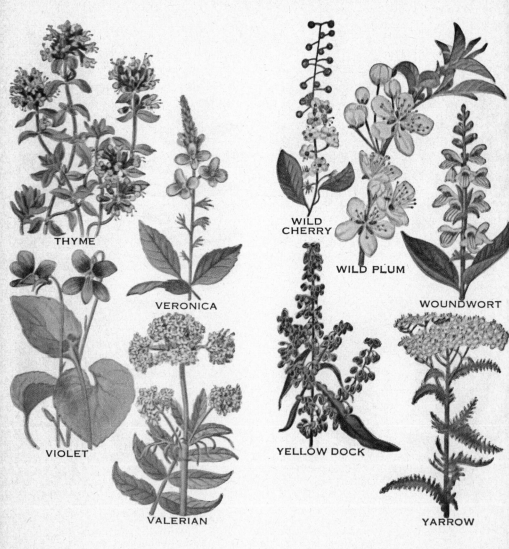

THYME

VERONICA

VIOLET

VALERIAN

WILD
CHERRY

WILD PLUM

WOUNDWORT

YELLOW DOCK

YARROW

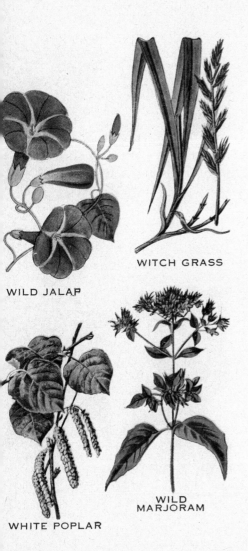

WILD JALAP

WITCH GRASS

WHITE POPLAR

WILD
MARJORAM

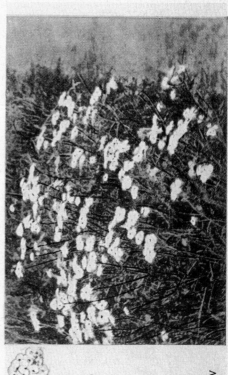

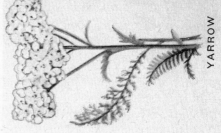

YARROW

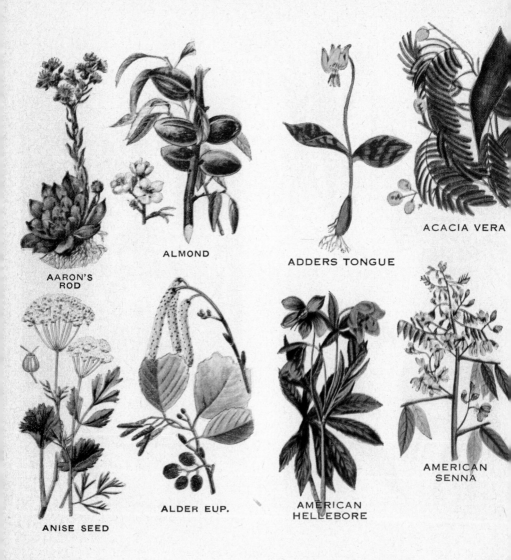

AARON'S
ROD

ALMOND

ADDERS TONGUE

ACACIA VERA

ANISE SEED

ALDER EUP.

AMERICAN
HELLEBORE

AMERICAN
SENNA

INDEX TO COLORED PLATES

GENERAL INDEX

287

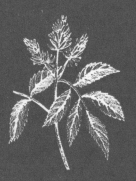

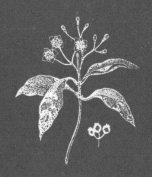

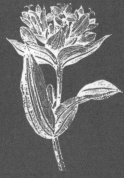

FLOWERING ASH.
FRAXINUS ORNUS.

PIMENTO, OR JAMAICA PEPPER
ALLSPICE.
MYRTUS PIMENTA.

PURPLE GENTIAN.
GENTIANA PURPUREA.

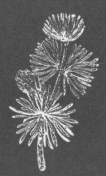

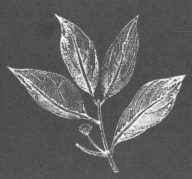

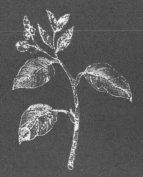

COMMON WHITE LARCH.
PINUS LARIX.

CAMPHOR TREE.
LAURUS CAMPHORA.

CASCARILLA.
CLUTIA ELUTERIA.

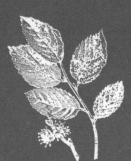

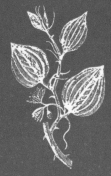

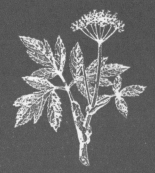

COMMON ELM.
ULMUS CAMPESTRIS.

SARSAPARILLA.
SMILAX SARSAPARILLA.

COMMON MASTERWORT
IMPERATORIA OSTRUTHIUM.